Attention Deficit Hyperactivity Disorder (ADHD)

Psychiatry- Theory, Applications, and Treatments Series

Attention Deficit Hyperactivity Disorder (ADHD)
Stuart M. Gordon and Aileen E. Mitchell
2009 ISBN: 978-1-60741-581-7

ATTENTION DEFICIT HYPERACTIVITY DISORDER (ADHD)

STUART M. GORDON
AND
AILEEN E. MITCHELL
EDITORS

Nova Biomedical Books
New York

For permission to use material from this book please contact us:
Telephone 631-231-7269; Fax 631-231-8175
Web Site: http://www.novapublishers.com

Library of Congress Cataloging-in-Publication Data

Attention deficit hyperactivity disorder (ADHD) / [edited by] Stuart M. Gordon and Aileen E. Mitchell.
p. ; cm.
Includes bibliographical references and index.
ISBN 978-1-60741-581-7 (hardcover)
1. Attention-deficit hyperactivity disorder. I. Gordon, Stuart M. II. Mitchell, Aileen E.
[DNLM: 1. Attention Deficit Disorder with Hyperactivity--physiopathology. 2. Adolescent. 3. Attention Deficit Disorder with Hyperactivity--drug therapy. 4. Child. 5. Dopamine Agents--therapeutic use. WS 350.8.A8 A88303 2009]
RJ506.H9A93135 2009, 618.92'8589--dc22 2009023561

Published by Nova Science Publishers, Inc. ✝ New York

Contents

Preface

Attention deficit hyperactivity disorder (ADHD) is a psychiatric condition affecting young children and adolescents, characterized by inappropriate high levels of hyperactivity, inattention and impulsivity. A strong genetic basis for ADHD has been documented by family, twin and adoption studies. Dopamine, a neurotransmitter, has been implicated to play an important role in ADHD since the most frequently prescribed drugs for ADHD are targeted at the dopaminergic system. Unfortunately, the disease continues into adulthood in 30-70% of patients. It has been proposed that ADHD may lead to memory deficits, delinquency, substance abuse, and problematic personality disorders, in addition to being one of the highest risk factors for other mental illnesses. This new book gathers the latest research from around the globe in this field.

Chapter 1 - Attention deficit hyperactivity disorder (ADHD) is a psychiatric condition affecting young children, characterized by inappropriate high levels of hyperactivity, inattention and impulsivity. Most children diagnosed with ADHD will be treated with stimulants and current prescribing trends indicate: 1) an increase in rates over the last 10-15 years; 2) treatment of children who are younger (preschoolers); 3) clinical preferences and recommendations over long-acting rather than short-acting preparations and continuous rather than intermittent usage. Since a child's brain continues to develop well into the second decade of life, the long-term use of such drugs during this critical phase of brain development could have important consequences on brain functioning, but surprisingly little is known about the developmental effects of these drugs. Ethical considerations preclude human experimentation to determine underlying drug effect mechanisms. This paper reviews evidence from the experimental animal literature on whether psychostimulants, such as methylphenidate (MPH), amphetamine (AMPH) and Adderall (ADD), administered peripubertally at clinically-relevant dosages, have any long-term neuroadaptive or enduring effects in adulthood. Advances in genetics and epigenetics have created a revolution in molecular neurobiology. These techniques, applied to animal models, permit the study of the effects of psychostimulants on gene expression as observed through different developmental periods across the lifespan. Several animal studies, utilizing clinically relevant MPH or amphetamine dosages indicate long-term neuroadaptive effects on expression of immediate early genes and peptides. The magnitude of such changes is also dependent on the developmental stage at which animals were exposed to psychostimulant treatment. There is a need for more intense developmental studies in animals to assist in understanding potential long-term neuroadaptations to low, oral doses of stimulants. Of greater concern is the recent emphasis on more chronic treatments in children that employ longer-acting oral preparations, as well as the newly-approved transdermal system.

Chapter 2 - ADHD and dysthymic disorder (DD) are common psychiatric disorders in children and adolescents with more males than females affected pre-puberty [1]. Further, both ADHD and DD are main drivers for oppositional defiant disorder [2], which is the most common reason for children and adolescents being referred to mental health services [3]. It is also known that ADHD and early onset depressive disorders such as DD have a 'greater than chance' association [4]. Indeed, impairing levels of inattentive type ADHD symptoms are a key symptom dimension within the nosological construct of DD. Yet, to date, there has been little or no systematic research examining the association between ADHD, inattentive type and DD using robust cognitive neuroscience probes with well defined brain behaviour relationships.

Chapter 3 - Attention-Deficit Hyperactivity Disorder (ADHD) is a developmental problem characterized by hyperactivity, sustained attention problems and impulsivity. Two main variants have been described, i.e. mesocortical (MC), with altered executive functions, and mesolimbic (ML) with delay aversion. The MC and ML variants are associated with altered MC and ML dopamine (DA) branches respectively. The Naples High Excitability rats (NHE) model the MC variant, whereas Spontaneously Hypertensive Rats (SHR) model the ML variant. Here, multiple behavioural, histochemical, pharmacological and molecular biology studies are reviewed as evidence for and against the MC hypothesis for NHE. Behavioural studies have included exposure to spatial novelties, i.e. Làt maze to monitor activity and non selective attention (NSA), and radial maze for NSA and selective spatial attention (SSA). In addition histochemical and molecular biology studies of Tyrosine Hydroxylase (TH), DAT, DA-D1 and DA-D2 receptors, and DA-related phosphoprotein 32 (DARPP32) as functional markers have been carried out in the forebrain. The results indicate that NHE rats feature the main aspects of the MC variant of ADHD, which is associated with hypertrophic and hyperfunctional MC DA branche, as assessed by larger A10 neurons, higher TH activity, and higher DAT and DARPP32 density in the ventral tegmental area. This profile was reverted by subchronic MPH (3 mg/kg). The MPH-induced changes in TH, DAT and DARPP32 in the PFC and striatum are consistent with a drug-induced reduction in MC activity. In addition, HPLC studies revealed high tissue content of excitatory amino acids (EAA) across the NHE forebrain. This, in turn, may lead to neurotoxicity and neurodegeneration in the striatum, as proposed for human ADHD by several fMRI studies. Finally the higher DA and EAA release in forebrain sites of NHE rats is likely to be associated with higher nitric oxide (NO) synthesis. In fact, behavioural studies with acute or subchronic inhibitors of NO synthesis reduced hyperactivity and increased NSA in NHE rats. These data may open new drug/no drug strategies for diagnosis and therapy of ADHD in humans.

Chapter 4 - Attention deficit hyperactivity disorder (ADHD) is one of the most common childhood onset neurobehavioral disorders characterized by a combination of developmentally inappropriate attention, hyperactivity, and impulsivity. A strong genetic basis for ADHD has been documented by family, twin, and adoption studies. Dopamine

(DA), a neurotransmitter, has been implicated to play an important role in ADHD since the most frequently prescribed drugs for ADHD are targeted at the dopaminergic system. For the same reason, dopaminergic system genes have long been considered as candidates for study. Two most widely explored dopaminergic genes are the DA transporter (*DAT1*) and DA receptor (*DRD4*) and it is hypothesized that specific alleles of these genes may alter DA transmission. For example, the 10-repeat allele of the *DAT1* gene is believed to be associated with faster re-uptake of DA while the 7-repeat allele of *DRD4* gene was found to generate a post-synaptic receptor with reduced binding affinity for DA. However, association studies between an allele and the disorder have yielded conflicting reports in different ethnic groups. Moreover, some of the ADHD patients failed to respond to the drugs targeted at the dopaminergic system and therefore others, like norepinephric, serotonergic systems etc., known to control the cognitive functions were also studied for association with the disorder. In the present investigation, the authors have looked into five candidate genes (*DAT1*, *DRD4*, *DBH*, *MAOA*, *SNAP25*) in nuclear families with ADHD probands belonging to the Indo-Caucasoid ethnicity. Genomic DNA isolated from leukocytes / buccal cells, donated by volunteers giving informed written consent, was used to study genetic polymorphisms. Data obtained were analyzed for family-based as well as population-based association tests to determine the risk of ADHD in this population. Analysis of five candidate genes revealed transmission of specific haplotypes to Indian ADHD cases from the parents, an information which could be useful while prescribing remedial medication to an ADHD proband.

Chapter 5 - Longitudinal research indicates that early emerging attention-deficit/hyperactivity disorder (ADHD) can mark the beginning of a developmental pathway that ends in antisocial behavior. Parent-child interactions characterized by coercive cycles of escalation—the tendency to match or exceed a partner's level of aversiveness—may contribute to children's progression along this pathway. In this study, the authors explored coercive escalation among preschoolers both with and without ADHD. Parent-child interactions during a laboratory task were coded for escalation, and oppositional behavior was assessed via parent report and observational ratings. Respiratory sinus arrhythmia (RSA), a physiological marker of emotion dysregulation, was also collected. Escalation by the child was correlated with oppositional behavior, with a stronger relationship found for observational ratings than for parent reports. Escalation was not correlated with RSA. However, low RSA was associated with observed emotion dysregulation and opposition. Thus, escalation and RSA emerged as independent correlates of oppositional behavior in this high risk sample.

Chapter 6 - Attention-deficit hyperactivity disorder (ADHD) is characterized by age-inappropriate inattention, impulsiveness, and hyperactivity. Experimental models, in addition to mimicking syndromal features, should resemble the clinical condition in pathophysiology, and predict potential new treatments. In this review, the authors summarized the different animal models of ADHD which are established from genetic and environmental alterations, and compared their similarities and differences to clinical ADHD. However, none is fully comparable to clinical ADHD. The pathophysiology involved varies, in this review the authors focused on the dopaminergic system in ADHD. Because, the most compelling evidence that dopaminergic mechanisms were involved in ADHD was pharmacological challenge in both animals and humans. However, the question was that whether any other central factors which regulated the process of dopaminergic neurotransmission involved in the origins of ADHD. The authors speculated that “synaptogenesis hypotheses” might be involved in ADHD. Above all, any improved models as well as further testing of their ability to predict treatment responses are required.

Chapter 7 - *Introduction:* An increasing number of parents turn to homeopathy for treatment of their children with attention defict hyperactivity disorder (ADHD). The Swiss ADHD-study aimed at obtaining scientific evidence for the effectiveness of homeopathy in hyperactive children by a randomized placebo controlled double blind trial, followed by five years of open label observation.

Methods: A total of 83 children, aged 6-16 years, with ADHD diagnosed using the Diagnostic and Statistical Mannual of Mental Disorders-IV (DSM-IV), were recruited. Their mean Conners Global Index (CGI)-rating was 19 points. Prior to the randomised double blind placebo controlled crossover study, they were treated with individually prescribed homeopathic medications (screening phase). 70 patients achieved an improvement of 50% or more in the CGI, which was confirmed by neuropsychological testing. 62 patients participated in the crossover trial. They were split into two groups and received either verum for 6 weeks followed by placebo for 6 weeks (group A), or vice versa (group B). CGI-evaluations were performed at the beginning of the trial and after each crossover period. The Conners Parent and Teacher Raing Scales were evaluated at diagnosis and again after the crossover trial, and CGI ratings were obtained at 18 and 60 months after treatment start.

Results: At the end of the open label *screening phase* cognitive performance such as visual global perception, impulsivity and divided attention, had improved significantly ($p<0.0001$). The comparison of suboptimal and optimal homeopathic prescriptions revealed a highly significant difference in the mean CGI-improvement per month ($p<0.0001$), showing that (optimal) remedies, which perfectly cover the patients symptoms, cause a much stronger improvement than (suboptimal) remedies with an insufficient coverage of the symptoms. During the *crossover trial* CGI parent-ratings were significantly lower under verum than under placebo ($p=0.0479$). Five years after treatment start mean CGI- ratings by parents reached 7 points (64% improvement, $p<0.0001$) in 28 patients who had continued homeopathy, and 9 points (53% improvement, $p=0.0001$) in 25 patients who had stopped any treatment. Seven participants had changed to Methylphenidate (MPD) after the crossover trial. Their final mean CGI-parent rating under MPD was 11 points.

Conclusion: The trial reveals specific effects of homeopathic treatment in ADHD, particularly in the areas of behavioural and cognitive functions. In longtime follow up 74% of all patients benefited from homeopathy without needing any other treatment.

Chapter 8 - ADHD symptoms are one of the most common psychiatric problems in children and adolescents [1]. On other hand, the magnitude of sleep problems in children and adolescents is high and it is a major public health concern [2]. The association of sleep and ADHD is still poorly recognized [3].

Chapter 9 - Since an emerging body of evidence is accumulating that endocrine disrupting chemicals exert their effects on the central nervous system, their neuronal risk assessment is now required. A previous study showed that a single intracisternal administration of bisphenol A, an endocrine disrupting chemical, into neonatal rats caused hyperactivity, seen in patients with attention deficit hyperactivity disorders(ADHD). To evaluate environmental contributions of bisphenol A to ADHD, it is very important to test the potential of the chemical via an environmental exposure route. In this study, the authors tested the hypothesis that oral exposure to bisphenol A would exhibit effects observed previously with direct instillation in the rat. Oral administration of 600 μg/pup/day bisphenol A into male Wistar rats aged 5 days to 3 weeks caused significant hyperactivity at 4-5 weeks of age. Treated rats were about 1.3 times as active in the nocturnal phase as were vehicle-treated control rats ($p < 0.005$). The long-term effects of the chemical resulted in a large reduction of immunoreactivity for tyrosine hydroxylase in the midbrain at 7 weeks of age, where terminal deoxynucleotidyl transferase-mediated dUTP nick end-labeling (TUNEL)-positive cells were detected. Furthermore, bisphenol A decreased gene expression levels of dopamine transporter in adult rats.

Chapter 10 - The psychostimulant methylphenidate (MPD) is the drug most often used to treat Attention Deficit Hyperactivity Disorder (ADHD), a common behavioral disorder of children. Psychostimulant exposure to children at the time of neuronal development can cause behavioral and physiological changes enduring during adulthood. Most of the studies on psychostimulant investigate short term effects of the drug, 5 to 120 minutes post injection. The objective of this study was to investigate whether acute or chronic exposure to MPD will modulate the circadian activity pattern. Maintaining the circadian activity pattern is a physiological process that regulates the internal homeostasis. Dose response protocol was used to study the effect of acute and chronic MPD in four groups of rats, each N=8, as follows: saline (control) group, and 0.6, 2.5, or 10.0 mg/kg i.p. MPD groups respectively. The experiment was performed over 11 consecutive days of continuous recording. All rats received saline on day 1, followed by saline or the assigned MPD dose (0.6, 2.5, or 10.0 mg/kg) on experimental days 2 through 7. After three washout days, a re-challenge of saline or MPD was injected. Each animal (of the MPD groups) received the same dose of MPD for re-challenge injection as the dose of MPD given on experimental day 2. The data evaluation was divided into four phases: acute, induction, washout and expression phases. There was a dose-dependent increase in the average locomotor activity. Analysis of the circadian rhythmic pattern of locomotion in the three dose groups demonstrated that only the 10.0 mg/kg MPD elicited significant changes in circadian pattern activity in the washout and the expression phase. In addition, this study showed that chronic MPD treatment elicits dose dependent withdrawal and behavioral sensitization in adolescent rats.

Chapter 11 - Attention deficit hyperactivity disorder (ADHD) is a neurobehavioral developmental disorder affecting several percent of the population, which usually presents itself during childhood, but can persist into adulthood or be diagnosed in adulthood also. Treatment of the male or female child, adolescent, young adult, or older adult with ADHD begins with a careful assessment to establish a correct diagnosis and what potential co-morbid conditions may also complicate the clinical picture. If a psychopharmacologic approach is chosen as part of the management strategy for this common conundrum, the clinician should understand that the medications noted by research to help many patients improve their attention dysfunction are stimulants, norepinephrine reuptake inhibitors, and antidepressants; alpha-2 agonists may improve the classic insomniac effect of stimulants. The most popular drugs and the ones with the most underlying research support are the stimulants, *methylphenidate* (available since 1957) and *amphetamine* (with observational data on its effectiveness starting in 1937). A number of newer, long-acting stimulants have been introduced in the past decade.

Chapter 12 - *Introduction*: Attention Deficit Hyperactivity Disorder (ADHD) is shown to be a disorder that is both familial as well as heritable. Over the last decade, and since the advent of advanced genotyping techniques, a lot of research has been done to uncover the genetic basis of ADHD. Trying to understand the genetics of ADHD helps us get a better understanding of its pathophysiology, its heritability and gives clues to any genetic subtypes that might exist. By realizing that diverse genetic variations might still produce the same clinical syndrome, the authors get a better understanding as to how individuals respond differently to the same medication.

Methods: The aim of this chapter is to educate those readers who have a basic understanding of the principles of genetics, by virtue of having a clinical background, but still need to be made familiar with recent advances in the genetics of ADHD, current trends and future directions. The chapter will begin with a brief introduction of genetic principles in psychiatric disorders and will involve discussion of basic physiology of the genetic targets where relevant. A glossary of relevant terms will be included. Discussion will include the challenges to conducting genetic research in psychiatric disorders. Only the most commonly researched genetic targets with the most compelling evidence to date will be discussed. The chapter will also include a section on pharmacogenetics – the genetic explanation of how individuals respond differently to the same medication. The chapter will explain how research in genetics is providing new insights into the disorder and what needs to be done to improve the quality of research.

Conclusion: Recent advances in bio-computational techniques and cheaper genotyping methods have led to a plethora of studies and a huge amount of information. Some of this information is changing the way people understand psychiatric disorders. However, clinicians find it difficult to keep pace with rapid advances and run the risk of not being able to understand what the new information means. This chapter aims to help clinicians who have an interest in ADHD get a better grip of this informational avalanche in the field of genetics.

Chapter 13 - Attention Deficit Hyperactivity Disorder (ADHD) is a common neuropsychiatric disorder with characteristics of inattention, hyperactivity and/or poor impulse control. Previous studies had also reported children with ADHD exhibit below average performance in adaptive functioning. In recent years, motor difficulties in children with ADHD have been addressed. Researchers found these children have poor postural adjustment, inadequate motor timing and force use. Given evidence of the deficits of adaptive functioning and motor ability, the aim of this study was to investigate the association between these two fields in children with ADHD.

The study group consisted of 25 children with ADHD, 19 males and 6 females, aged from 4.6 to 8.6 years (mean age 6.5 years, SD 1.2 years). The participants were recruited from a rehabilitation department of a teaching hospital. All the children were diagnosed by a pediatrician as meeting the Diagnostic and Statistical Manual of Mental Disorders-Fourth Edition Text Revision (DSM-IV) criteria for ADHD. The Movement Assessment Battery for Children (MABC), a standardized motor function assessment, was administrated by three physical therapists. MABC consists of three subtests: manual dexterity, ball skill, and static dynamic balance. The Chinese version of Adaptive Behavior Scales was used to assess the adaptive function of the children. This scale is a semi-structure parent-reported questionnaire, which consists of two parts for assessing adaptive behaviors in 10 life domains and mal-adaptive behaviors in other two life domains.

Nine (36%) children had significant motor impairments whereas seven (28%) children were in borderline. Ten (40%) children had definite adaptive problems in more than one adaptive domain. The children with impaired motor ability had significant poorer behaviors in the adaptive domains of communication and socialization. Regarding the subtest performances, children who had more impaired ability in manual dexterity performed worse behaviors in the adaptive domains of home living, socialization and self-direction. The results also showed children with poorer ball skill were associated with worse home-living behavior. Moreover, children who had more impaired balance exhibited poorer performance in the social behavior.

The results of this study offer evidences of motor problems and adaptive dysfunction in 25 children with ADHD. The authors found significant correlation between motor ability and adaptive functioning in these children, especially in the adaptive domains of self-direction, home-living and socialization. Identification of motor difficulties may have important implications for the type of support needed for effective management in the adaptive dysfunction in children with ADHD.

Chapter 14 - In this chapter the authors want to demonstrate a correlation between social skills and attention deficit hyperactivity disorder (ADHD) among adolescents with intellectual disability (ID). In a recent pilot study of adolescents dually diagnosed with mild intellectual disabilities and comorbid pathology of ADHD the authors defined three age-and IQ-match groups (males, n=12 in each group) with group I – composed of adolescent diagnosed with mild ID, group II - adolescents diagnosed with ADHD, and group III - adolescents diagnosed with ID and ADHD. The instruments used in the study were Wechsler Intelligence Scale for Children (WISC, according to the chronological age of the subjects) and the short version of the Developmental Behavior Checklist (DBC). The authors found that comorbidity was a factor differentiating. ADHD strongly increased the impairment of social skills, while behavioral disorders were less damaging in ID performance. The WISC and DBC instruments should be used with confidence in clinical and service settings, to allow a better assessment of co-occurrence morbidity in adolescents with ID. The interactions between intellectual disability and psychopathology behavior highlight the need to plan a more accurate diagnosis and appropriate rehabilitative intervention program, essential for improving the quality of life of the ID population.

In: Attention Deficit Hyperactivity Disorder (ADHD)
Editors: Stuart M. Gordon and Aileen E. Mitchell
ISBN 978-1-60741-581-7

Chapter 1

Psychostimulant–Induced Developmental Neuroadaptation: Implications for the Treatment of ADHD

***Normand Carrey*[*1,4], *Teena Chase*[2], *Jayne Katerina Allen*[3] *and Michael Wilkinson*[3,4,5]**

Department of Psychiatry[1], Department of Anatomy and Neurobiology[2], Department of Obstetrics and Gynaecology[3], Department of Physiology and Biophysics[4] and Division of Endocrinology and Metabolism[5],
Dalhousie University and IWK Health Centre, Faculty of Medicine,
Halifax, Nova Scotia, Canada

Abstract

Attention deficit hyperactivity disorder (ADHD) is a psychiatric condition affecting young children, characterized by inappropriate high levels of hyperactivity, inattention and impulsivity. Most children diagnosed with ADHD will be treated with stimulants and current prescribing trends indicate: 1) an increase in rates over the last 10-15 years; 2) treatment of children who are younger (preschoolers); 3) clinical preferences and recommendations over long-acting rather than short-acting preparations and continuous rather than intermittent usage. Since a child's brain continues to develop well into the second decade of life, the long-term use of such drugs during this critical phase of brain development could have important consequences on brain functioning, but surprisingly little is known about the developmental effects of these drugs. Ethical considerations preclude human experimentation to determine underlying drug effect mechanisms. This paper reviews evidence from the experimental animal literature on whether psychostimulants, such as methylphenidate (MPH), amphetamine (AMPH) and Adderall

[*] Correspondence: Dr Normand Carrey, Department of Psychiatry, IWK Health Centre
PO Box 9700, Halifax, Nova Scotia, Canada B3K 6R8, e-mail: Normand.carrey@iwk.nshealth.ca.

(ADD), administered peripubertally at clinically-relevant dosages, have any long-term neuroadaptive or enduring effects in adulthood. Advances in genetics and epigenetics have created a revolution in molecular neurobiology. These techniques, applied to animal models, permit the study of the effects of psychostimulants on gene expression as observed through different developmental periods across the lifespan. Several animal studies, utilizing clinically relevant MPH or amphetamine dosages indicate long-term neuroadaptive effects on expression of immediate early genes and peptides. The magnitude of such changes is also dependent on the developmental stage at which animals were exposed to psychostimulant treatment. There is a need for more intense developmental studies in animals to assist in understanding potential long-term neuroadaptations to low, oral doses of stimulants. Of greater concern is the recent emphasis on more chronic treatments in children that employ longer-acting oral preparations, as well as the newly-approved transdermal system.

1. Introduction

Although stimulants have been prescribed for many years for the treatment of ADHD, their putative long-term impact on the developing nervous system remains obscure (Andersen 2005; Carlezon and Konradi 2004). The last two decades have witnessed increased rates for stimulant prescriptions overall, for younger children and for longer periods of time (Zito et al 2000; Mayes et al 2008). Moreover there has been a remarkably steep increase in the number of prescriptions for amphetamine stimulants (Adderall; Dexedrine) at the same time as a decrease in the number for MPH (Swanson et al 2007). This transformation in clinical practice over the past two decades took place largely in the absence of long-term safety studies in children (Leckman and Young 2002). Difficulty in diagnoses, including overly inclusive criteria and non-specificity of symptoms in younger children, may result in inadvertent exposure to the long-term effect of psychostimulants (Teicher et al 1996). Moreover, there is a paucity of data from long-term animal studies despite clear indications that the developing brain is remarkably sensitive to changes in its macro- and micro-environment and that brain growth continues well into the second decade of life (Benes 1998). From a molecular biology point of view, it has generally been assumed that MPH interacts with the same brain pathways activated by drugs of abuse, producing increases in synaptic dopamine similar to cocaine and amphetamine (Swanson and Volkow 2002). Advances in molecular neuropharmacology allow the study, in developing animals, of the effect of psychostimulants on short- and long-term gene expression and subsequent neuroadaptation. Current human imaging and genomic studies are providing important insights into the effects of stimulant treatment but cannot provide the crucial developmental perspective across the life span available through animal models.

This chapter is intended to critically appraise those animal experiments focused on psychostimulants (MPH, d-amphetamine, d,l-amphetamine salts), which have as their experimental paradigm an emphasis on different developmental periods and that employed clinically relevant dosages. These latter studies include the effects of acute and chronic stimulant exposure on genetic and epigenetic mechanisms, and will contrast the prepubertal to the postpubertal period and possible enduring effects into adulthood. In a final section we will discuss the clinical implications of such studies.

At the outset it is important to address the main reasons why clinicians perceive that animal models are irrelevant to either their clinical work with children and youth with ADHD or its treatment by psychostimulants. The primary shortcoming is seen as the lack of a good animal model that exhibits the symptoms of ADHD. However it is clear that significant advances in our understanding of the neurochemistry of ADHD have been achieved with animal models, and several authoritative reviews outline the many advantages of using such experimental approaches (see e.g., Davids et al 2003; Russell 2007; Kostrzewa et al 2008). Nevertheless, although improved models are still required, it is not our intention to further debate this issue, but rather to critically examine another perceived shortcoming: i.e., that psychostimulant doses used in animal studies fail to simulate the treatment conditions normally seen in children within clinical practice.

1a. Blood Levels of MPH

Most of the earlier published experimental work devoted to the modeling of clinical psychostimulant treatment used high doses of, for example, MPH (10-100 mg/kg per day) usually administered via injection (Chase et al 2007). More recently efforts were made to use doses judged to be comparable to those used clinically. A comprehensive search of the literature revealed some interesting comparisons between treatments and serum levels in both animals and patients (Table 1). Children with ADHD are routinely treated with *oral* doses of MPH (< 1 mg/kg) via tablet, which yield peak plasma MPH levels of approximately 4-65 ng/ml (Table 1). A new method, using transdermal delivery, provided similar values in children (Pierce et al 2008). Overall, parallel results were observed in adult patients treated with MPH. However, in adult experimental rats injected with doses of MPH that were thought to be clinically relevant (0.5-10 mg/kg) we can see that serum levels of MPH varied between 100-6000 ng/ml. Thus on the basis of serum levels alone, the results of these rat experiments are unlikely to be clinically revealing. In contrast, several groups reported that treatment of adult rats with *oral* MPH yielded serum levels of MPH close to those seen in humans (Table 1). For example, oral MPH at doses of 0.5, 2, and 3.5 mg/kg yielded peak plasma MPH concentrations of 2, 36, and 62 ng/ml in the adult rat (Aoyama et al 1990a), and Bakhtiar and Tse (2003) reported serum levels ranging from 22-86 ng/ml in adult male rats given oral MPH (10 mg/kg).

There have been few efforts to establish blood levels of MPH in immature rats. Kuczenski and Segal (2002) treated adolescent rats with oral MPH (1-3 mg/kg) and determined that serum MPH levels varied from 7-11 ng/ml to 30-60 ng/ml. Additional reports from Wheeler et al (2007) and Chase et al (2007), including experiments with much younger rats, essentially confirmed and extended the earlier studies (Table 1). These investigations measured serum MPH levels following acute MPH (single dose). It is noteworthy that serum levels of MPH were only slightly higher following repeated oral dosing, at least in adult rats (2.5 mg/kg; 1.5 ng/ml vs. 5.5 ng/ml at week 13; Bakhtiar and Tse 2003). However, Beckman et al (2008a) reported the opposite effect in older rats; i.e., at higher doses (5-50 mg/kg per day), blood levels were reduced after 60 days of treatment (see Table 1).

Table 1. Blood levels of Methylphenidate

RATS: Injection of MPH				
Age	Dose (mg/kg); Route	Blood Level (ng/ml)	Sample Time	Reference
Adult	1; iv	500	1 hr	Patrick et al (1984)
Adult	0.5-5; iv	86-1090	2 hr	Aoyama et al (1990a)
Adult	50; ip	2000	15-30 min	Roberts et al (1994)
Adult	0.5; iv	424	1 hr	Aoyama et al (1977)
Adult	10; iv	6000	1 hr	Wargin et al (1983)
Adult	20; iv	6300	20 min	Huff & Davies (2002)
Adult	2, 5, 10; iv	1050, 2400, 5400	2 hr	Aoyama et al (1997)
Adult	7; ip	1000	8 hr	Thai et al (1999)
RATS: Oral Treatment with MPH				
Age (days)	Dose (mg/kg)	Blood Level (ng/ml)	Sample Time	Reference
7	5, 50, 100	144, 1736, 1917	1-3 hr	Beckman et al (2008)
70	5, 50, 100; multiple doses through 60 days	30, 213, 517	30-60 min	
15 & 40	1, 2 ,5	9, 15, 49	15 min	Wheeler et al (2007)
24	2.5, 5, 10	30, 150, 390	30 min	Chase et al (2007)
40	1 & 3	9, 30-60	15 min	Kuczenski & Segal (2002)

Table 1. (Continued)

RATS: Oral Treatment with MPH				
Age (days)	Dose (mg/kg)	Blood Level (ng/ml)	Sample Time	Reference
Adult	0.5, 2, 3.5, 5	2-259	15 min	Aoyama et al (1990a)
Adult	10	300-400	50 min	Wargin et al (1983)
Adult	1	45	10 min	Patrick et al (1984)
Adult	2.5, 10, 40	1.5, 22, 282	30-60 min	Bakhtiar & Tse (2003)
Pregnant	7, 25, 75	88, 293, 727	30-60 min	Bakhtiar & Tse (2004)
Adult	2	22	15 min	Berridge et al (2006)
MONKEY: MPH Treatment				
Age	Dose (mg/kg); Route	Blood Level (ng/ml)	Sample Time	Reference
Pre-adolescent	0.8-32; oral	approx 3.0 - 80	2 hrs	Wilcox et al (2008)
Peri-adolescent	1.2-1.6 x 2/day; 5 days/wk; 4 years plus challenge 3.0; oral	peak 16	60 min	Doerge et al (2000)
2.5 yrs	3; iv	peak 800	30 min	Wargin et al (1983)
MOUSE : Oral Treatment with MPH				
Age	Dose (mg/kg)	Blood Level (ng/ml)	Sample Time	Reference
Adult	3	30	15 min	Manjanatha et al (2008)

Table 1. (Continued)

HUMANS: MPH Treatment in Children				
Age	Dose (mg/kg); Route	Blood Level (ng/ml)	Sample Time	Reference
Children	0.34 and 0.65; oral	11 and 20	1.9-2.5 hr	Shaywitz et al (1982)
Children	0.25-0.68; oral	28-35	1-1.6 hr	Chan et al (1983)
Children	0.3; oral	10,8	1.5 hr	Wargin et al (1983)
Children	0.9; oral	20-33	100 min	Greenhill et al (2001)
Children	0.1-0.6; oral	14-17	2-9 hr	Teicher et al (2006)
Children	10-20 mg; bolus iv	60-100	0.5-2 hr	Chan et al (1980)
Male (12 yrs)	15 mg; oral bolus	65	30-60 min	Soldin et al (1979)
Children	5-15 mg x 3/day; oral bolus	peak approx 7, 8, 9	2, 5.5, 9.5 hr	Swanson et al (2003)
Children	15, 30, 45 mg/day; OROS sustained release	6-9	initial peak at 2 hr-10 hr	Swanson et al (2003)
Children	5, 10, or 20 mg; oral bolus	4, 11 and 16	2-10 hr	Quinn et al (2004)
Children	10-30 mg/9 hrs; transdermal	20-47	8 hr	Pierce et al (2008)
HUMANS: MPH Treatment in Adults				
Adult	0.15 & 0.3; oral	3.5-7.8	2 hr	Wargin et al (1983)
Adult	0.3; oral	15	2 hr	Zhu et al (2007)
Adult	0.5; oral	approx 10	1-2 hr	Silveri et al (2004)

Table 1. (Continued)

HUMANS: MPH Treatment in Adults				
Adult	50 mg; oral immediate release	21	2 hr	Parasrampuria et al (2007)
Adult	90 mg; oral immediate release	39	2 hr	
Adult	54 mg; oral osmotic release	9	7 hr	
Adult	108 mg; oral osmotic release	17	7 hr	
Adult	36 mg OROS; oral	approx 8-10	max 5 - 8 hr	Auiler et al (2002)
Adult	10 mg iv; bolus	60	0.5 hr	Srinivas et al (1993)
Adult	40 mg; oral bolus	15	2 hr	
Adult	40 mg; oral slow release	15	2-3 hr	
Adult	40 mg; oral chewable	2	2 hr	
Adult	40 mg; oral slow release	14	approx 2 hr	Wang et al (2004)
Adult	20 mg; oral bimodal release	approx 12-18	2 and 5 hr	Tuerck et al (2007)

A crucial question, important in any attempt to experimentally simulate MPH treatment in children, is whether the serum levels of MPH achieved in rats following oral treatment are biologically equivalent to similar levels seen in children. There is reason to think that this is not the case. Due to more rapid metabolism in rats it is possible that higher doses of MPH might be required to achieve a similar drug effect as that observed in humans (Gatley et al 1999; Gerasimov et al 2000). The maximal concentration of oral MPH in blood was estimated to peak by 15 min in the adult rat (Aoyama et al 1990a,b), and 1.5-2 hrs in children (Swanson and Volkow 2003; see Table 1), whereas the half-life for MPH in rat is 1 hr versus 2-3 hrs in humans (Volkow and Insel 2003). This suggests that any attempt to reproduce clinically relevant blood levels of MPH in rats may need to consider: 1) higher oral doses; 2) multiple oral treatments, or 3) a sustained release preparation, to maintain MPH concentrations over several hours. The latter approach is elegantly illustrated in the work of Swanson et al (2003) who showed that sustained release oral MPH (OROS methylphenidate), giving an initial rapid rise followed by a small further increase over 10 hrs, had the same clinical efficacy in children as three doses of oral MPH given through the day (Patrick et al 2008). One way to estimate "efficacy" in rats would be to quantify a biological response to oral MPH. For example, 5mg/kg oral MPH was the lowest dose able to significantly increase dopamine release in the nucleus (n.) accumbens of adolescent rats (Kuczenski and Segal 2002) though lower doses (1.0 mg/kg) caused secretion of norepinephrine from the hippocampus. These data indicate that low oral doses of MPH in young rats do have significant, albeit brief, biological effects in the brain. These authors also reported that three treatments with MPH (0.75-3.0 mg/kg, separated by 3 hrs, were effective in slightly *reducing* locomotor activity during the dark (active) phase. In similar experiments performed on adult rats in the light phase (Gerasimov et al 2000), *intragastric* MPH (5 mg/kg, but not 2 mg/kg) slightly, but significantly, increased dopamine secretion from n.accumbens. A similar change was also seen in locomotor activity. These two influential reports revealed that doses of oral MPH in the range 3.0-5.0 mg/kg might be the threshold for inducing a biological response in experimental rats (see Kuczenski and Segal 2005 for review). The different ages of the rats in these studies, and the obvious discrepancy in the time of day at which the experiments were carried out, make it difficult to draw firm conclusions as to the optimal oral dose of MPH.

We have used the localization of psychostimulant-induced gene expression as an alternative approach to establish this optimal dose. In earlier investigations we localized and quantified MPH-induced gene expression in multiple brain regions of prepubertal rats (Chase et al 2003, 2005a, b). In subsequent experiments we developed a clinically relevant method for administration of oral MPH to immature rats to more closely model the therapeutic treatment of children. We observed that prepubertal rats quickly learned to consume a bolus of chocolate drink, containing MPH, from a needle-free syringe without the need for restraint. This method allowed precise control over the amount that each rat consumed and enabled a rapid (within 30 sec) drug delivery, comparable to a child swallowing an MPH tablet. We also measured serum levels of MPH resulting from oral administration to determine whether these fell within the clinical range. Acute oral MPH at doses of 2.5, 5 and 10 mg/kg resulted in serum MPH levels of approximately 30, 150, and 390 ng/ml, respectively (Chase et al 2007). These values are similar to published data on oral treatment of adolescent or adult rats (see Table 1). A comparison with data from children is instructive;

i.e., oral doses of MPH (0.15-1.00 mg/kg) yielded plasma values of 3.5-40 ng/ml. These results imply that higher doses (approx 2.5-fold) are required in young rats to achieve the same blood levels of MPH as those seen in children. Employing the effector immediate early gene *arc* (*activity regulated cytoskeletal associated*) as a functional marker, we showed that acute oral MPH resulted in a dose-dependent elevation in striatal ARC-immunoreactivity (ir), and in *arc* mRNA, that was significant at the higher doses (7.5 and 10 mg/kg) compared with saline (no drug)). The distribution of staining was similar to that induced by MPH *injection* (Chase et al 2007). These data suggest that in prepubertal rats the threshold dose of oral MPH required to elicit an acute neural response in the brain is in the range 7.5-10 mg/kg. Similar results were obtained with *c-fos* expression as an end point (Chase et al; unpublished observations). This dose range is higher than that suggested by Kuczenski and Segal (2005) (see above), though this may reflect the younger age of our rats (PD 24 vs. PD 40), as well as performing our experiments in the light phase. Given that Kuczenski and Segal (2002) reported that three consecutive low doses of MPH, given at 3hr intervals, affected locomotor activity, it would be interesting to determine whether gene expression (e.g., *arc*) is also increased. Such an experiment would also simulate the therapeutic strategy outlined by Volkow and Swanson (2003). These authors emphasised the importance of avoiding the development of acute tolerance to MPH that is likely to develop when serum levels of MPH remain constant rather than increased at, for example, 3hr intervals.

1b. Blood Levels of Amphetamine

Given that the rate of prescriptions for Adderall has outstripped those for MPH (Swanson et al 2007), and the appearance of new amphetamine preparations such as Vyvance (lisdexamfetamine), the prodrug of dextroamphetamine, there is surprisingly little information available on blood levels of amphetamine in children or in young rats, particularly following oral intake of drug (see Table 2). Children and adolescents - variously treated with oral AMPH, mixed amphetamine salts (MAS) or ADD - have blood levels of AMPH in the range of 18-89 ng/ml and these studies also provided pharmacokinetic details for AMPH levels (Table 2).

A single study on prepubertal rats (PD 25), injected with a low dose of AMPH (0.5 mg/kg; sc), reported a maximum blood level of 85 ng/ml (5-15 min), with a plasma half-life of 60 min (Diaz Heijtz et al 2003). We have recently established a technique for administration of oral ADD to immature rats in an attempt to model the therapeutic treatment of children. The method is similar to that described for MPH (Chase et al 2007), and an acute oral dose of ADD (1.5 mg/kg; PD 24) gave blood levels of AMPH that approximated the clinical range over an extended time period (Figure 1). This preparation opens the way to a more complete study of the effects of chronic oral ADD on the developing brain.

More extensive investigations of AMPH blood levels have been published on oral ADD treatment in adults, and in general the data parallel those reported for children, with values between 30 and 100 ng/ml (Table 2).

Table 2. Blood Levels of Amphetamine

NON-HUMAN PRIMATES: Oral Treatment with AMPH			
Age	Dose (mg/kg)	Blood Level (ng/ml)	Reference
Adult Baboon	0.12-1.0; x 2/day; 4 weeks; 3:1 mixture d- and l- AMPH	approx 60-160	Ricaurte et al (2005)
Adult Squirrel Monkey	0.28-0.68; x 2/day; 4 weeks; 3:1 mixture d- and l- AMPH	approx 100-200	
RATS: Injection of AMPH			
Age	Dose (mg/kg); Route	Blood Level (ng/ml)	Reference
Prepubertal (PD 25-26)	0.5; sc	85	Diaz Heijtz et al (2003)
Adult	1.5; ip	100	Wolfe et al (1977)
Adult	5.0; ip	675	Honecker & Coper (1975)
HUMANS: AMPH Treatment in Children			
Age (years)	Dose; Route	Blood Level (ng/ml)	Reference
5-12	0.5 mg/kg; oral	70	Brown et al (1979)
5-12	0.5 mg/kg; oral; sustained release	70	Brown et al (1980)
7-12	10 mg x 2/day; oral bolus Adderall®	53	Greenhill et al (2003)
6-12	10, 20, or 30 mg bolus Adderall-XR®	29-89	McGough et al (2003)
	10 mg; bolus Adderall®	33	
13-17	10-60 mg; bolus; MAS	18-82	Kramer et al (2005)
HUMANS: AMPH Treatment in Adults			
Age (years)	Dose; Route	Blood Level (ng/ml)	Reference
29-47	0.25 mg/kg; oral d-AMPH	peak 50	Kupietz et al (1985)
18-55	20 mg bolus; extended-release Adderall®	peak 40	Tulloch et al (2002)

Table 2. (Continued)

HUMANS: AMPH Treatment in Adults			
Age (years)	Dose; Route	Blood Level (ng/ml)	Reference
18-50	20 mg bolus; Adderall-XR®	43	Auiler et al (2002)
18-55	20, 40 or 60 mg bolus; MAS	32-106	Clausen et al (2005)
21-50	37.5 mg bolus; triple bead MAS	50	Ermer et al (2007)
	25 mg MAS-XR plus 12.5 mg MAS-XR	49	
22-52	70 mg; oral bolus; LDX	60 (intact LDX)	Krishman et al (2008)
		80 (d-AMPH)	

PD; postnatal day
sc; subcutaneous
ip; intraperitoneal
XR; extended-release
MAS; mixed amphetamine salts
d-AMPH; dextroamphetamine
l-AMPH; levoamphetamine
LDX; lisdexamfetamine dimesylate (Vyvanse®; inactive prodrug converted to active metabolite d-amphetamine)

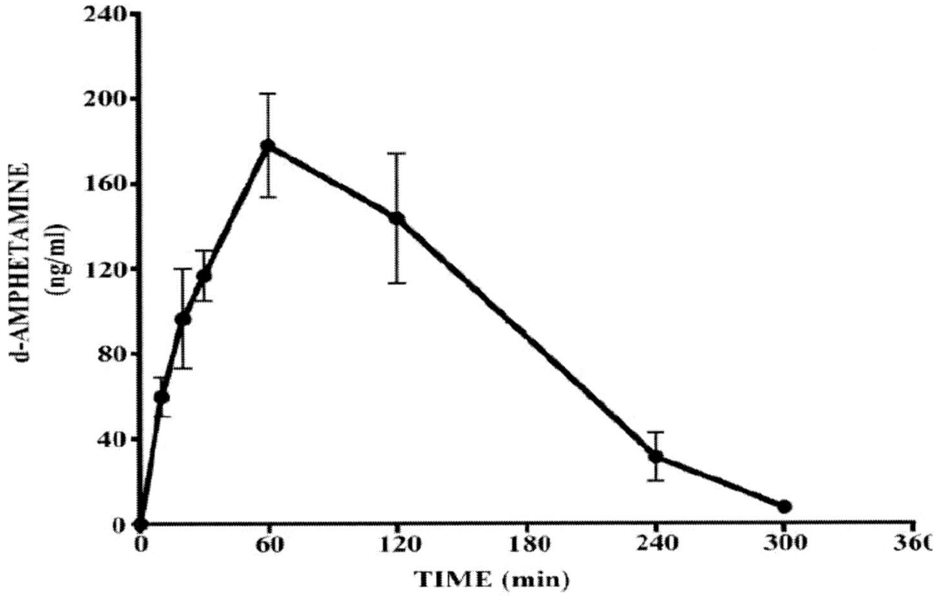

Figure 1. Blood levels of d-amphetamine following oral treatment with Adderall. Prepubertal rats (PD 24; n = 5 per group) were given a single dose of oral ADD (1.5 mg/kg). Serum was obtained at the indicated times, frozen at -70°c, and then analyzed for d-amphetamine by UPLC-mass spectrometry. Values are mean +/- sem.

In addition, an important study on adult non-human primates reported that oral doses of an amphetamine mixture (0.12-1.00 mg/kg), that approximated ADD, gave blood levels that varied from 60-200 ng/ml over a period of 4 weeks (Ricaurte et al 2005). Of great significance was their observation that this treatment appeared to be neurotoxic (see section 3b).

In conclusion, current and future experimental animal models in ADHD studies should strive to use clinically relevant oral doses of both MPH and AMPH. Researchers also need to calibrate biological responses, such as immediate early gene expression, to clinically relevant blood levels of stimulants.

2. Dopamine Signaling Pathways and Neuroadaptation

Neurons have the ability to respond and adapt to a range of external stimuli through altered structure and activity, often brought about by changes in gene expression. In developmental terms, changes in cellular function arise from an interaction of: (1) preprogrammed genetic and epigenetic factors, and (2) adaptive responses to the environment. In the short term neurons readily adapt to stimulation (neuroplasticity), but stimulation beyond physiological limits (e.g., addiction, trauma, drug treatment) can lead to both transient compensatory changes as well as permanent neuroadaptive changes (McClung and Nestler 2008). All psychostimulants such as MPH, amphetamines, and cocaine produce long term neuroadaptive changes in the fronto-striatal dopaminergic system, the main neurotransmitter pathway involved in cognition, movement and reward/punishment. An important question is whether these drugs, given orally at low levels, on a chronic basis, during sensitive periods of development, produce neuroadaptive changes in gene expression.

Psychostimulant-induced dopaminergic stimulation begins with binding at dopamine receptors, most probably of the D1 subtype (Yano et al 2006; Diaz Heijtz and Castellanos 2006; Cho et al 2007) followed by activation of G-proteins and intracellular messengers. A major intracellular target is now known to be DARPP-32 (*dopamine and cAMP-regulated phosphoprotein,* Mr32kDa), which is enriched in dopamine-sensitive neurons. The phosphorylation of DARPP-32 is essential for mediating the effects of psychostimulants (Svenningsson et al 2004; Bateup et al 2008) and it seems likely from this work that MPH, like cocaine, acts through DARPP-32 in striatonigral, rather than striatopallidal, neurons. Little work has been done however on the effects of MPH on DARPP-32. Fukui et al (2003) showed that *in vitro*, striatal slices from prepubertal mice did not respond to MPH with phosphorylation of DARPP-32 whereas slices from older mice responded with a significant increase of thr75 phosphorylation. Since both young and old mice responded to methamphetamine with activation of DARRP-32, the authors concluded that prepubertal mice did not possess a functional mechanism for MPH-induced release of vesicular dopamine. This seems inconsistent with the known stimulatory effects of MPH on *cfos* expression in neonatal and prepubertal mice (Penner et al 2002). On the other hand, recent studies in young rats by Souza et al (2008) indicated that neither acute nor repeated MPH treatment (PD 25; 1 or 2 mg/kg; ip; acute injections or x 28 daily injections) was effective in modifying absolute levels of DARPP-32; i.e., phosphorylation of DARPP-32 was not investigated. Similar results were seen in older rats. In contrast, small inhibitory changes were observed in hippocampus and cerebellum in rats of both ages. It remains unknown whether MPH or ADD might affect phosphorylation of DARPP-32 in immature rat brain, and this is an obvious experiment to carry out.

Dopaminergic stimulation also modulates immediate early gene (IEG) expression. IEGs such as *cfos*, *fosb*, *zif 268*, and *jun* are expressed at low levels in the unstimulated brain, and are induced in response to many external stimuli, such as psychostimulants, heat shock, feeding/fasting, fluctuations in the light/dark cycle, drug-induced seizure and stress (Morgan and Curran 1991; Hughes and Dragunow 1995; Herdegen and Leah 1998; McClung et al 2004). During development IEGs are implicated in normal cellular growth and differentiation (Curran and Morgan 1994), and analysis of their expression provides a revealing window into developmental processes. Thus, amphetamine, cocaine and MPH all acutely increase *cfos* expression in brain, but the level of stimulation appears to decrease developmentally between weanling, adolescence and adulthood (Andersen 2005; Andersen and Navalta 2004). Thus the effects of stimulants on IEGs appear to be more robust in younger animals, perhaps indicating greater plasticity and sensitivity (Andersen et al 2001). However this might be an oversimplification since more recent studies in discrete striatal nuclei (e.g., ventral caudate-putamen) revealed the opposite to be true; i.e., the effects of cocaine on *cfos* increase with age (Cao et al 2007). Nevertheless the localization/quantification of IEG activation is a valuable tool for investigating possible long-term effects of psychostimulants. In addition recent microarray expression studies revealed that MPH regulates a multiplicity of genes related to synaptic plasticity, including those involved in formation, maturation, and stabilization of new neural circuitry (Adriani et al 2006a, b). These data suggest the possibility that the young brain responds readily to MPH with widespread changes in gene expression. It also seems likely that treatment with ADD will induce similar modifications in the immature brain (Yuferov et al 2005).

Nurr1 is a remarkable immediate early gene that is critical for the development of dopamine neurons (Perlmann and Wallen-Mackenzie 2004) and has been implicated in the etiology of ADHD (Smith et al 2005). Moreover, *nurr1* heterozygous (+/-) mutant mice are hyperactive in a novel environment (Rojas et al 2007) and *nurr1* appears to be a regulator of the human DAT gene (Sacchetti et al 2001) and of the dopamine vesicular monoamine transporter VMAT2 (See Section *7c*; Jankovic et al 2005). It is presently unknown whether *nurr1* might be regulated by psychostimulants such as MPH and amphetamine, but human *nurr1* expression is reduced in dopamine neurons of cocaine abusers (Bannon et al 2002) and in cocaine-treated rats (Leo et al 2007). These data suggest that *nurr1* should be the focus of future work into long-term effects of MPH and Adderall.

3. Developmental Neurochemistry

In order to anticipate possible psychostimulant-induced changes in brain development, we should consider the normal chain of developmental events. The same basic sequence of maturational events such as neurogenesis, neural migration/pathfinding, apoptosis, synapse production and elimination, and myelination occurs in humans, primates and rodents (Andersen 2003). Developmental neuroplasticity involves neuronal and glial modifications in response to stimuli or experiences. These include alterations in dendritic tree formation, connections within and between regions, neurotransmitters, receptors and transporters, synaptic sprouting, axon growth and synapse formation (Andersen and Navalta 2004). Serotonin, norepinephrine, and dopamine neurons are born early in the course of brain development and are among the first afferents to colonize the cortex (Insel 2000). In many instances, receptors for these transmitters are present early at higher levels than in the adult and specific receptor subunits may be exclusively present during the developmental period, suggesting that they serve developmentally different functions than in the mature brain (Vaccarino and Leckman 2000; Carrey and Kutcher 1998).

In humans there are two developmental periods during which dramatic synaptic modification and rearrangements occur (Andersen 2003). The first is between the time of birth to the first 2-3 years of life, and from 7-15 years (periadolescence) there is another stage of extensive overproduction followed by a "pruning" of synapses and receptors reaching adult levels by 18-22 years (Andersen 2005). During this process of fine-tuning an estimated 40-50% of synaptic connections are established and eliminated during periadolescence to young adulthood in boys, and to a lesser extent in girls (Andersen 2003). In the rat, the peak period of synaptogenesis in striatal medium spiny neurons occurs during the prepubertal period (PD 15-30) (Wang and Pickel 2004). Both of these sensitive periods - peripuberty in rats and adolescence in children - are precisely those most studied for the effects of MPH.

Synaptic overproduction and pruning parallel developmental changes in dopamine receptors (D1R and D2R) and the dopamine transporter (DAT). In male rats the density of D1R and D2R increases sharply from PD 20 to a peak by PD 40-60 (the peripubertal period representing the elimination phase), and then steadily declines (55%) to adulthood (PD 60-80) in the striatum, though levels remain elevated in n.accumbens (Andersen et al 1997). In the prefrontal cortex (PFC) there is more overproduction of DRs than in the striatum, in addition to delayed pruning (Andersen and Teicher 2000). This parallels the peak in DR production and elimination through the childhood-adolescent period in humans (Seeman et al 1987). Developmental differences in the levels of cyclic AMP were increased in the striatum and n.accumbens of peripubertal male rats, compared to adults (Andersen 2002). Thus, the pre/peripubertal period represents an important critical time of neuronal growth and differentiation in human and rodent brain (Andersen 2005).

The density of DATs steadily increased through puberty (PD 25-50), and then declined in adulthood (Moll et al 2000) with parallel upregulation of postsynaptic receptors and second messengers (Andersen 2005), changes found in humans as well (Haycock et al 2003). Subsequently rats in the periadolescent period show greater activity in response to novel environments, a marker of dopaminergic stimulation (Laviola et al 2003) as they transition to adulthood levels of stable behavioral responses. In this sense they appear to be similar to children with ADHD.

Regions of the brain mature at different times, implying that each region has a critical, sensitive period during which drug exposure may alter the course of development. Based on phylogeny, older structures, like the striatum and motor cortex, mature earlier than higher order regions, such as the cingulate and frontal cortices (Thompson et al 2000). This different time-course of development means that the effect of a drug on a particular region will depend on the time-period and duration of drug exposure (Andersen 2005). The enhanced plasticity of the prepubertal brain makes it more vulnerable to stimuli, and this vulnerability appears to be lost following puberty (Andersen 2003). Andersen (2003) suggested that changes in the mature brain in response to a stimulus are adaptive or compensatory to maintain homeostasis, but changes in the immature brain cause alterations in the course of development that affect the maturation of neuronal structure, connections, and excitability (Andersen 2005).

3a. Psychostimulant-Induced Structural Modifications Of Immature Brain

As outlined already, during certain maturational periods the developing brain may be exquisitely sensitive to stimulation with dopaminergic drugs such as MPH, and this could have detrimental consequences in the adult brain (Stanwood and Levitt 2004). However the obverse of this could also be true, that MPH or amphetamine might exert trophic support of developing neurons. Few studies have been reported in these areas, though in adult rats a single, relatively low, dose of amphetamine (2mg/kg; ip) induced a small but significant increase in dendritic spine density in n.accumbens (Robinson and Kolb 2004). Of greater significance is that this treatment, when extended, prevents the ability of later experience to modify synaptic plasticity, perhaps leading to behavioral deficits (Kolb et al 2003). Such data may have significance in the possible consequences of treatment of young animals or children with MPH or ADD.

Experiments in the peripubertal rat (PD 22-45) revealed that injections of MPH (1 and 5 mg/kg) induced the growth of larger and more complex dendritic trees in pyramidal neurons of the anterior cingulate cortex (Zehle et al 2007). Morshedi et al (2009) made similar observations in the immature rat medial prefrontal cortex following repeated injections of amphetamine (1.5 and 3 mg/kg). These findings are consistent with previous reports (e.g., Diaz Heijtz et al 2003) on amphetamine-induced increases in dendritic length and branches of pyramidal neurons in immature rats treated with a low dose of amphetamine (0.5 mg/kg; x 2 per day; sc; PD 22-34). Treatment of younger rats (PD 10-14) with a higher dose of amphetamine (2 mg/kg; sc; PD10, 12 and 14) induced dendritic growth in dopaminergic neurons of the ventral tegmental area (Mueller et al 2006). Diaz Heijtz et al (2003) also speculated that such changes occurred at glutamatergic synapses. In an attempt to delineate possible neurochemical changes that might accrue from MPH treatment, Gray et al (2007) investigated the effects of MPH (5 mg/kg; x 2 per day; ip; PD 7-35) on dopamine, norepinephrine, serotonin and acetylcholine systems. The medial prefrontal cortex (mPFC) of rats given MPH showed 55% greater immunoreactivity for the catecholamine marker tyrosine hydroxylase (TH), 60% more Nissl-stained cells, and 40% less norepinephrine transporter (NET)-ir density. In the dentate gyrus, MPH-treated rats showed a 51% decrease in NET-ir density and a 61% expanded distribution of the new-cell marker PSA-NCAM (polysialylated form of neural cell adhesion molecule). In medial striatum, TH-ir decreased by 21%, and in hypothalamus, neuropeptide Y-ir increased by 10% in MPH-exposed rats. In total these data revealed a marked trophic effect of MPH in brain areas related to motivated behaviour and cognition. Three important questions are: 1) would such changes still be evident using lower, clinically relevant doses? 2) would they occur following oral treatment? and 3) would there be eventual compensatory biochemical downregulation in response to a chronic treatment regimen?

3b. Psychostimulant-Induced Neurotoxicity

The questions posed above apply equally well to investigations aimed at evaluating whether MPH or AMPH is neurotoxic. It has long been assumed that this is not the case in the rodent brain, though these conclusions were reached following high dose treatment of *adult* animals (Yuan et al 1997; Zaczek et al 1989). Also, fairly low doses of injected MPH (1, 2 and 10 mg/kg; ip) in young rats (PD 25-53) increased levels of creatine kinase in prefrontal cortex and striatum, an effect the authors concluded was unlikely to be neurotoxic (Scaini et al 2008). In terms of possible adverse neurochemical effects of MPH in the developing brain, Martins et al (2006) reported that injected MPH (1-10 mg/kg), given chronically (PD 25-53), significantly increased lipid peroxidation in prefrontal cortex, striatum, hippocampus and cerebellum, even at the lowest doses. This group also found that the same doses of MPH induced DNA damage in peripheral blood cells and in the striatum (Andreazza et al 2007). On the other hand, MPH exerts countervailing effects on antioxidant enzymes that may prevent the adverse effects of oxidative stress (Gomes et al 2008). This group also speculated that since MPH increases the activity of mitochondrial respiratory enzymes and metabolic activity, especially in cerebellum, this may also induce oxidative stress (Fagundes et al 2007). Neuronal death (apoptosis) was also detected in neonatal (PD 5) mouse striatum, but not cortex, following injection of MPH even at low doses (0.5-50 mg/kg; Husson et al 2004). In marked contrast, MPH was reported to be neuroprotective against a neurotoxic insult in neonatal mice, and in neuronal cells *in vitro* (Husson et al 2004; Ludolph et al 2006). A more recent study by Lagace et al (2006) provided some support for the stimulation of apoptosis by MPH. This group demonstrated that MPH treatment in young rats (2 mg/kg; ip x 2 per day; PD 20-35) decreased neurogenesis in the adult hippocampus, possibly via stimulation of apoptosis. We should conclude from these investigations that MPH, at least at high injected doses, has unanticipated effects in the developing brain, perhaps independently of the involvement of dopamine. These data have implications for the treatment of very young children with MPH. In fact, DNA damage was described in peripheral lymphocytes from children treated with MPH (El-Zein et al 2005), though this result could not be replicated in other studies that included amphetamine treatment (Stopper et al 2008; Witt et al 2008). An extensive study in mice also showed a lack of effect of oral MPH on mutagenicity (Manjanatha et al 2008). Two extensive and authoritative reviews of the possible developmental toxicity of MPH in humans and animals were recently published (Golub et al 2005; Beckman et al 2008a, b).

As a final point concerning general toxicity, rather than neurotoxicity, there are suggestions that chronic oral MPH may have deleterious effects on other systems such as heart, kidney, thymus, bladder, cornea and retina in rats and mice (Tunc et al 2008; Take et al 2008; Manjanatha et al 2008).

Although there is an extensive literature on the adverse influence of amphetamine *abuse* on the brain (Frey et al 2006; Yamamoto et al 2005; Advokat 2007), there are few reports on the possibility that prolonged amphetamine/Adderall treatment in children, or in young laboratory animals, may have neurotoxic consequences. For example, short-term treatment of adult rats even with low doses of amphetamine (1 or 2 mg/kg; ip; x 7 days) significantly increased oxidative stress in prefrontal cortex and hippocampus (Frey et al 2006). An elegant study in adult non-human primates (baboon and squirrel monkey) revealed a significant neurotoxic effect of oral amphetamine (Ricaurte et al 2005). These animals showed significant reductions in biochemical markers of dopaminergic neuron terminals. For example, striatal levels of dopamine, DAT and VMAT2 were all attenuated. Of particular note were the efforts to establish clinically-relevant blood levels of amphetamine following oral treatment with an amphetamine mixture that approximated ADD (see Table 2). These data strongly suggest that the possible adverse neural effects of Adderall, especially in its extended release form, should be investigated in young animals.

4. Stimulant–Induced Modification of Immediate Early Gene (IEG) Expression in the Developing Brain

An extensive series of molecular studies by several groups, including our own, has made it clear that the major, but not exclusive, site of action of MPH is the striatum (Yano and Steiner 2007). However, numerous other brain regions are also sensitive to psychostimulants, including amphetamine. As noted in Section 3, much of this work focused on immediate early genes such as *cfos*. In the present section we will briefly review this evidence but also outline more recent work that implicates other neuroplasticity-related genes in the acute and long-term effects of Ritalin and Adderall in the developing brain. Note that all of the data to be described herein were obtained from animals *injected* with stimulants. As emphasized in Section 1 it is now critical to reevaluate some of these results and to investigate the response of central genes to *oral* treatment with stimulants.

In general IEGs function to couple short-term signals received by cells to long-term changes in phenotype and function (Morgan and Curran 1995). The encoded proteins from IEGs act as transcription factors, binding to AP1 sites in the promoter region of downstream genes to regulate expression of various signaling molecules such as Substance P, dynorphin, enkephalin, cell cycle proteins, neurotrophins, interleukins, cytoskeletal matrix proteins, ion channels, receptors and transporters (Morgan and Curran 1995). In addition to the striatum, dopamine-modulated transcription factors are expressed in multiple areas of the brain such as cortex and n.accumbens.

4a. Acute Psychostimulant-Induced Regulation of IEGs

Psychostimulant-induced changes in gene regulation are particularly pronounced in the striatum. Moreover, experiments in *cfos*-knockout mice clearly revealed the necessity of *cfos* expression to mediate dopamine-induced neuronal activity in, for example, the n.accumbens (Hu et al 2008; Xu 2008). Psychostimulants and DA receptor agonists alter the expression of many IEGs/transcription factors and peptides in striatal neurons (Yano and Steiner 2007). The subsequent molecular cascade of events that may lead to permanent neuroadaptation has been studied closely with a series of drugs (cocaine, amphetamine, and MPH) all of which bind to the dopamine transporter. One important difference between them is that MPH has low affinity for the serotonin transporter, whereas all three drugs bind to both the norepinephrine transporter, as well as the DAT (Kuczenski and Segal 1997). However a further critical difference between the actions of MPH and amphetamine lies in the ability of the latter to increase the secretion of dopamine from neuron terminals (Gainetdinov et al 2002). Thus amphetamine is 4- to10-fold more potent than MPH in increasing extracellular dopamine levels (Schiffer et al 2006; Easton et al 2007). In terms of possible long-term effects of psychostimulants it may be prudent to consider that chronic treatment with amphetamine (or ADD) and MPH may have quite different consequences in terms of cell signaling and neuroadaptation.

Expression of the *cfos* family of transcription factors is widespread and developmentally regulated in the rodent brain (Alcantara and Greenough 1993). MPH-induced *cfos* expression in striatum changes postnatally from a patchy to a homogeneous adult pattern by PD 28 in the mouse (Penner et al 2002) and the rat (Kosofsky et al 1995). A valuable, detailed topographical map of MPH-induced *cfos* induction in adult rat striatum was produced by Yano and Steiner (2005). *cFos* responds readily to acute MPH in multiple regions of the adolescent rat brain (Chase et al 2005a). Thus the cerebral cortex, the Islands of Calleja, the piriform cortex and n.accumbens are all targets for MPH whereas induction of *fos*B was restricted to the striatum. These data suggest that *fosB* is not regulated by acute MPH treatment to the same degree as *cfos*. The relevance of *fosB* to an interpretation of long-term effects of MPH will be discussed below (see section 4c).

Other IEGs have been investigated using developmental paradigms. These include *zif 268*, a zinc finger protein transcription factor that shows robust cortical changes after dopaminergic stimulation and *Homer 1a*, a scaffolding protein located at the post-synaptic density (Yano and Steiner 2007; Cotterly et al 2007). The effects of MPH on *Homer 1a* are particularly interesting since this protein is implicated in some aspects of synaptic restructuring and turnover, and the *Homer 1* knockout mouse has learning deficits and is spontaneously hyperactive (Szumlinski et al 2006). In contrast, selective overexpression of *Homer 1a* in striatal medium spiny neurons resulted in a reduction of open-field activity, and amphetamine increased their behavioural response (Tappe and Kuner 2006). Taken together, these data indicate that *Homer 1a* is a critical gene in the striatal response to stimulants and in the control of locomotor behaviour. In addition, and of great significance, are recent gene expression profiles that implicate several plasticity-related gene families - e.g., synapse organization, synaptogenesis, morphogenesis and cytoskeletal organization - in the response of the immature brain to repeated stimulation with MPH (Adriani et al 2006b).

cAMP response element binding protein (CREB) is, like FOS, a transcription factor crucial for stimulus-transcription coupling in neurons. CREB is bound to DNA sequences called *cAMP response elements* (CRE) and is activated by phosphorylation to increase or decrease the transcription of certain genes, including growth factors and structural proteins.

CREB activation is therefore thought to be intimately involved in long-term changes in plasticity (McLung and Nestler 2008). Compared to studies in adult rodents, little attention has been paid to the effects of MPH or amphetamine on CREB in the immature brain. For example, in n.accumbens of adult rats previously treated with MPH prepubertally (PD 20-35, 2 mg/kg x 2 per day; ip) levels of CREB expression were elevated by 50% over controls (Andersen et al 2002). These adult rats also demonstrated a reduced sensitivity to cocaine. Thus MPH treatment in the adolescent period has enduring behavioral and neurochemical effects. A subsequent extensive microarray study essentially replicated these findings (Adriani et al 2006b). In investigations more easily compared to the results from *cfos* expression studies (see above), amphetamine also affects CREB signaling in striatum (Choe et al 2002; Shaw-Lutchman et al 2003), though such an effect has not been reported in the immature brain. Further research is needed to elucidate the developmental impact of chronic stimulants, including MPH and ADD, on CREB in immature animals.

4b. Gene Expression Changes Following Repeated Doses of MPH

In efforts to simulate therapeutic drug treatment of children with ADHD, several groups investigated the effects of repeated doses of MPH on gene expression. Note that in all cases the drug was given by injection. In contrast to the stimulatory effect of a single injection of MPH, repeated MPH *down-regulated* several IEGs, including *cfos,* in peripubertal rats and mice (see Yano and Steiner 2007 for review). Notably, the MPH-induced decline in FOS protein production was selective and occurred only in the striatum and Islands of Calleja, but not in frontal cortex and n.accumbens, where levels of cFOS-ir remained elevated following multiple injections (Chase et al 2005a). An important developmental difference was that *cfos* was down-regulated by a high dose of chronic MPH (10 mg/kg) in the *adult* rat striatum, but a lower dose (2 mg/kg), effective in the peripubertal rat, was ineffective, demonstrating increased sensitivity of the immature brain. This downregulation of striatal *cfos* expression remained detectable following MPH challenge in adulthood (30 days following the last MPH injection) (Chase et al 2005a).

4c. The Response of FOSB to Repeated Treatment with MPH

Important new studies have begun to investigate the effects of MPH on *fos*B expression. The significance of this work lies in the fact that *fos*B encodes not only FOSB, but a splice variant, ΔFOSB, that is reported to accumulate in striatal substance P/dynorphin-expressing neurons following chronic cocaine treatment. ΔFOSB is very stable in brain, with a half-life of 4 to 7 days (Chen et al 1997). Whereas *cfos* expression is down-regulated by repeated cocaine treatment, ΔFOSB-ir gradually increases, specifically in the striatum of adult rats (Hope et al 1994). ΔFOSB is considered to be a "molecular switch" that regulates long-term changes in drug-induced neuroadaptation and may be part of a possible mechanism for the development of addiction following chronic drug exposure (Chen et al 1997; Nestler et al 1999; Kelz and Nestler 2000; McClung et al 2004). For this reason we hypothesised that chronic treatment with MPH or ADD might increase *fosB* expression. Little work has been reported on the effects of stimulants on ΔFOSB in immature, prepubertal, animals. Repeated high doses of amphetamine (5 mg/kg; ip) elevated levels of ΔFOSB-ir in the striatum and n.accumbens of prepubertal, but not older, mice (Ehrlich et al 2002). In contrast we showed that a low dose of MPH (2 mg/kg; sc) stimulated striatal *fosB* expression in prepubertal rats, though not to the same extent as *cfos* (Chase et al 2005a, b). However, compared to its effect on *cfos*, repeated MPH did not inhibit the normal *fosB* response; i.e., FOSB-ir remained elevated in the prepubertal rat striatum following chronic MPH treatment at both doses of MPH (2 and 10 mg/kg; sc)(Chase et al. 2005a, b). Large increases in FOSB-ir were seen in frontal and piriform cortices following multiple treatments with high dose MPH (Chase et al 2005a). Thus, these data indicate that the developing brain is sensitive to repeated doses of MPH in terms of an accumulation of *fosB*-encoded protein(s). Whether this immunoreactivity represents ΔFOSB remains to be determined. Perotti et al (2008) recently reported a new approach to localize ΔFOSB-ir and demonstrated that chronic cocaine treatment strongly increased striatal ΔFOSB-ir.

4d. Amphetamine-Stimulated Gene Expression

It should already be clear that little attention has been paid to the possible long-term influence of amphetamine on gene expression in the immature brain, though differences in gene expression through development are observed in response to acute amphetamine. Snyder-Keller and Keller (1998) found that acute amphetamine (2 or 5 mg/kg) induced cFOS-ir in the striatum of PD 1-7 rats, with staining becoming more homogeneous as the rats aged. Andersen et al (2001) reported that a single dose of AMPH (1 and 5 mg/kg; i.p.) elevated striatal and cortical cFOS-ir in rats more significantly at PD 21 than PD 35 and 60. Similar to our results with oral ADD (see below), doses as low as 1 mg/kg stimulated cFOS expression. These studies indicate that the degree and pattern of expression of IEGs depends on age and developmental period of the animal with the more immature brain being more plastic in its response.

Similar investigations with ADD, a mixture of amphetamine salts, and in particular its extended release form, ADD-XR, are urgently needed because of the recent rapid rise in prescriptions for this drug (Swanson et al 2007). Preliminary data from our laboratory indicates that *cfos* is very sensitive to the acute effects of low doses of *oral* ADD-XR (0.6 mg/kg) in the immature rat, when compared to MPH (Allen et al. unpublished data). Moreover, we demonstrated that chronic treatment with oral ADD-XR not only severely down-regulated *cfos* expression in prepubertal rat striatum, but did so at a daily dose (1.5 mg/kg; x 14 days; Figure. 2) that was without effect with MPH; i.e.; oral MPH has no effect on *cfos* expression below 7.5 mg/kg (Chase et al; unpublished data).

Perhaps of equal significance is our finding that ADD-induced increases in FOS-ir were seen in the cerebral cortex at oral doses lower than the threshold dose necessary to stimulate *cfos* expression in the striatum (Allen et al; unpublished observations). This raises the possibility that the effects of Adderall-XR in children with ADHD could conceivably be mediated via a non-striatal mechanism, or at least through a process that does not regulate *cfos* expression in striatum. Our data suggest that the extended release form of ADD should be the focus of more extensive gene expression studies.

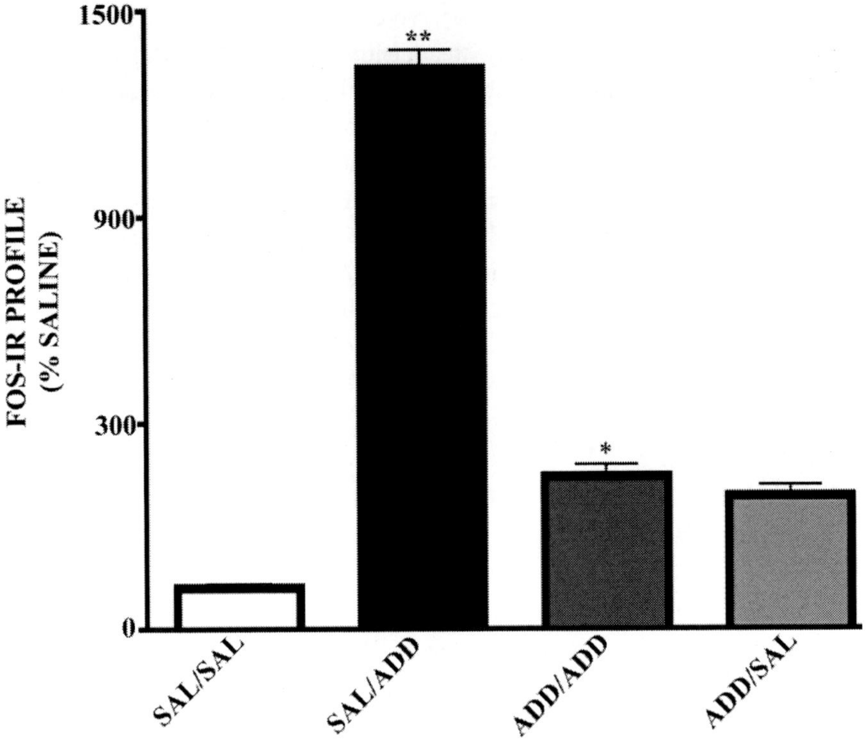

Figure 2. Densitometric analysis of oral ADD-induced FOS-IR in prepubertal rat striatum. Graph shows significant downregulation of FOS-immunoreactivity (ir) following repeated treatment with oral ADD (PD24-PD38 ; 1.5 mg/kg; x 1 per day; 14 days). Rats were sacrificed by perfusion-fixation 2 hrs following the final treatment. Immunohistochemistry for FOS-IR employed a Santa Cruz polyclonal antiserum (# SC-52; 1:40,000; Chase et al 2005a). SAL/SAL = 13 days of saline (SAL) treatment followed by a single challenge dose of saline on day 14 (n = 4); SAL/ADD = 13 days of SAL followed by a challenge dose of oral ADD on day 14 (1.5 mg/kg; n = 5); ADD/ADD = 13 days of oral ADD followed by a challenge dose of oral ADD on day 14 (1.5 mg/kg; n = 5); ADD/SAL = 13 days of oral ADD (1.5 mg/kg) followed by a challenge dose of SAL on day 14 (n = 4); $**p<0.001$ versus saline; $*p<0.001$ versus an acute dose. Bars represent mean (+/- sem) number of FOS+ nuclear profiles per treatment group.

In summary, there are differential effects of developmental period on stimulant-induced IEG expression. Acute MPH, amphetamine and ADD elevated cFOS-ir in a dose-dependent manner in both the neonatal, prepubertal, and peripubertal rat striatum and cortex. MPH stimulated both *cfos and fosB* expression in the striatum and several extra-striatal regions of the developing rat brain. In juveniles and adults chronic MPH treatment blunted the *cfos* response to a challenge dose, though this effect was significant only at the higher dose for adults, indicating a greater sensitivity in the younger animals. Downregulation of striatal *cfos* expression remained detectable following MPH challenge in adulthood, though only after repeated high-dose stimulation with MPH in the immature rat. In contrast to the effect on *cfos*, repeated MPH treatment induced an elevation in FOSB-ir compared to acute treatment in the immature rat striatum.

The stimulant-induced downregulation of *cfos*, and elevation of FOSB-ir, and possibly ΔFOSB, in specific regions of the brain, may represent different roles for these IEGs in the response of the immature brain to chronic treatment with stimulants. The expression of *cfos* may reflect short-term adaptation across several brain regions to excessive dopaminergic stimulation whereas *fosb and* ΔFOSB expression may be more involved in the long-term changes in neuroplasticity induced by chronic stimulation (Kelz and Nestler 2000; McClung et al 2004). Psychostimulant-induced changes in IEG expression may result in altered expression of downstream genes regulated by IEGs, including cocaine-induced *cyclin dependent kinase 5 (cdk5)*, a gene affecting dendritic tree formation in medium spiny neurons of n.accumbens and striatum (Bibb et al 2001; Norrholm et al 2003). Indeed, recent studies in pubertal rats revealed that low doses of injected AMPH (1,2 and 4 mg/kg; ip) transiently increased the expression of the cdk5 activator, p25, in striatum (Mlewski et al 2008).

5. Stimulant- Induced Changes in Effector Immediate Early Genes: *Arc* and *Bdnf*

In view of our evidence that chronic treatment of prepubertal male rats with MPH or ADD may lead to persistent changes in *cfos* and *fosB*/ΔFOSB expression, we next examined two genes already implicated in stimulant-induced neuroplasticity. These so-called "effector" IEGs, such as *arc* (activity regulated cytoskeletal associated) or *bdnf* (brain-derived neurotrophic factor), are considered to be markers of stimulus-induced structural modifications (Steward and Worley 2002; Tzingounis and Nicoll 2006; Yin et al 2002). *Arc* mRNA and protein are localized to synapses (dendritic spines) following neuronal activation in adult rats (Steward and Worley 2002), and by cocaine in striatal cell bodies and dendrites in adult rats (Fosnaugh et al 1995). In striatum, ARC protein was localized to synaptic sites on dendrites during prepubertal development (PD15-30) (Wang and Pickel 2004). In the developing rat forebrain, basal *arc* mRNA and protein expression was detected as early as PD 8, reached peak levels at PD 21, remained elevated to adulthood (PD 56), and then decreased by 3 months old (Lyford et al 1995). Maximum levels of *arc* expression, localized to dendritic spines and shafts of medium spiny neurons, parallels the peak period of synaptogenesis (PD 15-30)(Wang and Pickel 2004). These data suggest that *arc* is involved in striatal neuroplasticity throughout development and during normal alterations in synaptic structure and function in the adult brain. Of significance to the present paper, cocaine (10-20 mg/kg; ip) and amphetamine (3-5 mg/kg; ip) -induced *arc* expression following acute (Fosnaugh et al 1995; Tan et al 2000; Klebaur et al 2002; Samaha et al 2004) and chronic (Fumagalli et al 2006; Ujike et al 2002) treatment, particularly in the striatum and cortical regions of the adult rat brain. Our studies in prepubertal rats revealed that treatment with acute MPH (2 and 10 mg/kg; sc.) induced a dose-dependent increase in *arc* expression (ARC-ir) in striatum and to a lesser extent in frontal cortex (Chase et al 2007). The elevation in ARC-ir induced by acute MPH was significantly attenuated in prepubertal rat striatum chronically treated with MPH (2 and 10 mg/kg; 14 days), but not in the frontal cortex. The

MPH-induced desensitization of *arc* expression observed in the prepubertal striatum; i.e., in response to a challenge dose of MPH, remained detectable following a drug-free period of 4 weeks, indicative of an enduring response into adulthood.

There is speculation that abnormal BDNF levels could be implicated in the etiology of ADHD (Tsai 2003). BDNF provides trophic support for the survival and differentiation of dopaminergic neurons in the mammalian brain (Hyman et al 1991; Huang and Reichardt 2003). Conversely, dopaminergic stimulation increases bdnf expression in striatal and cortical neurons (Kuppers and Beyer 2001; Meredith et al 2002). In addition, *bdnf*, like *arc*, is implicated in activity-dependent synaptic plasticity (Bramham and Messaoudi 2005). Abundant BDNF-ir was localized to many regions of the adult rat brain (Friedman et al 1998), but was undetectable in the striatum in the unstimulated rat brain. However, cocaine and amphetamine increased BDNF protein levels in the striatum of adult rats and in neuronal cell cultures, possibly via D_1 dopamine receptors (Kuppers and Beyer 2001; Meredith et al 2002; Zhang et al 2002; Fang et al 2003). *Bdnf* mRNA was elevated by a single dose of cocaine (20 mg/kg) in the frontal and parietal cortex of adult rats (Le Foll et al 2005), and in the striatum of young adult mice following a single dose of methamphetamine (Thomas et al. 2004). These data implicate psychostimulants as regulators of *bdnf* expression. Moreover *bdnf* (+/-) knockout mice are reported to be hyperactive (Kernie et al 2000), a study confirmed using conditional *bdnf* (-/-) and *trkB* knockouts (Rios et al 2001; Zorener et al 2003).

In contrast to these data, little attention has been given to the possible effects of MPH or amphetamine on *bdnf* expression in the developing brain. This is doubly surprising given that BDNF regulates *arc* expression (Yin et al 2002; Alder et al 2003). We recently reported (Chase et al 2007) that neither acute (2 or 10 mg/kg) nor repeated MPH (10 mg/kg; 14 days; sc.) was effective in significantly altering *bdnf* mRNA in the striatum or frontal cortex of peripubertal (PD 38) rats. However a single dose of MPH (10 mg/kg) resulted in a small but significant inhibition of hypothalamic *bdnf* mRNA and repeated MPH (2 and 10 mg/kg) also significantly attenuated hypothalamic *bdnf*. Recent unpublished studies by Banerjee and Zetterstrom (2008a, b) also detected significant (> 30%) MPH-induced downregulation of *bdnf* mRNA in hippocampus and parietal cortex in prepubertal rats (2 mg/kg x 2 per day; ip; 14 days). Thus *bdnf* expression in the immature brain, and especially in non-striatal areas, might be vulnerable to inhibition by psychostimulants. This may have consequences for normal brain development. The study of psychostimulant effects on effector IEGs should be further pursued to establish the links between underlying programmed development, activity-dependent stimulation, chronic stimulants and neuroplasticity.

6. Stimulant-Induced Modification of Chromatin

As we have outlined, there is now considerable literature devoted to the influence of MPH and amphetamine on gene transcription in the developing brain. These studies have been invaluable in localizing the effects of psychostimulants in specific brain areas. However, there is a need for a new approach in order to probe possible longer-term changes in transcriptional regulation. Epigenetic mechanisms: "the structural adaptation of chromosomal regions so as to register, signal or perpetuate altered activity states" (Bird 2007) offer just such a means to examine long-term effects of MPH in the immature brain. For example, cocaine and amphetamine influence neurons by modifying chromatin structure via ΔFOSB and acetylation, methylation and phosphorylation of histones (Renthal and Nestler 2008; Jiang et al 2008). Recent studies by Renthal et al (2008) revealed that chronic treatment of adult rats with amphetamine (4 mg/kg; ip) induced downregulation of striatal *cfos* expression via ΔFOSB and histone deacetylase1. This result led us to speculate that our recent demonstration of MPH-induced downregulation of *cfos* activation in immature rat brain, and the concomitant stimulation of *fosB* expression (Chase et al 2005a) might also be mediated through changes in histone acetylation. Our preliminary results demonstrated that low doses of ADD (oral) and MPH (sc) stimulate histone phosphorylation in immature rat striatum and Islands of Calleja (Figure 3 and 4).

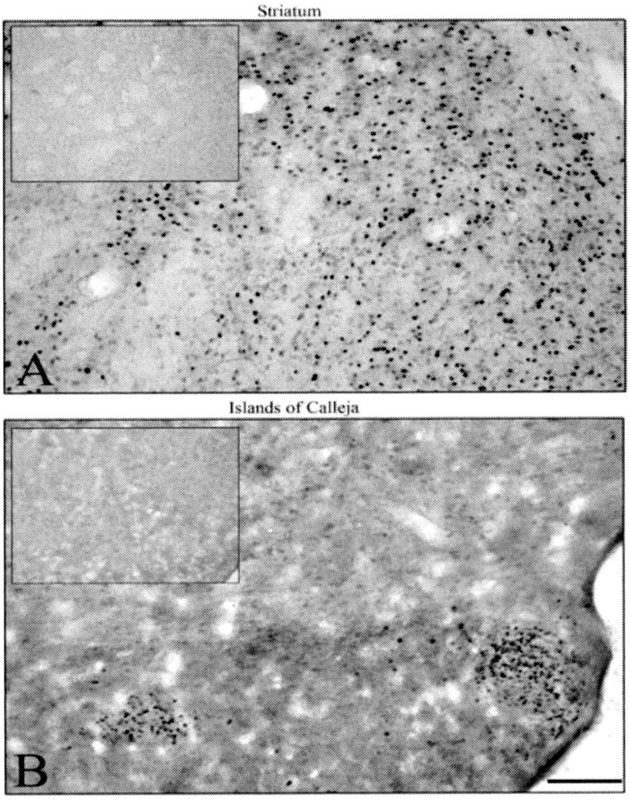

Figure 3. Oral Adderall-induced increase in histone H3 phosphorylation. Representative photomicrographs of oral ADD-induced histone H3 (phospho S10) immunoreactivity (Abcam; 1:30,000) in striatum (A) and Islands of Calleja (B). Male rats (PD 24) were treated with a single oral dose of ADD (1.5 mg/kg) and sacrificed by perfusion-fixation at 60 minutes post-administration. Dark nuclear staining is readily seen in many cells in the dorsomedial aspect of the striatum (A). Inset shows the absence of nuclear-ir in saline-treated controls. In (B) note the dense staining in cell nuclei of the Islands of Calleja. Scale bar = 100μm.

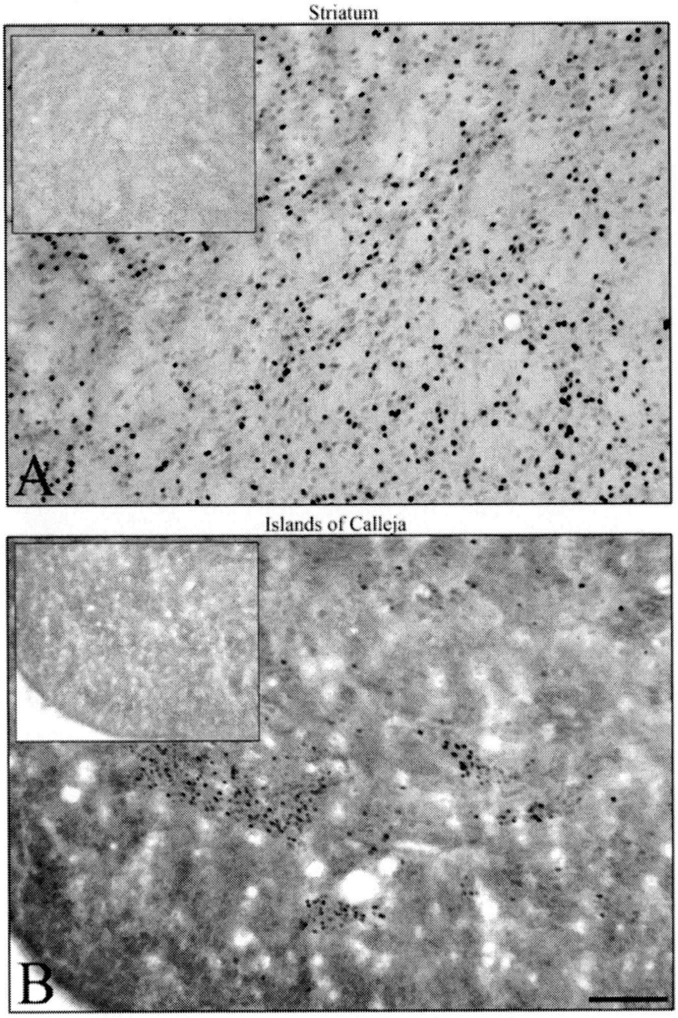

Figure 4. Methylphenidate-induced increase in histone H3 phosphorylation. Representative photomicrographs of injected MPH-induced histone H3 (phospho S10) immunoreactivity. (Abcam; 1:30,000) in striatum (A) and Islands of Calleja (B). Male rats (PD 24) were treated with MPH (5 mg/kg; sc) and sacrificed by perfusion-fixation at 30 minutes post-injection. Dark nuclear staining is apparent in many cells in the dorsomedial aspect of the striatum (A). Inset shows the absence of nuclear-ir in saline-treated controls. In (B) note the dense staining in cell nuclei of the Islands of Calleja. Scale bar = 100μm.

Our conclusion is that psychostimulant treatment especially in the prepubertal rat acts, at least in part, via an epigenetic mechanism. A similar implication can be taken from the work of Black et al (2006) who treated adolescent rats with ascending doses of cocaine to produce an increased response to cocaine as adults and an overall decrease in histone H3 methylation. In contrast, acute cocaine leads to a transient increase in striatal histone acetylation at the *cfos* promoter (Kumar et al 2005).

In total these studies indicate that the effects of MPH and amphetamine on chromatin remodelling in the developing brain should be an important focus of future research. Also, since environmental influences during sensitive periods of development influence histone modification (Meaney and Szyf 2005) it would be prudent to consider the possibility that psychostimulants and environmental influences may interact in yet unknown ways to affect long-term neuroadaptation, especially since very young children in all kinds of settings are now being treated with MPH and ADD.

7. Stimulant-Induced Changes in Peptides, Neurotransmitters and Transporters

7a. Striatal Peptides

Striatal projection neurons under dopaminergic control express several neuropeptides that are differentially expressed between neurons of the two striatal output pathways. Neurons projecting to the entopeduncular nucleus or substantia nigra (direct pathway) express substance P and dynorphin whereas neurons that project to the globus pallidus (indirect pathway) express enkephalin (Steiner and Gerfen 1998; McGinty 2007). These peptides may act as negative feedback or compensatory factors to regulate striatal output on the system when there is excessive dopamine stimulation. Upregulated expression of dynorphin in the striatum is a well-established long-term effect of cocaine and amphetamine stimulation (Brandon and Steiner 2003). However, although acute amphetamine treatment increases substance P and dynorphin levels, with more subtle effects on enkephalin, acute MPH (adult rats; 2-10 mg/kg; ip) increased substance P expression with little effect on dynorphin and no effect on enkephalin. In adolescent rats chronic treatment with high dose MPH resulted in significant blunting of substance P expression following a cocaine challenge. In contrast, a modest increase for dynorphin (Brandon and Steiner 2003) and no change for enkephalin expression, was observed following repeated MPH (2 to 10 mg; sc) (Yano and Steiner 2007).

There seems to be little effect of MPH on opioids in young rats, and substance P is only affected at high doses. Nonetheless, before any definitive conclusions can be reached, more work needs to be done in younger age groups and on several brain areas (including striatal, cortical and accumbal regions). More importantly there are no data on whether amphetamine salts (e.g., ADD) affect striatal peptides in the immature brain, although a low dose of d-amphetamine (Dexedrine; 2.5 mg/kg; ip) increased striatal preproenkephalin and preprodynorphin mRNA levels, albeit in adult rats (Shi and McGinty 2006). Other neuropeptides, such as neurotensin and cholecystokinin, are implicated in striatal function and should also be investigated as targets for psychostimulant action in the immature brain (Ferraro et al 2007; Loonam et al 2003; Dobner et al 2003).

7b. Excitatory and Inhibitory Striatal Neurotransmitters

Glutamate and GABA are the most abundant neurotransmitters in the mammalian brain and the functional interaction between dopaminergic transmission and glutamatergic modulation plays a critical integrational role in striatal output (David et al 2005). The balance between glutamatergic and GABAergic tone is also pivotal in the modulation of synaptic plasticity (Collingridge et al 2004), and as noted already in the discussion on CREB, these systems are implicated in the mechanism of action of addictive psychostimulants (McLung and Nestler 2008). In addition, proteins such as Homer, whose expression is regulated by MPH (see Section 4a) anchor and link glutamate receptors - such as the NMDA and type-1 metabotropic GluR subtypes - to cytoskeletal elements and signalling pathways (Szumlinski et al 2006). Nevertheless, few reports exist on attempts to implicate glutamate transmission in the effects of MPH. For example, Gaytan et al (2000) reported that blockade of the NMDA receptor with the antagonist MK-801 was able to prevent the development of sensitization to the locomotor effects of MPH in adult rats. Pascoli et al (2005) used adult mice to show that both MPH and amphetamine increased the phosphorylation of GLUR1 receptors in the prefrontal cortex. This effect was only seen at high doses. The possible involvement of GLU/GABA transmission in the long-term effects of MPH in the developing brain has so far been investigated by two groups. In their continuing investigations into developmental influences of MPH treatment, Andersen et al (2002) reported that MPH (PD 20-35; 2 mg/kg; ip; x 2 per day), had no effect on the levels of glutamate receptor proteins GluR1, GluR2/3 or NMDA in n.accumbens. In contrast, a large increase in GluR2/3 level was observed in adult rats treated with MPH. Adriani et al (2006a, b), in their pioneering microarray studies in adolescent rats (PD 30; 2 mg/kg/day; ip; x 14 days) reported that more than 700 genes were upregulated in the striatum, including two subunits of the GABA A receptor ($\gamma 1$ and $\beta 3$) and the ionotropic glutamate receptor, GluR6. These two reports emphasise that further attention should be directed towards elucidating the involvement of glutamate and GABA in the effects of MPH. Striatal glutamate and glutamate receptors are also firmly implicated in the mechanism of action of amphetamine (Nestler 2005; Wang et al 2006), providing a further focus to pursue an understanding of the potential long-term effects of ADD on the developing brain.

7c. Stimulants and Dopamine Transporters

Because of the efficacy of methylphenidate and amphetamine in the treatment of ADHD, it is generally assumed that the dopamine transporter is the primary site of action of these drugs. Indeed, multiple brain imaging studies established that ADHD patients possess abnormal dopaminergic frontostriatal circuits (Krause 2008). Most reports suggest that DAT levels are elevated in ADHD, though this view is not without its detractors (Swanson et al 2007). Nevertheless, there is agreement that treatment of ADHD patients with MPH results in lower DAT availability (Krause 2008). It remains important to investigate possible long-term effects of MPH or amphetamine on the DAT, particularly since both of these drugs have profound behavioural and neurochemical effects in mutant mice that lack the DAT (Gainetdinov and Caron 2003). For example MPH and amphetamine have a calming effect on these hyperactive mice, and a very high dose of MPH (30 mg/kg; ip) remains capable of inducing *cfos* expression in some brain areas despite the absence of the DAT. There is also evidence that MPH and amphetamine affect other transporters such as those for norepinephrine and serotonin (e.g., see Yano and Steiner 2007). The evidence is clear that MPH treatment reduces the number of DAT sites detectable by binding in both human and rodent brain (Krause 2008; Swanson et al 2007; Dresel et al 1998; Nikolaus et al 2007). Whether this reduction represents a true downregulation of DAT expression, or is simply a reflection of occupancy of the binding site, remains to be determined. An important study by Feron et al (2005) indicated that in children treated for many months with MPH, DAT levels appear to largely return to normal within 4 weeks following cessation of drug treatment. Investigations of this type need to be confirmed. In a similar study in rats, Moll et al (2001) reported that striatal DAT levels decreased by 25% in MPH-exposed prepubertal rats (age 25 days ; 2 mg/kg; oral; 14 days) and further decreased to 50% by adulthood, one month following cessation of MPH treatment. A similar study, extending the exposure period to 8 months, revealed a biphasic effect on the expression of striatal dopamine D2 receptors (Thanos et al 2007); i.e., levels of D2 receptor availability were reduced at 2 months of treatment but were increased at 8 months. Although this group did not acknowlege the earlier work by Moll et al (2001), a possible explanation for their data might be that alterations in DAT levels caused dopamine-induced changes in dopamine receptors. It is highly unlikely that MPH remained bound to the DAT, and a reasonable conclusion is that DAT expression is permanently down-regulated or that the normal developmental increase in dopaminergic innervation is compromised. An important difference in the respective methods could also have influenced the results; i.e., the rats used by Thanos et al (2007) were forced to drink the MPH quickly, in a water-restriction regime, whereas the animals used by Moll et al (2001) were allowed free access to the MPH/water. These data suggest that more work is needed to establish whether DAT levels are a useful marker for long-term effects of MPH. Also, given that amphetamine is a well-described neurotoxin (Advokat 2007), and that the number of prescriptions for ADD is rapidly increasing (Swanson et al 2007) , investigation of the possible adverse effects of ADD on DAT expression in the developing brain is urgently required.

MPH is assumed to increase synaptic dopamine levels by inhibiting reuptake of dopamine via the DAT. In contrast amphetamine is transported into nerve terminals through the DAT and subsequently binds to the vesicular monoamine transporter, VMAT2, where it induces the release of vesicular dopamine and facilitates its release into the synapse (Fleckenstein and Hanson 2003). However, new evidence suggests that MPH may also affect dopaminergic terminals by redistributing the VMAT2 protein in a manner distinct from that of amphetamine. MPH redistributes synaptic vesicles from the terminal membrane into the cytoplasm to increase transport of dopamine into the vesicles (Riddle et al 2007). At the same time, a population of vesicles that remain at the membrane increase their uptake of dopamine, via VMAT2, and increase the releasable pool of dopamine (Volz et al 2007). Thus MPH and amphetamine, at low doses, interact with VMAT2 to reduce, and increase, respectively, the cytoplasmic levels of dopamine. It is possible that VMAT2 could represent a useful therapeutic target, though an additional important question is whether chronic treatment with either of these psychostimulants might cause dysregulation of VMAT2 expression (Fleckenstein et al 2008).

7d. Effects on Dopamine Receptors

Molecular genetic studies have associated ADHD with variants in the dopamine D2, D3, D4 and D5 receptor genes (Faraone et al 2005; Thapar et al 2005; Davis et al 2008; Nyman et al 2007). Animal experiments have also focused on the relevance of dopamine and adrenergic receptor function in investigations into the mode of action of psychostimulants. For example, MPH and AMPH regulate gene expression via D1 as well as the α2 receptor (Yano et al 2006; Arnsten et al 2005). The importance of dopamine receptors (DAR) in mediating the therapeutic effects of MPH and ADD is therefore clear. However, even though striatal DAR production and pruning undergo significant changes through puberty and adolescence (Teicher et al 1995), no concerted effort has been made to determine whether DAR gene expression might be affected by long term treatment with MPH or ADD. The microarray studies of Adriani et al (2006a, b) indicated that D1 and D2 gene expression was unaltered by MPH (PD 30-44; 2 mg/kg; ip), though experiments on younger rats might be more informative. Andersen et al (2008) reported that D3 mRNA levels, but not those for D1, D2, D4 and D5, were reduced in prefrontal cortex of young rats following MPH treatment (PD 20-35; 2 mg/kg; x 2 per day; ip). They observed no effect of the treatment on striatal or n.accumbens DAR mRNA. In a similar study, Souza et al (2008) reported that MPH (PD 25-53; 1, 2 and 10 mg/kg; ip) increased the levels of NCS-1 protein in cortex, but not in striatum. NCS-1 is a dopamine interacting protein thought to be involved in neuronal plasticity.

This limited evidence suggests that, at least in young rats, MPH appears to be ineffective in changing DAR gene expression, particularly since the dosages used would have given very high serum levels of drug (see Table 1). Nonetheless it would be informative to perform similar experiments with ADD, and to determine whether DAR gene expression might be altered in discrete brain nuclei using in situ hybridization.

8. Behavioral Paradigms of Reinforcing or Aversive Properties of Stimulants: Enduring Effects in Adulthood

Experimental animal paradigms that include behavioral measures have the advantage of correlating gene expression more directly to the upstream neural loops that underlie behavioral expression. In this review we have elaborated on a variety of neurochemical changes that may accrue from chronic treatment of prepubertal animals with MPH or amphetamine. Investigations into some of the possible consequences of such changes can be accomplished through behavioral studies. Such a developmental perspective is particularly important because of the clinical concern that stimulant exposure during a critical phase of brain development may predispose to enduring effects in adulthood (Wilens et al 2003). In essence, this approach seeks to determine if early exposure to psychostimulants leads to the reinforcing or aversive properties of the same, or similar, drug in adulthood. As noted earlier, the numerous published studies in the rat are likely to be compromised because of the high doses of MPH normally used in these investigations, and may therefore be of little clinical significance (Volkow and Insel 2003). Also, from the earliest work by Brandon et al (2001), it is apparent that the degree of brain maturation, at the time of initial treatment with MPH, may dictate the subsequent behavioral actions of cocaine. For example, treatment of adolescent rats (PD 35-42) with daily, single injections of MPH (2-10 mg/kg; ip) induced an enhanced sensitivity to, and an increase in self-administration of, cocaine when tested 14 days later (Brandon et al 2001). In marked contrast, four later reports, all using similar treatment (MPH; 2 mg/kg; x 2 per day; ip; PD 20-35) (Andersen et al 2002; Carlezon et al 2003; Mague et al 2005)), or a modification (Adriani et al 2006b) arrived at the opposite conclusion. In addition, Bolanos et al (2003) used the same paradigm to show that MPH treatment decreased the sensitivity to rewarding stimuli such as sucrose and sex. An intriguing addition to this literature is the demonstration that spontaneously hyperactive rats (SHR) given MPH (2.5 mg/kg; ip; PD 35-45) also showed a reduced rewarding effect of cocaine (Augustyniak et al 2006).

Some of these studies also raised concerns that early exposure to MPH could lead to an increase in depressive-like behaviour, anxiety and poor stress tolerance in adults exposed to MPH treatment in the pre- and periadolescent period (Bolanos et al 2003; Carlezon et al 2003; Bolanos et al 2008). In contrast, a more extended prepubertal treatment with MPH (PD 7-35; 5 mg/kg; ip; x 2 per day) induced a state of reduced anxiety-like behavior (Gray et al 2007).

Two studies in mice again produced conflicting results. Chronic treatment with high doses of MPH (10 mg/kg; i.p; 7 days) during the prepubertal period (PD 26-32) resulted in decreased reward effects of a cocaine challenge in adulthood (Achat-Mendes et al 2003). However, following this cocaine challenge the mice developed a sensitized response to cocaine-induced reward. In a second study in mice, MPH (PD 15-28; 1, 5 and 10 mg/kg; ip; Guerriero et al 2006) did not increase the liability for cocaine abuse in adulthood.

There are several reasons for the lack of consistency in some of the results obtained from these studies: (a) the use of different ages of immature rats exposed to MPH; (b) variations in MPH pretreatment time (7, 15 days, 2-8 months); (c) different behavioral measures studied (self-administration (i.v.) versus conditioned place preference (CPP) and intracranial self-stimulation); and (d) daily versus twice daily MPH injections. For example, the different responses seen in older rats (PD 35-42; Brandon et al 2001), compared to those seen in the younger groups (PD 20-35; e.g., Andersen et al 2002), might be due to the much higher levels of testosterone in the more mature PD 35 rats. The dose of MPH used in all these experiments is also a problem (see also Kuczenski and Segal 2005). As we emphasised in Section 1, the blood levels of MPH reached after injection of the drug are far from clinically relevant. The behavioral experiments described here used approximately 2 mg/kg of MPH (ip). Given that an *oral* dose of 2.5 mg/kg MPH in prepubertal rats gave blood levels within the clinical range (30 ng/ml; see Table 1), it seems likely that 2 mg/kg ip would yield far higher values than those seen in children. Indeed, we used mass spectrometry to show that in infant rats given MPH (2 mg/kg; sc; PD10) blood levels of the drug reached values in excess of 300 ng/ml (Unpublished observations). Efforts to determine possible behavioral effects of MPH following oral treatment are so far limited. Kuczenski and Segal (2002) treated adolescent rats with oral MPH (PD 41-69; 0.75 and 3 mg/kg; x 3 per day) but found no evidence of an increase in sensitization to a methamphetamine challenge. Their conclusion was that MPH did not produce an increase in abuse liability. In a second study, Thanos et al

(2007) attempted to simulate clinical treatment by including MPH in the drinking water of young rats (PD30; 2 month or 8 month exposures; 1-2 mg/kg). The authors reported effects on striatal dopamine receptors (D2R lower at 2 months, but higher at 8 months compared to controls) but found no evidence for an increase in cocaine self-administration following 8 months of oral MPH.

MPH's differential effect may not be similar to early cocaine exposure or induce a later susceptibility to cocaine's rewarding effects. It nonetheless does produce enduring effects on future behavior some of which may be adaptive (reduced sensitivity to cocaine reward) while other behaviors are deleterious (depressive like states) (Carlezon et al 2003). These data may have some relevance to the growing abuse of MPH (Swanson and Volkow 2008), but not to the clinically relevant lower dose treatment of ADHD children.

9. Conclusion

We can draw the following conclusions from this review: 1) commonly prescribed stimulants such as MPH, and ADD, administered chronically to animals at low dosages produce reliable and measurable neuroadaptive changes in dopaminergic signalling systems; 2) differential effects of stimulants become obvious depending on the developmental period; the prepubertal brain appears to be more sensitive to stimulants than the adult brain; the peripubertal or "adolescent brain" appears to have a transitional period from pre- to postpubertal neuroadaptive functioning; 3) preliminary evidence exists for "enduring effects" which linger into adulthood with early exposure to stimulants given pre- or peripubertally; 4) there exists a "threshold" for a biological response and below this threshold gene expression changes appear to be transient; 5) the threshold for a meaningful gene expression change is affected by route of administration; i.e., higher oral doses are required compared to those used for intraperitoneal or subcutaneous treatments, and 6) there is preliminary evidence for qualitative and quantitative differential effects on gene expression between commonly used psychostimulants.

Changes in the immature brain occur as a result of exposure to chronic but clinically relevant dosages of the commonly prescribed stimulants, and these effects are observed at all levels of the dopaminergic signaling pathways, from early short-term responses (changes in DAR, IEGs, CREB, DAT) to longer term downstream genes involved in peptidergic control, structural synaptic modification (effector IEGs) and epigenetic chromatin-histone acetylation and phosphorylation. The results on the effects of stimulants outlined in this review are complementary to the growing body of knowledge concerning the influence of commonly prescribed psychotropics on various neurotransmitter systems of the developing brain. For example Wegerer et al (1999) found that prepubertal rats treated with fluoxetine had persistently increased density of serotonin transporters in the frontal cortex as adults. Dopamine antagonists such as neuroleptics administered to pregnant or nursing rat mothers had enduring changes in dopamine receptors of their offspring (Rosengarten and Friedhoff 1979; Duncan et al 1987). For example, if neonates are deprived of dopamine stimulation they do not show the compensatory increase in D2 receptors seen in adults receiving neuroleptics (Duncan et al 1987). The response varies according to developmental stage;

periadolescent rats appear to be more sensitive to the behavioral (cataleptic) effects of catecholamine antagonists while at the same time displaying hyposensitivity to dopamine agonists (Spear and Brake 1983). Carrey et al (2002) found that postpubertal rats, pretreated prepubertally with the antidepressants desipramine and sertraline, reacted differently to a neuroendocrine challenge than did control animals.

The effects of MPH, ADD and Dexedrine treatment are often compared with those of other stimulants associated with abuse potential, such as cocaine. However although these comparisons are fruitful, too often this debate has prevented investigations into the manner through which *orally* administered stimulants affect neuroplasticity and subsequent neuroadaptation (Volkow and Insel 2003; Yano and Steiner 2007). Especially relevant here is the work of Robinson and coworkers (Samaha et al 2004) who have proposed that the rate of cocaine administration will determine changes in gene expression and neural plasticity. Thus a careful study of gene expression resulting from oral (slow) administration of ADD or MPH is likely to be different to that seen after injection (fast). Also, the lion's share of the debate has focused on comparisons between MPH and cocaine (Yano and Steiner 2007), and relatively little attention has been paid to the effects of oral Dexedrine (d-amphetamine) and mixed amphetamine salts such as ADD, two medications that potentially have more enduring effects than MPH. As the biochemical and behavioral long-term studies, with follow-up in adulthood, have demonstrated, although MPH may not have the same long-term effects as cocaine, nonetheless enduring neuroadaptations occur, possibly mediated by downregulation of *cfos* expression, and upregulation of CREB and substance P in n.accumbal and striatal projection neurons. It is now critical that researchers focus attention on the quantifiable effects of clinically relevant oral dosages, and the precise parameters around the threshold necessary to produce a meaningful biological response in gene expression. As molecular technology advances, more and more probes will become available to pinpoint changes in signaling pathways which have either neuroadaptive, salutary effects (neurogenesis, proteins associated with enhanced synaptic transmission) or deleterious effects (CREB upregulation, chronically elevated compensatory ΔFOSB or peptide changes). However developmental timing is everything; even what appears to be a salutary change on the surface (e.g., amphetamine-mediated growth in dendritic arborization), may compromise underlying finely tuned genetic programs of growth and development.

The biological basis of putative enduring effects of early exposure to stimulants may be permanent yet subtle and hence difficult to measure experimentally. One possible mechanism for these lasting effects may be chemical imprinting in a developing brain (Andersen and Navalta 2004; Anderson 2005) where early drug exposure influences neuronal activity, even when the drug itself is no longer present, by programing or re-programing the course of development. Imprinting is not necessarily produced by toxic destruction of neurons but could influence sensitivity to subsequent drug challenge by redirecting maturation during sensitive periods (Andersen 2003). These neuroplastic changes, initially regulated by IEGs in striatal and accumbal neurons, may become chronic through downstream modulation of genes involved in several aspects of neuron functioning such as synaptic plasticity and/or peptide expression. Epigenetic changes in histone acetylation/phosphorylation and methylation provide other pathways that may influence short- to long-term changes but may also mediate early environmental influences acting through other neurotransmitter systems (serotonergic) or other brain areas (HPA axis).

9a. Limitations

There are obvious methodological challenges that make comparisons between investigations difficult, and extrapolation to humans at this point must be cautious. Nonetheless, promising studies are already underway that seek to control for: a) developmental period; b) clinically-relevant oral dosing, with accompanying blood level determination and, c) dose response curves to determine threshold values and biobehaviorally relevant end point responses. An additional practical issue concerns the lack of availability of several of the marketed psychostimulants in their pure form (e.g., MPH, d-amphetamine or d,l- amphetamine salts) to allow comparison with the effects of, for example, ADD within the same experiment. Access to these compounds is often difficult for proprietary reasons.

A recurring criticism of basic science investigations aimed at understanding stimulant effects in ADHD patients is focussed on the usefulness of conducting most experiments in normal animals. As we noted in the Introduction, there are many animal models of ADHD (Davids et al 2003), each with their own advantages and disadvantages, but it is probably true to say that an ideal model is yet to be developed. Until such time as this might occur, much work needs to be done on the possible long-term influences of stimulant action in the developing brain. This becomes doubly important when one considers that there are likely to be large numbers of normal children incorrectly diagnosed with ADHD who are subsequently treated with stimulants for long periods of time.

9b. Implications for Clinicians

The paradox of investigating the effect of chronic exposure to oral stimulants on gene expression is that clinicians are seeking ADHD treatments with long-term therapeutic changes in certain dopaminergic systems (enhanced attention through frontally mediated pathways). These must be based on extended modification of neuroplasticity in order to be permanent while hoping to avoid other deleterious changes in other DA pathways (e.g., CREB-mediated dynorphin-based dysphoria in n.accumbens neurons). In the future, better designed biobehavioral experimental studies could guide the clinician to individualize treatment by considering several factors across the lifespan when he or she must make a decision about when and how to recommend a chronic course of stimulant treatment. For example: 1) *Consideration of developmental stage*. If stimulants are necessary then there may be an optimal period to introduce them without attendant risks for the very young or adolescents, since both of these periods are characterized by intense synaptic activity (synaptogenesis in the very young, and pruning in adolescence). Alternatively, when very young children have severe side effects to even low dosages of stimulants, this may indicate a lower threshold for sensitivity and should be a consideration in delaying initiation of stimulant treatment; 2) *Consideration of developmental effects of exposure to chronic high levels of oral stimulants*. Currently, when a medication loses its effect (tolerance) clinicians use clinical judgement to impose escalating doses of stimulants that exceed recommended guidelines resulting in a group of children exposed over long periods of time to high levels of stimulants. There may be a threshold effect where escalating doses of chronic stimulants lead to permanent neuroadaptive changes; 3) *The imperative for longer daily coverage*. Even though there is a clinical logic for having extended coverage, higher daily levels of stimulants may lead to more permanent neuroadaptive changes through disruptive effects on clock genes and circadian rhythms; 4) *Drug holidays*. Clinical studies are needed to establish whether long-term (years) continuous treatments are warranted or whether periodic discontinuation of treatment could recalibrate neuroplasticity; alternatively drug holidays may inadvertently lead to sensitization to future exposure to stimulants; 5) *Not all stimulants are created equal*. Neuroadaptations in different gene expression pathways may depend on specific stimulant preparations, including differences between families of stimulants (direct agonists vs DAT blockers) and within a family (different isomers); 6) *Consider other drug interactions (nicotine, alcohol, marijuana, antidepressants, antipsychotics)* for their potential interactions with stimulants leading to neuroadaptive changes; 7) *Consider other co-morbid conditions* that could possibly modify underlying response to neuroadaptive changes (e.g., FAS); 8) *In children and adolescence* consider other environmental influences, especially chronic family stress, PTSD and early maternal environment as interacting with stimulant effects on epigenetic mechanisms.

Acknowledgments

The studies carried out in our laboratory were funded by CIHR/NSHRF/IWK (Regional Partnership Program), the IWK Health Centre, the Scottish Rite Charitable Foundation of Canada and the Atlee Endowment of the Department of Obstetrics and Gynaecology. The authors gratefully acknowledge the assistance of D.A Wilkinson and P.M.H Wilkinson in this work. Dr Evelyn Soo and Joseph Hui generously carried out the determination of blood levels of amphetamine.

References

Achat-Mendes C, Anderson KL, Itzhak Y (2003) Methylphenidate and MDMA adolescent exposure in mice: long-lasting consequences on cocaine-induced reward and psychomotor stimulation in adulthood. *Neuropharmacology* 45:106-115.

Adriani W, Leo D, Guarino M, Natoli A, Di Consiglio E, De Angelis G, Traina E, Testai E, Perrone-Capano C, Laviola G (2006a) Short-term effects of adolescent methylphenidate exposure on brain striatal gene expression and sexual/endocrine parameters in male rats. *Ann. N Y Acad. Sci.* 1074:52-73.

Adriani W, Leo D, Greco D, Rea M, di Porzio U, Laviola G, Perrone-Capano C (2006b) Methylphenidate administration to adolescent rats determines plastic changes on reward-related behavior and striatal gene expression. *Neuropsychopharmacology* 31:1946-1956.

Advokat C (2007) Update on amphetamine neurotoxicity and its relevance to the treatment of ADHD. *J. Atten. Disord.* 11:8-16.

Alcantara AA, Greenough WT (1993) Developmental regulation of Fos and Fos-related antigens in cerebral cortex, striatum, hippocampus, and cerebellum of the rat. *J. Comp. Neurol.* 334:75-85.

Alder J, Thakker-Varia S, Bangasser DA, Kuroiwa M, Plummer MR, Shors TJ, Black IB (2003) Brain-derived neurotrophic factor-induced gene expression reveals novel actions of VGF in hippocampal synaptic plasticity. *J. Neurosci.* 23:10800-10808.

Andersen SL, Rutstein M, Benzo JM, Hostetter JC, Teicher MH (1997) Sex differences in dopamine receptor overproduction and elimination. *Neuroreport* 8:1495-1498.

Andersen SL, Teicher MH (2000) Sex differences in dopamine receptors and their relevance to ADHD. *Neurosci. Biobehav. Rev.* 24:137-141.

Andersen SL, LeBlanc CJ, Lyss PJ (2001) Maturational increases in c-fos expression in the ascending dopamine systems. *Synapse* 41:345-350.

Andersen SL (2002) Changes in the second messenger cyclic AMP during development may underlie motoric symptoms in attention deficit/hyperactivity disorder (ADHD). *Behav. Brain Res.* 130:197-201.

Andersen SL, Arvanitogiannis A, Pliakas AM, LeBlanc C, Carlezon WA, Jr. (2002) Altered responsiveness to cocaine in rats exposed to methylphenidate during development. *Nat Neurosci.* 5:13-14.

Andersen SL (2003) Trajectories of brain development: point of vulnerability or window of opportunity? *Neurosci. Biobehav. Rev.* 27:3-18.

Andersen SL, Navalta CP (2004) Altering the course of neurodevelopment: a framework for understanding the enduring effects of psychotropic drugs. *Int. J. Dev. Neurosci.* 22:423-440.

Andersen SL (2005) Stimulants and the developing brain. Trends Pharmacol Sci 26:237-243.

Andersen SL, Napierata L, Brenhouse HC, Sonntag KC (2008) Juvenile methylphenidate modulates reward-related behaviors and cerebral blood flow by decreasing cortical D3 receptors. *Eur. J. Neurosci.* 27:2962-2972.

Andreazza AC, Frey BN, Valvassori SS, Zanotto C, Gomes KM, Comim CM, Cassini C, Stertz L, Ribeiro LC, Quevedo J, Kapczinski F, Berk M, Goncalves CA (2007) DNA damage in rats after treatment with methylphenidate. *Prog. Neuropsychopharmacol. Biol. Psychiatry* 31:1282-1288.

Aoyama T, Kotaki H, Iga T (1990a) Dose-dependent kinetics of methylphenidate enantiomers after oral administration of racemic methylphenidate to rats. *J. Pharmacobiodyn.* 13:647-652.

Aoyama T, Kotaki H, Honda Y, Nakagawa F (1990b) Kinetic analysis of enantiomers of threo-methylphenidate and its metabolite in two healthy subjects after oral administration as determined by a gas chromatographic-mass spectrometric method. *J. Pharm. Sci.* 79:465-469.

Arnsten AF, Dudley AG (2005) Methylphenidate improves prefrontal cortical cognitive function through alpha2 adrenoceptor and dopamine D1 receptor actions: Relevance to therapeutic effects in Attention Deficit Hyperactivity Disorder. *Behav. Brain Funct.* 1:2.

Augustyniak PN, Kourrich S, Rezazadeh SM, Stewart J, Arvanitogiannis A (2006) Differential behavioral and neurochemical effects of cocaine after early exposure to methylphenidate in an animal model of attention deficit hyperactivity disorder. *Behav. Brain Res.* 167:379-382.

Auiler JF, Liu K, Lynch JM, Gelotte CK (2002) Effect of food on early drug exposure from extended-release stimulants: results from the Concerta, Adderall XR Food Evaluation (CAFE) Study. *Curr. Med. Res. Opin.* 18:311-316.

Bakhtiar R, Tse FL (2003) Toxicokinetic assessment of methylphenidate (Ritalin(R)) in a 13-week oral (gavage) toxicity study in rats using an enantiomeric liquid chromatography/tandem mass spectrometry assay. *Rapid Commun. Mass Spectrom.* 17:2160-2162.

Banerjee PS, Zetterstrom TSC (2008a) Chronic methylphenidate administration inhibits brain-derived neurotrophic factor gene expression in juvenile rat brain. In: Proceedings of the British Pharmacological Society. Cited from www.pA2online.org/abstracts/Vol5Issue2abst007P.pdf

Banerjee PS, Zetterstrom TS (2008b) Effects of methylphenidate on Brain-derived Neurotrophic Factor protein levels in juvenile rat brain. Program No. 746.6/X8. In: 2008 Neuroscience Meeting Planner. Washington, DC: Society for Neuroscience, 2008. Online.

Bannon MJ, Pruetz B, Manning-Bog AB, Whitty CJ, Michelhaugh SK, Sacchetti P, Granneman JG, Mash DC, Schmidt CJ (2002) Decreased expression of the transcription factor NURR1 in dopamine neurons of cocaine abusers. *Proc. Natl. Acad. Sci. U S A* 99:6382-6385.

Bateup HS, Svenningsson P, Kuroiwa M, Gong S, Nishi A, Heintz N, Greengard P (2008) Cell type-specific regulation of DARPP-32 phosphorylation by psychostimulant and antipsychotic drugs. *Nat. Neurosci.* 11:932-939.

Beckman DA, Schneider M, Youreneff M, Tse FL (2008a) Juvenile toxicity assessment of d,l-methylphenidate in rats. *Birth Defects Res. B Dev. Reprod. Toxicol.* 83:48-67.

Beckman DA, Schneider M, Youreneff M, Tse FL (2008b) Developmental toxicity assessment of d,l-methylphenidate and d-methylphenidate in rats and rabbits. *Birth Defects Res. B Dev. Reprod Toxicol.* 83:489-501.

Benes FM (1998) Brain development, VII. Human brain growth spans decades. *Am. J. Psychiatry* 155:1489.

Bibb JA, Chen J, Taylor JR, Svenningsson P, Nishi A, Snyder GL, Yan Z, Sagawa ZK, Ouimet CC, Nairn AC, Nestler EJ, Greengard P (2001) Effects of chronic exposure to cocaine are regulated by the neuronal protein Cdk5. *Nature* 410:376-380.

Bird A (2007) Perceptions of epigenetics. *Nature* 447:396-398.

Black YD, Maclaren FR, Naydenov AV, Carlezon WA, Jr., Baxter MG, Konradi C (2006) Altered attention and prefrontal cortex gene expression in rats after binge-like exposure to cocaine during adolescence. *J. Neurosci.* 26:9656-9665.

Bolanos CA, Barrot M, Berton O, Wallace-Black D, Nestler EJ (2003) Methylphenidate treatment during pre- and periadolescence alters behavioral responses to emotional stimuli at adulthood. *Biol. Psychiatry* 54:1317-1329.

Bolanos CA, Willey MD, Maffeo ML, Powers KD, Kinka DW, Grausam KB, Henderson RP (2008) Antidepressant treatment can normalize adult behavioral deficits induced by early-life exposure to methylphenidate. *Biol. Psychiatry* 63:309-316.

Bramham CR, Messaoudi E (2005) BDNF function in adult synaptic plasticity: The synaptic consolidation hypothesis. *Prog. Neurobiol.* 76:99-125.

Brandon CL, Marinelli M, Baker LK, White FJ (2001) Enhanced reactivity and vulnerability to cocaine following methylphenidate treatment in adolescent rats. *Neuropsychopharmacology* 25:651-661.

Brandon CL, Steiner H (2003) Repeated methylphenidate treatment in adolescent rats alters gene regulation in the striatum. *Eur. J. Neurosci.* 18:1584-1592.

Brown GL, Hunt RD, Ebert MH, Bunney WE, Jr., Kopin IJ (1979) Plasma levels of d-amphetamine in hyperactive children. Serial behavior and motor responses. *Psychopharmacology* (Berl) 62:133-140.

Brown GL, Ebert MH, Mikkelsen EJ, Hunt RD (1980) Behavior and motor activity response in hyperactive children and plasma amphetamine levels following a sustained release preparation. *J. Am. Acad. Child Psychiatry* 19:225-239.

Cao J, Lotfipour S, Loughlin SE, Leslie FM (2007) Adolescent maturation of cocaine-sensitive neural mechanisms. *Neuropsychopharmacology* 32:2279-2289.

Carlezon WA, Jr., Mague SD, Andersen SL (2003) Enduring behavioral effects of early exposure to methylphenidate in rats. *Biol. Psychiatry* 54:1330-1337.

Carlezon WA, Jr., Konradi C (2004) Understanding the neurobiological consequences of early exposure to psychotropic drugs: linking behavior with molecules. *Neuropharmacology* 47 Suppl 1:47-60.

Carrey N, Kutcher S (1998) Developmental pharmacodynamics: implications for child and adolescent psychopharmacology. J. *Psychiatry Neurosci.* 23:274-276.

Carrey NJ, Dursun S, Clements R, Renton K, Waschbusch D, MacMaster FP (2002) Noradrenergic and serotonergic neuroendocrine responses in prepubertal, peripubertal, and postpubertal rats pretreated with desipramine and sertraline. *J. Am. Acad. Child. Adolesc. Psychiatry* 41:999-1006; discussion 1007-1009.

Chase TD, Brown RE, Carrey N, Wilkinson M (2002) Repeated ritalin attenuates Fos-ir in the rat striatum. *Soc. Neurosci. Abstr.* 28:808.805.

Chase TD, Brown RE, Carrey N, Wilkinson M (2003) Repeated methylphenidate attenuates *c-fos* expression in the striatum of prepubertal rats. *Neuroreport* 14:769-772.

Chase TD, Carrey N, Brown RE, Wilkinson M (2005a) Methylphenidate regulates c-fos and fosB expression in multiple regions of the immature brain. *Brain Res. Dev. Brain Res.* 156:1-12.

Chase TD, Carrey N, Brown RE, Wilkinson M (2005b) Methylphenidate differentially regulates c-fos and fosB expression in the developing rat striatum. *Brain Res. Dev. Brain Res* .157:181-191.

Chase T, Carrey N, Soo E, Wilkinson M (2007) Methylphenidate regulates activity regulated cytoskeletal associated but not brain-derived neurotrophic factor gene expression in the developing rat striatum. *Neuroscience* 144:969-984.

Chen J, Kelz MB, Hope BT, Nakabeppu Y, Nestler EJ (1997) Chronic Fos-related antigens: stable variants of deltaFosB induced in brain by chronic treatments. *J. Neurosci.* 17:4933-4941.

Cho DI, Quan W, Oak MH, Choi HJ, Lee KY, Kim KM (2007) Functional interaction between dopamine receptor subtypes for the regulation of c-fos expression. *Biochem. Biophys. Res. Commun.* 357:1113-1118.

Choe ES, Chung KT, Mao L, Wang JQ (2002) Amphetamine increases phosphorylation of extracellular signal-regulated kinase and transcription factors in the rat striatum via group I metabotropic glutamate receptors. *Neuropsychopharmacology* 27:565-575.

Clausen SB, Read SC, Tulloch SJ (2005) Single- and multiple-dose pharmacokinetics of an oral mixed amphetamine salts extended-release formulation in adults. *CNS Spectr.* 10:6-15.

Collingridge GL, Isaac JT, Wang YT (2004) Receptor trafficking and synaptic plasticity. *Nat. Rev. Neurosci.* 5:952-962.

Cotterly L, Beverley JA, Yano M, Steiner H (2007) Dysregulation of gene induction in corticostriatal circuits after repeated methylphenidate treatment in adolescent rats: differential effects on zif 268 and homer 1a. *Eur. J. Neurosci* .25:3617-3628.

Curran T, Morgan J (1994) Fos: an immediate-early transcription factor in neurons. *J. Neurobiol.* 26:403-412.

David HN, Ansseau M, Abraini JH (2005) Dopamine-glutamate reciprocal modulation of release and motor responses in the rat caudate-putamen and nucleus accumbens of "intact" animals. *Brain Res. Brain Res. Rev.* 50:336-360.

Davids E, Zhang K, Tarazi FI, Baldessarini RJ (2003) Animal models of attention-deficit hyperactivity disorder. *Brain Res. Brain Res. Rev* .42:1-21.

Davis C, Patte K, Levitan RD, Carter J, Kaplan AS, Zai C, Reid C, Curtis C, Kennedy JL (2008) A psycho-genetic study of associations between the symptoms of binge eating disorder and those of attention deficit (hyperactivity) disorder. *J. Psychiatr. Res.*

Diaz Heijtz R, Kolb B, Forssberg H (2003) Can a therapeutic dose of amphetamine during pre-adolescence modify the pattern of synaptic organization in the brain? *Eur. J. Neurosci. 1*8:3394-3399.

Diaz Heijtz R, Castellanos FX (2006) Differential effects of a selective dopamine D1-like receptor agonist on motor activity and c-fos expression in the frontal-striatal circuitry of SHR and Wistar-Kyoto rats. *Behav. Brain Funct.* 2:18.

Dobner PR, Deutch AY, Fadel J (2003) Neurotensin: dual roles in psychostimulant and antipsychotic drug responses. *Life Sci.* 73:801-811.

Dresel SH, Kung MP, Plossl K, Meegalla SK, Kung HF (1998) Pharmacological effects of dopaminergic drugs on in vivo binding of [99mTc]TRODAT-1 to the central dopamine transporters in rats. *Eur. J. Nucl. Med.* 25:31-39.

Duncan GE, Criswell HE, McCown TJ, Paul IA, Mueller RA, Breese GR (1987) Behavioral and neurochemical responses to haloperidol and SCH-23390 in rats treated neonatally or as adults with 6-hydroxydopamine. *J. Pharmacol. Exp. Ther.* 243:1027-1034.

Easton N, Steward C, Marshall F, Fone K, Marsden C (2007) Effects of amphetamine isomers, methylphenidate and atomoxetine on synaptosomal and synaptic vesicle accumulation and release of dopamine and noradrenaline in vitro in the rat brain. *Neuropharmacology* 52:405-414.

Ehrlich ME, Sommer J, Canas E, Unterwald EM (2002) Periadolescent mice show enhanced DeltaFosB upregulation in response to cocaine and amphetamine. *J. Neurosci.* 22:9155-9159.

El-Zein RA, Abdel-Rahman SZ, Hay MJ, Lopez MS, Bondy ML, Morris DL, Legator MS (2005) Cytogenetic effects in children treated with methylphenidate. *Cancer Lett.* 230:284-291.

Ermer JC, Shojaei A, Pennick M, Anderson CS, Silverberg A, Youcha SH (2007) Bioavailability of triple-bead mixed amphetamine salts compared with a dose-augmentation strategy of mixed amphetamine salts extended release plus mixed amphetamine salts immediate release. *Curr. Med. Res. Opin.* 23:1067-1075.

Fagundes AO, Rezin GT, Zanette F, Grandi E, Assis LC, Dal-Pizzol F, Quevedo J, Streck EL (2007) Chronic administration of methylphenidate activates mitochondrial respiratory chain in brain of young rats. *Int .J. Dev. Neurosci* .25:47-51.

Fang H, Chartier J, Sodja C, Desbois A, Ribecco-Lutkiewicz M, Walker PR, Sikorska M (2003) Transcriptional activation of the human brain-derived neurotrophic factor gene promoter III by dopamine signaling in NT2/N neurons. *J. Biol. Chem.* 278:26401-26409.

Faraone SV, Perlis RH, Doyle AE, Smoller JW, Goralnick JJ, Holmgren MA, Sklar P (2005) Molecular genetics of attention-deficit/hyperactivity disorder. *Biol. Psychiatry* 57:1313-1323.

Feron FJ, Hendriksen JG, van Kroonenburgh MJ, Blom-Coenjaerts C, Kessels AG, Jolles J, Weber WE, Vles JS (2005) Dopamine transporter in attention-deficit hyperactivity disorder normalizes after cessation of methylphenidate. *Pediatr. Neurol.* 33:179-183.

Ferraro L, Tomasini MC, Fuxe K, Agnati LF, Mazza R, Tanganelli S, Antonelli T (2007) Mesolimbic dopamine and cortico-accumbens glutamate afferents as major targets for the regulation of the ventral striato-pallidal GABA pathways by neurotensin peptides. *Brain Res. Rev.* 55:144-154.

Fleckenstein AE, Hanson GR (2003) Impact of psychostimulants on vesicular monoamine transporter function. *Eur. J. Pharmacol* .479:283-289.

Fleckenstein AE, Volz TJ, Hanson GR (2008) Psychostimulant-induced alterations in vesicular monoamine transporter-2 function: Neurotoxic and therapeutic implications. *Neuropharmacology.*

Fosnaugh JS, Bhat RV, Yamagata K, Worley PF, Baraban JM (1995) Activation of arc, a putative "effector" immediate early gene, by cocaine in rat brain. *J. Neurochem.* 64:2377-2380.

Frey BN, Valvassori SS, Gomes KM, Martins MR, Dal-Pizzol F, Kapczinski F, Quevedo J (2006) Increased oxidative stress in submitochondrial particles after chronic amphetamine exposure. *Brain Res.* 1097:224-229.

Friedman WJ, Black IB, Kaplan DR (1998) Distribution of the neurotrophins brain-derived neurotrophic factor, neurotrophin-3, and neurotrophin-4/5 in the postnatal rat brain: an immunocytochemical study. *Neuroscience* 84:101-114.

Fukui R, Svenningsson P, Matsuishi T, Higashi H, Nairn AC, Greengard P, Nishi A (2003) Effect of methylphenidate on dopamine/DARPP signalling in adult, but not young, mice. *J. Neurochem* .87:1391-1401.

Fumagalli F, Bedogni F, Frasca A, Di Pasquale L, Racagni G, Riva MA (2006) Corticostriatal up-regulation of activity-regulated cytoskeletal-associated protein expression after repeated exposure to cocaine. *Mol. Pharmacol.* 70:1726-1734.

Gainetdinov RR, Sotnikova TD, Caron MG (2002) Monoamine transporter pharmacology and mutant mice. *Trends Pharmacol. Sci.* 23:367-373.

Gainetdinov RR, Caron MG (2003) Monoamine transporters: from genes to behavior. *Annu Rev. Pharmacol. Toxicol. 4*3:261-284.

Gatley SJ, Volkow ND, Gifford AN, Fowler JS, Dewey SL, Ding YS, Logan J (1999) Dopamine-transporter occupancy after intravenous doses of cocaine and methylphenidate in mice and humans. *Psychopharmacology* (Berl) 146:93-100.

Gerasimov MR, Franceschi M, Volkow ND, Gifford A, Gatley SJ, Marsteller D, Molina PE, Dewey SL (2000) Comparison between intraperitoneal and oral methylphenidate administration: A microdialysis and locomotor activity study. *J. Pharmacol. Exp. Ther.* 295:51-57.

Golub M, Costa L, Crofton K, Frank D, Fried P, Gladen B, Henderson R, Liebelt E, Lusskin S, Marty S, Rowland A, Scialli J, Vore M (2005) NTP-CERHR Expert Panel Report on the reproductive and developmental toxicity of methylphenidate. *Birth Defects Res. B Dev .Reprod. Toxicol.* 74:300-381.

Gomes KM, Petronilho FC, Mantovani M, Garbelotto T, Boeck CR, Dal-Pizzol F, Quevedo J (2008) Antioxidant enzyme activities following acute or chronic methylphenidate treatment in young rats. *Neurochem. Res .3*3:1024-1027.

Gray JD, Punsoni M, Tabori NE, Melton JT, Fanslow V, Ward MJ, Zupan B, Menzer D, Rice J, Drake CT, Romeo RD, Brake WG, Torres-Reveron A, Milner TA (2007) Methylphenidate administration to juvenile rats alters brain areas involved in cognition, motivated behaviors, appetite, and stress. *J. Neurosci.* 27:7196-7207.

Greenhill LL, Swanson JM, Steinhoff K, Fried J, Posner K, Lerner M, Wigal S, Clausen SB, Zhang Y, Tulloch S (2003) A pharmacokinetic/pharmacodynamic study comparing a single morning dose of adderall to twice-daily dosing in children with ADHD. J Am *Acad .Child Adolesc. Psychiatry* 42:1234-1241.

Guerriero RM, Hayes MM, Dhaliwal SK, Ren JQ, Kosofsky BE (2006) Preadolescent methylphenidate versus cocaine treatment differ in the expression of cocaine-induced locomotor sensitization during adolescence and adulthood. *Biol. Psychiatry* 60:1171-1180.

Haycock JW, Becker L, Ang L, Furukawa Y, Hornykiewicz O, Kish SJ (2003) Marked disparity between age-related changes in dopamine and other presynaptic dopaminergic markers in human striatum. *J. Neurochem.* 87:574-585.

Herdegen T, Leah JD (1998) Inducible and constitutive transcription factors in the mammalian nervous system: control of gene expression by Jun, Fos and Krox, and CREB/ATF proteins. *Brain Res. Brain Res. Rev.* 28:370-490.

Honecker H, Coper H (1975) Kinetics and metabolism of amphetamine in the brain of rats of different ages. N*aunyn Schmiedebergs Arch. Pharmacol.* 291:111-121.

Hope BT, Nye HE, Kelz MB, Self DW, Iadarola MJ, Nakabeppu Y, Duman RS, Nestler EJ (1994) Induction of a long-lasting AP-1 complex composed of altered Fos-like proteins in brain by chronic cocaine and other chronic treatments. *Neuron* 13:1235-1244.

Hu XT, Nasif FJ, Zhang J, Xu M (2008) Fos regulates neuronal activity in the nucleus accumbens. *Neurosci. Lett.* 448:157-160.

Huang EJ, Reichardt LF (2003) Trk receptors: roles in neuronal signal transduction. *Annu. Rev. Biochem.* 72:609-642.

Hughes P, Dragunow M (1995) Induction of immediate-early genes and the control of neurotransmitter-regulated gene expression within the nervous system. *Pharmacol. Rev.* 47:133-178.

Husson I, Mesples B, Medja F, Leroux P, Kosofsky B, Gressens P (2004) Methylphenidate and MK-801, an N-methyl-d-aspartate receptor antagonist: shared biological properties. *Neuroscience* 125:163-170.

Hyman C, Hofer M, Barde YA, Juhasz M, Yancopoulos GD, Squinto SP, Lindsay RM (1991) BDNF is a neurotrophic factor for dopaminergic neurons of the substantia nigra. *Nature* 350:230-232.

Insel TR (2000) Gene discovery and the future of psychiatry. CNS Spectr 5:17.

Jankovic J, Chen S, Le WD (2005) The role of Nurr1 in the development of dopaminergic neurons and Parkinson's disease. *Prog. Neurobiol.* 77:128-138.

Jiang Y, Langley B, Lubin FD, Renthal W, Wood MA, Yasui DH, Kumar A, Nestler EJ, Akbarian S, Beckel-Mitchener AC (2008) Epigenetics in the nervous system. *J. Neurosci.* 28:11753-11759.

Kelz MB, Nestler EJ (2000) deltaFosB: a molecular switch underlying long-term neural plasticity. *Curr. Opin. Neurol.* 13:715-720.

Kernie SG, Liebl DJ, Parada LF (2000) BDNF regulates eating behavior and locomotor activity in mice. *Embo J.* 19:1290-1300.

Klebaur JE, Ostrander MM, Norton CS, Watson SJ, Akil H, Robinson TE (2002) The ability of amphetamine to evoke arc (Arg 3.1) mRNA expression in the caudate, nucleus accumbens and neocortex is modulated by environmental context. *Brain Res.* 930:30-36.

Kolb B, Gorny G, Li Y, Samaha AN, Robinson TE (2003) Amphetamine or cocaine limits the ability of later experience to promote structural plasticity in the neocortex and nucleus accumbens. *Proc. Natl. Acad .Sci. U S A* 100:10523-10528.

Kosofsky BE, Genova LM, Hyman SE (1995) Postnatal age defines specificity of immediate early gene induction by cocaine in developing rat brain. *J. Comp. Neurol* 351:27-40.

Kramer WG, Read SC, Tran BV, Zhang Y, Tulloch SJ (2005) Pharmacokinetics of mixed amphetamine salts extended release in adolescents with ADHD. CNS Spectr 10:6-13.

Krause J (2008) SPECT and PET of the dopamine transporter in attention-deficit/hyperactivity disorder. *Expert. Rev. Neurother.* 8:611-625.

Krishnan SM, Pennick M, Stark JG (2008) Metabolism, distribution and elimination of lisdexamfetamine dimesylate: open-label, single-centre, phase I study in healthy adult volunteers. *Clin. Drug Investig.* 28:745-755.

Kuczenski R, Segal DS (1997) Effects of methylphenidate on extracellular dopamine, serotonin, and norepinephrine: comparison with amphetamine. *J. Neurochem.* 68:2032-2037.

Kuczenski R, Segal DS (2002) Exposure of adolescent rats to oral methylphenidate: preferential effects on extracellular norepinephrine and absence of sensitization and cross-sensitization to methamphetamine. *J. Neurosci.* 22:7264-7271.

Kuczenski R, Segal DS (2005) Stimulant actions in rodents: implications for attention-deficit/hyperactivity disorder treatment and potential substance abuse. Biol Psychiatry 57:1391-1396.

Kumar A, Choi KH, Renthal W, Tsankova NM, Theobald DE, Truong HT, Russo SJ, Laplant Q, Sasaki TS, Whistler KN, Neve RL, Self DW, Nestler EJ (2005) Chromatin remodeling is a key mechanism underlying cocaine-induced plasticity in striatum. *Neuron* 48:303-314.

Kupietz SS, Bartlik B, Angrist B, Winsberg BG (1985) Psychostimulant plasma concentration and learning performance. *J. Clin. Psychopharmacol.* 5:293-295.

Kuppers E, Beyer C (2001) Dopamine regulates brain-derived neurotrophic factor (BDNF) expression in cultured embryonic mouse striatal cells. *Neuroreport* 12:1175-1179.

Lagace DC, Yee JK, Bolanos CA, Eisch AJ (2006) Juvenile administration of methylphenidate attenuates adult hippocampal neurogenesis. *Biol. Psychiatry* 60:1121-1130.

Laviola G, Macri S, Morley-Fletcher S, Adriani W (2003) Risk-taking behavior in adolescent mice: psychobiological determinants and early epigenetic influence. *Neurosci. Biobehav. Rev.* 27:19-31.

Le Foll B, Diaz J, Sokoloff P (2005) A single cocaine exposure increases BDNF and D3 receptor expression: implications for drug-conditioning. *Neuroreport* 16:175-178.

Leckman J, Young C (2002) Commentary: Noradrenergic and serotonergic neuroendocrine responses in prepubertal, pubertal, and postpubertal rats pretreated with Desipramine and Sertaline. *J. Am. Acad. Child Adolesc. Psychiatry* 41:1007-1009.

Leo D, di Porzio U, Racagni G, Riva MA, Fumagalli F, Perrone-Capano C (2007) Chronic cocaine administration modulates the expression of transcription factors involved in midbrain dopaminergic neuron function. *Exp. Neurol.* 203:472-480.

Loonam TM, Noailles PA, Yu J, Zhu JP, Angulo JA (2003) Substance P and cholecystokinin regulate neurochemical responses to cocaine and methamphetamine in the striatum. *Life Sci.* 73:727-739.

Ludolph AG, Schaz U, Storch A, Liebau S, Fegert JM, Boeckers TM (2006) Methylphenidate exerts no neurotoxic, but neuroprotective effects in vitro. *J. Neural. Transm.* 113:1927-1934.

Lyford GL, Yamagata K, Kaufmann WE, Barnes CA, Sanders LK, Copeland NG, Gilbert DJ, Jenkins NA, Lanahan AA, Worley PF (1995) Arc, a growth factor and activity-regulated gene, encodes a novel cytoskeleton-associated protein that is enriched in neuronal dendrites. *Neuron* 14:433-445.

Mague SD, Andersen SL, Carlezon WA, Jr. (2005) Early developmental exposure to methylphenidate reduces cocaine-induced potentiation of brain stimulation reward in rats. *Biol. Psychiatry* 57:120-125.

Manjanatha MG, Shelton SD, Dobrovolsky VN, Shaddock JG, McGarrity LG, Doerge DR, Twaddle NW, Lin CJ, Chen JJ, Mattison DR, Morris SM (2008) Pharmacokinetics, dose-range, and mutagenicity studies of methylphenidate hydrochloride in B6C3F1 mice. *Environ. Mol. Mutagen* 49:585-593.

Martins MR, Reinke A, Petronilho FC, Gomes KM, Dal-Pizzol F, Quevedo J (2006) Methylphenidate treatment induces oxidative stress in young rat brain. *Brain Res.* 1078:189-197.

Mayes R, Bagwell C, Erkulwater J (2008) ADHD and the rise in stimulant use among children. *Harv. Rev. Psychiatry* 16:151-166.

McClung CA, Ulery PG, Perrotti LI, Zachariou V, Berton O, Nestler EJ (2004) DeltaFosB: a molecular switch for long-term adaptation in the brain. *Brain Res. Mol. Brain Res.* 132:146-154.

McClung CA, Nestler EJ (2008) Neuroplasticity mediated by altered gene expression. *Neuropsychopharmacology* 33:3-17.

McGinty JF (2007) Co-localization of GABA with other neuroactive substances in the basal ganglia. *Prog. Brain Res.* 160:273-284.

McGough JJ, Biederman J, Greenhill LL, McCracken JT, Spencer TJ, Posner K, Wigal S, Gornbein J, Tulloch S, Swanson JM (2003) Pharmacokinetics of SLI381 (ADDERALL XR), an extended-release formulation of Adderall. *J. Am. Acad. Child Adolesc. Psychiatry* 42:684-691.

Meaney MJ, Szyf M (2005) Maternal care as a model for experience-dependent chromatin plasticity? *Trends Neurosci*. 28:456-463.

Meredith GE, Callen S, Scheuer DA (2002) Brain-derived neurotrophic factor expression is increased in the rat amygdala, piriform cortex and hypothalamus following repeated amphetamine administration. *Brain Res.* 949:218-227.

Mlewski EC, Krapacher FA, Ferreras S, Paglini G (2008) Transient enhanced expression of Cdk5 activator p25 after acute and chronic d-amphetamine administration. *Ann. N Y Acad. Sci.* 1139:89-102.

Moll GH, Mehnert C, Wicker M, Bock N, Rothenberger A, Ruther E, Huether G (2000) Age-associated changes in the densities of presynaptic monoamine transporters in different regions of the rat brain from early juvenile life to late adulthood. *Brain Res. Dev. Brain Res.* 119:251-257.

Moll GH, Hause S, Ruther E, Rothenberger A, Huether G (2001) Early methylphenidate administration to young rats causes a persistent reduction in the density of striatal dopamine transporters. *J. Child Adolesc. Psychopharmacol.* 11:15-24.

Morgan JI, Curran T (1991) Stimulus-transcription coupling in the nervous system: involvement of the inducible proto-oncogenes fos and jun. *Annu. Rev. Neurosci.* 14:421-451.

Morgan JI, Curran T (1995) Immediate-early genes: ten years on. Trends Neurosci 18:66-67.

Morshedi MM, Rademacher DJ, Meredith GE (2009) Increased synapses in the medial prefrontal cortex are associated with repeated amphetamine administration. *Synapse* 63:126-135.

Mueller D, Chapman CA, Stewart J (2006) Amphetamine induces dendritic growth in ventral tegmental area dopaminergic neurons in vivo via basic fibroblast growth factor. *Neuroscience* 137:727-735.

Nestler EJ, Kelz MB, Chen J (1999) DeltaFosB: a molecular mediator of long-term neural and behavioral plasticity. *Brain Res.* 835:10-17.

Nestler EJ (2005) Is there a common molecular pathway for addiction? *Nat. Neurosci.* 8:1445-1449.

Nikolaus S, Antke C, Beu M, Kley K, Larisch R, Wirrwar A, Muller HW (2007) In-vivo quantification of dose-dependent dopamine transporter blockade in the rat striatum with small animal SPECT. *Nucl. Med. Commun* 28:207-213.

Norrholm SD, Bibb JA, Nestler EJ, Ouimet CC, Taylor JR, Greengard P (2003) Cocaine-induced proliferation of dendritic spines in nucleus accumbens is dependent on the activity of cyclin-dependent kinase-5. *Neuroscience* 116:19-22.

Nyman ES, Ogdie MN, Loukola A, Varilo T, Taanila A, Hurtig T, Moilanen IK, Loo SK, McGough JJ, Jarvelin MR, Smalley SL, Nelson SF, Peltonen L (2007) ADHD candidate gene study in a population-based birth cohort: association with DBH and DRD2. *J. Am. Acad Child Adolesc Psychiatry* 46:1614-1621.

Patrick KS, Straughn AB, Perkins JS, Gonzalez MA (2008) Evolution of stimulants to treat ADHD: transdermal methylphenidate. *Hum. Psychopharmacol.*

Penner MR, McFadyen MP, Pinaud R, Carrey N, Robertson HA, Brown RE (2002) Age-related distribution of c-fos expression in the striatum of CD-1 mice after acute methylphenidate administration. *Brain Res. Dev. Brain Res.* 135:71-77.

Perlmann T, Wallen-Mackenzie A (2004) Nurr1, an orphan nuclear receptor with essential functions in developing dopamine cells. *Cell Tissue Res.* 318:45-52.

Perrotti LI, Weaver RR, Robison B, Renthal W, Maze I, Yazdani S, Elmore RG, Knapp DJ, Selley DE, Martin BR, Sim-Selley L, Bachtell RK, Self DW, Nestler EJ (2008) Distinct patterns of DeltaFosB induction in brain by drugs of abuse. *Synapse* 62:358-369.

Pierce D, Dixon CM, Wigal SB, McGough JJ (2008) Pharmacokinetics of methylphenidate transdermal system (MTS): results from a laboratory classroom study. *J. Child Adolesc. Psychopharmacol.* 18:355-364.

Renthal W, Carle TL, Maze I, Covington HE, 3rd, Truong HT, Alibhai I, Kumar A, Montgomery RL, Olson EN, Nestler EJ (2008) Delta FosB mediates epigenetic desensitization of the c-fos gene after chronic amphetamine exposure. *J. Neurosci.* 28:7344-7349.

Renthal W, Nestler EJ (2008) Epigenetic mechanisms in drug addiction. *Trends Mol. Med.* 14:341-350.

Ricaurte GA, Mechan AO, Yuan J, Hatzidimitriou G, Xie T, Mayne AH, McCann UD (2005) Amphetamine treatment similar to that used in the treatment of adult attention-deficit/hyperactivity disorder damages dopaminergic nerve endings in the striatum of adult nonhuman primates. *J. Pharmacol. Exp. Ther.* 315:91-98.

Riddle EL, Hanson GR, Fleckenstein AE (2007) Therapeutic doses of amphetamine and methylphenidate selectively redistribute the vesicular monoamine transporter-2. *Eur. J. Pharmacol.* 571:25-28.

Rios M, Fan G, Fekete C, Kelly J, Bates B, Kuehn R, Lechan RM, Jaenisch R (2001) Conditional deletion of brain-derived neurotrophic factor in the postnatal brain leads to obesity and hyperactivity. *Mol. Endocrinol.* 15:1748-1757.

Robinson TE, Kolb B (2004) Structural plasticity associated with exposure to drugs of abuse. *Neuropharmacology 47 Suppl.* 1:33-46.

Rojas P, Joodmardi E, Hong Y, Perlmann T, Ogren SO (2007) Adult mice with reduced Nurr1 expression: an animal model for schizophrenia. *Mol. Psychiatry* 12:756-766.

Rosengarten H, Friedhoff AJ (1979) Enduring changes in dopamine receptor cells of pups from drug administration to pregnant and nursing rats. *Science* 203:1133-1135.

Russell VA (2007) Neurobiology of animal models of attention-deficit hyperactivity disorder. *J. Neurosci. Methods* 161:185-198.

Sacchetti P, Brownschidle LA, Granneman JG, Bannon MJ (1999) Characterization of the 5'-flanking region of the human dopamine transporter gene. *Brain. Res. Mol Brain Res.* 74:167-174.

Sacchetti P, Mitchell TR, Granneman JG, Bannon MJ (2001) Nurr1 enhances transcription of the human dopamine transporter gene through a novel mechanism. *J. Neurochem.* 76:1565-1572.

Samaha AN, Mallet N, Ferguson SM, Gonon F, Robinson TE (2004) The rate of cocaine administration alters gene regulation and behavioral plasticity: implications for addiction. *J. Neurosci.* 24:6362-6370.

Scaini G, Fagundes AO, Rezin GT, Gomes KM, Zugno AI, Quevedo J, Streck EL (2008) Methylphenidate increases creatine kinase activity in the brain of young and adult rats. *Life Sci.* 83:795-800.

Schiffer WK, Volkow ND, Fowler JS, Alexoff DL, Logan J, Dewey SL (2006) Therapeutic doses of amphetamine or methylphenidate differentially increase synaptic and extracellular dopamine. *Synapse* 59:243-251.

Seeman P, Bzowej NH, Guan HC, Bergeron C, Becker LE, Reynolds GP, Bird ED, Riederer P, Jellinger K, Watanabe S, et al. (1987) Human brain dopamine receptors in children and aging adults. *Synapse* 1:399-404.

Shaw-Lutchman TZ, Impey S, Storm D, Nestler EJ (2003) Regulation of CRE-mediated transcription in mouse brain by amphetamine. *Synapse* 48:10-17.

Shi X, McGinty JF (2006) Extracellular signal-regulated mitogen-activated protein kinase inhibitors decrease amphetamine-induced behavior and neuropeptide gene expression in the striatum. *Neuroscience* 138:1289-1298.

Smith KM, Bauer L, Fischer M, Barkley R, Navia BA (2005) Identification and characterization of human NR4A2 polymorphisms in attention deficit hyperactivity disorder. *Am. J. Med. Genet B Neuropsychiatr. Genet.* 133B:57-63.

Snyder-Keller A, Keller RW, Jr. (1998) Stimulant-mediated c-fos induction in striatum as a function of age, sex, and prenatal cocaine exposure. *Brain Res.* 794:88-95.

Souza RP, Soares EC, Rosa DV, Souza BR, Gomes KM, Valvassori SS, Reus GZ, Inacio CG, Martins MR, Gomez MV, Quevedo J, Romano-Silva MA (2008a) Cerebral DARPP-32 expression after methylphenidate administration in young and adult rats. *Int. J. Dev. Neurosci.*

Souza RP, Soares EC, Rosa DV, Souza BR, Reus GZ, Barichello T, Gomes KM, Gomez MV, Quevedo J, Romano-Silva MA (2008b) Methylphenidate alters NCS-1 expression in rat brain. *Neurochem. Int* 53:12-16.

Spear LP, Brake SC (1983) Periadolescence: age-dependent behavior and psychopharmacological responsivity in rats. *Dev. Psychobiol.* 16:83-109.

Stanwood GD, Levitt P (2004) Drug exposure early in life: functional repercussions of changing neuropharmacology during sensitive periods of brain development. *Curr. Opin. Pharmacol.* 4:65-71.

Steiner H, Gerfen CR (1998) Role of dynorphin and enkephalin in the regulation of striatal output pathways and behavior. *Exp. Brain Res.* 123:60-76.

Steward O, Worley P (2002) Local synthesis of proteins at synaptic sites on dendrites: role in synaptic plasticity and memory consolidation? *Neurobiol. Learn. Mem* .78:508-527.

Stopper H, Walitza S, Warnke A, Gerlach M (2008) Brief review of available evidence concerning the potential induction of genomic damage by methylphenidate. *J. Neural. Transm.* 115:331-334.

Svenningsson P, Nishi A, Fisone G, Girault JA, Nairn AC, Greengard P (2004) DARPP-32: an integrator of neurotransmission. *Annu. Rev. Pharmacol. Toxicol.* 44:269-296.

Swanson JM, Volkow ND (2002) Pharmacokinetic and pharmacodynamic properties of stimulants: implications for the design of new treatments for ADHD. *Behav. Brain. Res.* 130:73-78.

Swanson JM, Volkow ND (2003) Serum and brain concentrations of methylphenidate: implications for use and abuse. *Neurosci. Biobehav. Rev.* 27:615-621.

Swanson J, Gupta S, Lam A, Shoulson I, Lerner M, Modi N, Lindemulder E, Wigal S (2003) Development of a new once-a-day formulation of methylphenidate for the treatment of attention-deficit/hyperactivity disorder: proof-of-concept and proof-of-product studies. *Arch. Gen. Psychiatry* 60:204-211.

Swanson JM, Kinsbourne M, Nigg J, Lanphear B, Stefanatos GA, Volkow N, Taylor E, Casey BJ, Castellanos FX, Wadhwa PD (2007) Etiologic subtypes of attention-deficit/hyperactivity disorder: brain imaging, molecular genetic and environmental factors and the dopamine hypothesis. *Neuropsychol. Rev.* 17:39-59.

Swanson JM, Volkow ND (2008) Increasing use of stimulants warns of potential abuse. *Nature* 453:586.

Szumlinski KK, Kalivas PW, Worley PF (2006) Homer proteins: implications for neuropsychiatric disorders. *Curr. Opin. Neurobiol.* 16:251-257.

Take G, Bahcelioglu M, Oktem H, Tunc E, Gozil R, Erdogan D, Calguner E, Helvacioglu F, Giray SG, Elmas C (2008) Dose-dependent immunohistochemical and ultrastructural changes after oral methylphenidate administration in rat heart tissue. *Anat. Histol. Embryol.* 37:303-308.

Tan A, Moratalla R, Lyford GL, Worley P, Graybiel AM (2000) The activity-regulated cytoskeletal-associated protein arc is expressed in different striosome-matrix patterns following exposure to amphetamine and cocaine. *J. Neurochem.* 74:2074-2078.

Tappe A, Kuner R (2006) Regulation of motor performance and striatal function by synaptic scaffolding proteins of the Homer1 family. Proc Natl Acad Sci U S A 103:774-779.

Teicher MH, Andersen SL, Hostetter JC, Jr. (1995) Evidence for dopamine receptor pruning between adolescence and adulthood in striatum but not nucleus accumbens. *Brain Res. Dev. Brain. Res.* 89:167-172.

Teicher MH, Ito Y, Glod CA, Barber NI (1996) Objective measurement of hyperactivity and attentional problems in ADHD. *J. Am. Acad .Child Adolesc. Psychiatry* 35:334-342.

Thanos PK, Michaelides M, Benveniste H, Wang GJ, Volkow ND (2007) Effects of chronic oral methylphenidate on cocaine self-administration and striatal dopamine D2 receptors in rodents. *Pharmacol. Biochem. Behav .87*:426-433.

Thapar A, O'Donovan M, Owen MJ (2005) The genetics of attention deficit hyperactivity disorder. Hum Mol Genet 14 Spec No. 2:R275-282.

Thomas DM, Francescutti-Verbeem DM, Liu X, Kuhn DM (2004) Identification of differentially regulated transcripts in mouse striatum following methamphetamine treatment--an oligonucleotide microarray approach. *J. Neurochem.* 88:380-393.

Thompson PM, Giedd JN, Woods RP, MacDonald D, Evans AC, Toga AW (2000) Growth patterns in the developing brain detected by using continuum mechanical tensor maps. *Nature* 404:190-193.

Tsai SJ (2003) Attention-deficit hyperactivity disorder and brain-derived neurotrophic factor: a speculative hypothesis. *Med. Hypotheses* 60:849-851.

Tulloch SJ, Zhang Y, McLean A, Wolf KN (2002) SLI381 (Adderall XR), a two-component, extended-release formulation of mixed amphetamine salts: bioavailability of three test formulations and comparison of fasted, fed, and sprinkled administration. *Pharmacotherapy* 22:1405-1415.

Tunc E, Erdogan D, Gozil R, Bahcelioglu M, Calguner E, Take G, Caglar G, Oktem H (2008) Dose-Dependent Immunohistochemical Changes in Rat Cornea and Retina after Oral Methylphenidate Administration. *Anat Histol. Embryol.*

Tzingounis AV, Nicoll RA (2006) Arc/Arg3.1: linking gene expression to synaptic plasticity and memory. *Neuron* 52:403-407.

Ujike H, Takaki M, Kodama M, Kuroda S (2002) Gene expression related to synaptogenesis, neuritogenesis, and MAP kinase in behavioral sensitization to psychostimulants. *Ann. N. Y Acad. Sci* 965:55-67.

Vaccarino F, Leckman J (2000) Molecular neurobiology of development. In: Pharmacology: the Fourth Generation of Progress (Revised) (Bloom F, Kupfer D, eds). New York: Raven Press. Cited from www.acnp.org/g4/GN401000080/CH.html.

Volkow ND, Insel TR (2003) What are the long-term effects of methylphenidate treatment? *Biol .Psychiatry* 54:1307-1309.

Volkow ND, Swanson JM (2003) Variables that affect the clinical use and abuse of methylphenidate in the treatment of ADHD. *Am. J. Psychiatry* 160:1909-1918.

Volz TJ, Farnsworth SJ, King JL, Riddle EL, Hanson GR, Fleckenstein AE (2007) Methylphenidate administration alters vesicular monoamine transporter-2 function in cytoplasmic and membrane-associated vesicles. *J. Pharmacol. Exp. Ther* .323:738-745.

Wang H, Pickel VM (1998) Dendritic spines containing mu-opioid receptors in rat striatal patches receive asymmetric synapses from prefrontal corticostriatal afferents. *J. Comp. Neurol.* 396:223-237.

Wang H, Pickel VM (2004) Activity-regulated cytoskeleton-associated protein arc is targeted to dendrites and coexpressed with mu-opioid receptors in postnatal rat caudate-putamen nucleus. *J. Neurosci. Res.* 77:323-333.

Wang JQ, Liu X, Zhang G, Parelkar NK, Arora A, Haines M, Fibuch EE, Mao L (2006) Phosphorylation of glutamate receptors: a potential mechanism for the regulation of receptor function and psychostimulant action. *J. Neurosci. Res.* 84:1621-1629.

Wegerer V, Moll GH, Bagli M, Rothenberger A, Ruther E, Huether G (1999) Persistently increased density of serotonin transporters in the frontal cortex of rats treated with fluoxetine during early juvenile life. *J. Child Adolesc. Psychopharmacol.* 9:13-24; discussion 25-16.

Wheeler TL, Eppolito AK, Smith LN, Huff TB, Smith RF (2007) A novel method for oral stimulant administration in the neonate rat and similar species. *J. Neurosci. Methods* 159:282-285.

Wilens TE, Faraone SV, Biederman J, Gunawardene S (2003) Does stimulant therapy of attention-deficit/hyperactivity disorder beget later substance abuse? A meta-analytic review of the literature. *Pediatrics* 111:179-185.

Witt KL, Shelby MD, Itchon-Ramos N, Faircloth M, Kissling GE, Chrisman AK, Ravi H, Murli H, Mattison DR, Kollins SH (2008) Methylphenidate and amphetamine do not induce cytogenetic damage in lymphocytes of children with ADHD. *J. Am. Acad. Child. Adolesc. Psychiatry* 47:1375-1383.

Wolfe GW, Bousquet WF, Schnell RC (1977) Circadian variations in response to amphetamine and chlorpromazine in the rat. *Commun. Psychopharmacol.* 1:29-37.

Xu M (2008) c-Fos is an intracellular regulator of cocaine-induced long-term changes. *Ann. N Y Acad. Sci* .1139:1-9.

Yamamoto BK, Bankson MG (2005) Amphetamine neurotoxicity: cause and consequence of oxidative stress. *Crit. Rev. Neurobiol.* 17:87-117.

Yano M, Steiner H (2005) Topography of methylphenidate (ritalin)-induced gene regulation in the striatum: differential effects on c-fos, substance P and opioid peptides. *Neuropsychopharmacology* 30:901-915.

Yano M, Beverley JA, Steiner H (2006) Inhibition of methylphenidate-induced gene expression in the striatum by local blockade of D1 dopamine receptors: interhemispheric effects. *Neuroscience* 140:699-709.

Yano M, Steiner H (2007) Methylphenidate and cocaine: the same effects on gene regulation? *Trends Pharmacol. Sci* .28:588-596.

Yin Y, Edelman GM, Vanderklish PW (2002) The brain-derived neurotrophic factor enhances synthesis of Arc in synaptoneurosomes. *Proc. Natl. Acad. Sci. U S A* 99:2368-2373.

Yuan J, McCann U, Ricaurte G (1997) Methylphenidate and brain dopamine neurotoxicity. *Brain Res.* 767:172-175.

Yuferov V, Nielsen D, Butelman E, Kreek MJ (2005) Microarray studies of psychostimulant-induced changes in gene expression. *Addict Biol.* 10:101-118.

Zaczek R, Battaglia G, Contrera JF, Culp S, De Souza EB (1989) Methylphenidate and pemoline do not cause depletion of rat brain monoamine markers similar to that observed with methamphetamine. *Toxicol. Appl. Pharmacol.* 100:227-233.

Zehle S, Bock J, Jezierski G, Gruss M, Braun K (2007) Methylphenidate treatment recovers stress-induced elevated dendritic spine densities in the rodent dorsal anterior cingulate cortex. *Dev. Neurobiol.*67:1891-1900.

Zhang D, Zhang L, Lou DW, Nakabeppu Y, Zhang J, Xu M (2002) The dopamine D1 receptor is a critical mediator for cocaine-induced gene expression. *J. Neurochem.* 82:1453-1464.

Zito JM, Safer DJ, dosReis S, Gardner JF, Boles M, Lynch F (2000) Trends in the prescribing of psychotropic medications to preschoolers. *Jama* 283:1025-1030.

Zorner B, Wolfer DP, Brandis D, Kretz O, Zacher C, Madani R, Grunwald I, Lipp HP, Klein R, Henn FA, Gass P (2003) Forebrain-specific trkB-receptor knockout mice: behaviorally more hyperactive than "depressive". *Biol. Psychiatry* 54:972-982.

In: Attention Deficit Hyperactivity Disorder (ADHD)
Editors: Stuart M. Gordon and Aileen E. Mitchell
ISBN 978-1-60741-581-7

Chapter 2

ADHD and Dysthymic Disorder in Children and Adolescents: Recent Insights From Cognitive Neuroscience And Functional Magnetic Resonance Imaging

Alasdair Vance*

Head Academic Child Psychiatry, Department of Paediatrics, University of Melbourne
Royal Children's Hospital, Melbourne, Australia

Introduction

ADHD and dysthymic disorder (DD) are common psychiatric disorders in children and adolescents with more males than females affected pre-puberty [1]. Further, both ADHD and DD are main drivers for oppositional defiant disorder [2], which is the most common reason for children and adolescents being referred to mental health services [3]. It is also known that ADHD and early onset depressive disorders such as DD have a 'greater than chance' association [4]. Indeed, impairing levels of inattentive type ADHD symptoms are a key symptom dimension within the nosological construct of DD. Yet, to date, there has been little or no systematic research examining the association between ADHD, inattentive type and DD using robust cognitive neuroscience probes with well defined brain behaviour relationships.

Study one addresses this by examining visuospatial memory and working memory and their association with impairing levels of inattention in children and adolescents with DD. Study two then investigates well characterized visuospatial working memory neural networks via mental rotation functional magnetic resonance imaging (fMRI) paradigms and their association with impairing levels of inattention in children and adolescents with DD. Data

* South East Building, Gatehouse Street, Parkville, Melbourne VIC 3052, Australia, Phone: 61 3 9345-4666, Fax: 61 3 9345-6002, email: avance@unimelb.edu.au.

from a cross-sectional study of (a) visuospatial memory and (b) visuospatial working memory in pre-pubertal, medication-naïve children with DD and age-, gender- and 'performance IQ'-matched healthy control participants are presented in Study one. In addition, Study two outlines data from a cross sectional study of a visuospatial working memory mental rotation fMRI paradigm in (a) post-pubertal adolescents with DD and (b) pre-pubertal children with DD and age-, gender-, handedness- and 'performance IQ'-matched healthy control participants. Children with DD demonstrate impairment in visuospatial memory that is delay-independent, which suggests dysfunction of encoding aspects linked to inattention, rather than retention and recall aspects of visuospatial memory. They also demonstrate impairment in visuospatial working memory (VSWM), including impairment in the spatial span and strategy components of VSWM. Inattentive symptoms are significantly associated with the VSWM impairment. The adolescent DD participants evince decreased right fronto-parietal activation with the fMRI VSWM probe while the pre-pubertal DD children demonstrate decreased activation of right fronto-striatal-temporal-parietal brain regions along with the right insula region. Key clinical and research implications of these findings are explored.

Study One

Visuospatial Memory

DD is the most prevalent depressive disorder in pre-pubertal children and a major risk factor for the development of major depressive disorder (MDD) [4] with low psychosocial functioning that persists into adolescence and adulthood [5]. Currently, it is unknown whether there are developmental stage-dependent neurobiological risk factors underlying DD.

In children and adolescents, DD is associated with impairing levels of inattention that manifest as clinically observed cognitive symptoms, including 'concentration difficulties', 'poor attention' and difficulties with 'decision making' [4,6-8]. These symptoms have been associated with deficits in neuropsychological measures of attention, short-term memory and working memory [9,10]. Recently, we have explored the association between cognitive symptoms of inattention and visuospatial memory encoding and retrieval in children with Attention Deficit Hyperactivity Disorder, combined type (ADHD-CT) [10]. Our study found that observable visuospatial memory deficits may be due to deficits in the attentional aspect of information encoding, rather than deficits in information retention and recall. These findings implied dysfunction of fronto-striatal neurocognitive systems associated with the encoding of stimuli, rather than dysfunction to medial temporal lobe-linked neural networks associated with retention and recall aspects of visuospatial memory [11-13].

To date, DD has been associated with deficits in verbal memory in pre-pubertal children [14,15]. However, verbal abilities are also known to be impaired in DD, which may confound the investigation of verbal memory in this group of children [16]. Also, children and adolescents with MDD were included in the samples studied rather than DD alone.

Taken together, these findings suggest that visuospatial memory may be a better way of exploring memory ability in children with DD. In our prior study, we used the delayed matching-to-sample (DMTS) visuospatial memory task from the Cambridge Neuropsychological Test Automated Battery (CANTAB) [10,17]. This task allows the separation of deficits in encoding from retrieval aspects of visuospatial memory, providing a measure of the extent to which encoding deficits contribute to observed retention and recall deficits [18]. The task achieves the separation of deficits because: (1) The memory demand of the task can be increased by increasing the delay between the presentation of the target stimulus and the presentation of the exemplars. Increasing the delay makes the representation of the encoded stimulus vulnerable to decay, which increases the demand on retention and recall processes. (2) The presentation of the choice exemplars while the target stimulus is still visible (a matching to sample (MTS) condition) allows the memory demands of the task to be removed. The MTS condition provides a control to determine the extent to which factors influencing encoding, such as attention differences, may contribute to deficits in target stimulus recognition or recall.

Furthermore, the types of strategies that participants use to make memory-based decisions may be analysed through the manipulation of the exemplars [12], such that they share some, but not all, of the target features (for example, the same colour as the target but a different shape). Responses to the DMTS task can be made manually and pictorial stimuli can be used, reducing the effect of any language impairment on performance. This is relevant to studies of children and adolescents with depressive disorders, given an association of deficits in verbal functioning with DD and MDD observed in children and adolescents [16]. Finally, the MTS and DMTS conditions are randomised, with all conditions identical until after stimulus presentation [10,19].

Therefore, to examine whether memory deficits *per se* are associated with DD in children and adolescents, the present study examined the association of DD with visuospatial memory in pre-pubertal children aged 6 to 12 years. To achieve this, medication-naïve, pre-pubertal children with carefully defined DD performed the CANTAB DMTS task. The DMTS task conditions were used to measure visuospatial memory retention and recall ability, while the MTS task condition was used to measure visuospatial information encoding ability. Given the impairing levels of inattention associated with DD, taken together with recent findings of the association between inattention and encoding aspects of visuospatial memory, it was hypothesised that visuospatial memory encoding ability, will be impaired in the DD group compared to a healthy control group.

Method

Participants

Twenty-six male and female pre-pubertal (Tanner stage I [20]) children aged 6 to 12 years [9.96 (1.73) years] were identified with medication naïve DD (DSM-IV [21]) during their initial clinical evaluation. The cases were recruited from primary health practitioners in primary schools in metropolitan Melbourne. DD was defined through separate semi-structured clinical interviews with parent(s) and child (Anxiety Disorders Interview Schedule for Children (A-DISC) [22]). Symptoms of DD were also evaluated dimensionally using parent report (Child Behaviour Checklist (CBCL) anxiety depression subscale [23]) and child report (Children's Depression Inventory (CDI) total depression scale [24]), where clinical level DD symptoms were observed to be greater than 1.5 standard deviations above the mean for a child's age and gender (Table 1). Patients also exhibited inattentive symptoms (Child Behaviour Checklist (CBCL) attention subscale [23]). These twenty-six patients had no other known medical, neurological or endocrine disorders, MDD, Attention Deficit Hyperactivity Disorder, combined type, Conduct Disorder, Developmental Coordination Disorder or reading/spelling learning disorders (Wide Range Achievement Test, 3rd Edition, [25]).

Twenty-eight pre-pubertal (Tanner stage I [20]) healthy control participants, who did not meet criteria for any psychiatric, neurological or endocrine disorder, were again defined through a semi-structured clinical interview (A-DISC) [22] with their parent(s) and with each child, and by the parent (CBCL, anxiety depression subscale [23]) and child (CDI, total depression scale [24]) reports. They did not differ from the DD group in age, gender or 'performance IQ', as assessed by the perceptual reasoning index from the Wechsler Intelligence Test for Children, 4th edition [26] (Table 1).

Measures

Computerised Neuropsychological Tasks

Visuospatial memory was assessed through measurement of performance on the DMTS task selected from the CANTAB [17]. The DMTS test assessed the ability to recall a complex target stimulus (an abstract pattern), presented on the screen for 4 seconds. There were four conditions, each with 10 trials presented randomly. In the MTS condition, the target stimulus remained on the screen with the choice exemplars. In the DMTS delay conditions, the target stimulus was removed followed by a 0, 4, or 12 second delay before the choice exemplars were presented. In all trials, participants were required to choose the target stimulus in a four-alternative forced choice procedure between the correct pattern, and three 'distractor' patterns.

Performance was measured according to the number of correct responses at the simultaneous and each of the delay levels. Further analysis examined three types of possible errors at each level of the task. 1) a "colour error" was committed when the participant selected the wrong coloured pattern but the correct shape; 2) a "shape error" was committed when the participant selected an incorrectly shaped pattern that was the correct colour, and 3) an "distractor error" was committed when the incorrect pattern was selected that was both the wrong colour and shape.

Statistical Analysis

Both the (1) accuracy and (2) latency of responses on the DMTS task were compared between groups using repeated measures analysis of variance (ANOVA). Given the known sensitivity of visuospatial memory measures to the effects of age and/or 'performance IQ' [10,27,28], ANCOVA, co-varying for the effects of age and/or 'performance IQ', was performed when either/both of these variables had a significant independent association with the dependent variable under investigation. To investigate the effect of encoding ability on retention and recall ability, ANCOVA was also performed to analyse the accuracy across delay conditions (0, 4, and 12 seconds) co-varying for performance on the MTS condition. Differences between groups in the types of errors made on the DMTS task, including distractor, shape and colour errors, were analysed using a 2 (group) x 4 (condition) x 3 (error type) repeated measures ANOVA. To estimate effect sizes, Cohen's d calculation for unequal sample sizes was used to examine differences between group performance on both accuracy and latency measures. Finally, the strength of the association between parent and child reported depressive symptoms, inattention symptoms and DMTS total accuracy scores was explored using Pearson's product moment correlation coefficients.

Results

Descriptive Statistics

Table 1 shows the mean age and 'performance IQ' for the healthy control group and the DD group. Independent samples t-tests showed that the two groups did not differ significantly with respect to mean 'performance IQ', $t(52) = -1.67$, $p = .10$, and age, $t(52) = -0.36$, $p = .72$. Pearson chi-square tests showed that the two groups did not differ significantly with respect to gender, $\chi 2(1) = 1.64$, $p = .20$. In the DD group, 77% of participants were male and 23% were female. In the healthy control group, 61% of participants were male and 39% were female. DD patients exhibited significantly higher depressive symptoms, according to both parent, $t(52) = 7.13$, $p < 0.0005$, and child, $t(52) = 14.66$, $p < 0.0005$, reports, as well as higher inattentive symptoms, $t(52) = 9.43$, $p < 0.0005$ (Table 1).

Table 1. Group characteristics

	DD (n = 26) M (SD)	Control (n = 28) M (SD)	t (52)	p
Age	9.96 (1.73)	10.11 (1.26)	-0.36	.72
Gender (M,F)	20,6	17,11	1.64#	.20
'Performance IQ'	100.08 (11.12)	105.43 (12.33)	-1.67	.10
CBCL anx/dep	73.00 (11.04)	54.12 (7.77)	7.13	<.0005
CDI	69.69 (5.82)	41.48 (7.98)	14.66	<.0005
CBCL att	70.88 (9.75)	52.00 (3.05)	9.43	<.0005

M=male, F=female; 'performance IQ' = perceptual reasoning index using the Wechsler Intelligence Scale for Children, version 4; CBCL anx/dep=Child Behaviour Checklist anxiety depression subscale; CDI=Children's Depression Inventory total depression scale; CBCL att=Child Behaviour Checklist attention subscale; # χ^2 test used for categorical variables

Accuracy on the Delayed Matching to Sample Task

Differences between groups in the number of correct responses on the DMTS task were analysed using repeated measures ANOVA. There was a significant effect of condition, Wilks' $\lambda = .26$, $F(3,49) = 46.16$, $p < .0005$, and diagnostic group $F(1,51) = 15.83$, $p < .0005$, partial $\eta^2 = .24$, on the number of correct responses. Figure 1 shows that the number of correct responses was lower for the DD group than for the healthy control group. Cohen's *d* (1.09) showed a large effect size. There was a significant interaction between condition and diagnostic group, Wilks' $\lambda = .86$, $F(3,49) = 2.74$, $p = .05$. *Post hoc t*-tests revealed that the DD group performed worse than the healthy control participants at the simultaneous [DD: mean=9.08, S.D.=1.08; control: mean=9.64, S.D.=0.83; t (51)= -2.15, p=.04] and the three delay conditions [0 second delay: DD: mean=6.40, S.D.=2.04; control: mean=8.39, S.D.=1.50; t (51)= -4.08, p<.0005; 4 second delay: DD: mean=7.08, S.D.=1.71; control: mean=8.14, S.D.=1.51; t (51)= -2.41, p=.02; 12 second delay DD: mean=5.20, S.D.=1.89; control: mean=6.89, S.D.=2.10; t (51)= -3.07, p=.003].

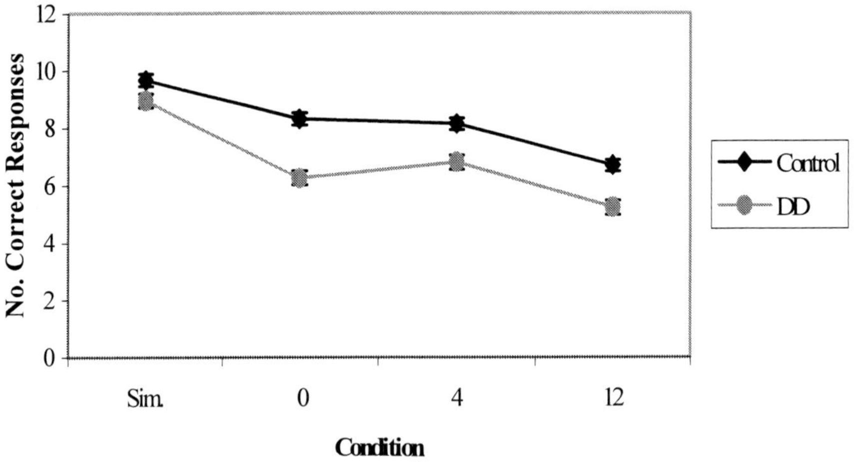

Figure 1. Number of correct responses for each condition of the Delayed Matching to Sample task (standard error bars included).

To control for the effect of encoding ability on retention and recall ability, the MTS condition was included as a covariate in a repeated measures ANCOVA analysis of the number of correct responses on the DMTS task delay conditions (0, 4 and 12). There was no significant effect of condition, Wilks' $\lambda = .98$, $F(2,49) = 0.44$, $p = .65$, on the number of correct responses. There was a significant effect of diagnostic group $F(1,50) = 10.12$, $p = .003$, partial $\eta^2 = .17$, after co-varying for the simultaneous MTS condition, $F(1,50) = 6.02$, $p = .02$, partial $\eta^2 = .11$, which had a significant independent association with the accuracy of performance on the delay conditions. According to the estimated marginal means, the DD group (M = 6.38, SE = .29) again made fewer correct responses than the healthy control group (M = 7.67, SE = .27). Cohen's *d* (1.11) showed a large effect size. No significant interaction was found between condition and group, Wilks' $\lambda = .91$, $F(2,49) = 2.35$, $p = .11$, and condition and the MTS condition, Wilks' $\lambda = .96$, $F(2,49) = 1.05$, $p = .36$.

Types of errors on the Delayed Matching to Sample Task

Differences between groups in the types of errors made on the DMTS task, including distractor, shape and colour errors, were analysed using a 2 (group) x 4 (condition) x 3 (error type) repeated measures ANOVA. Although there was no significant effect of condition (type of error), Wilks' $\lambda = .93$, $F(2,50) = 1.94$, $p = .16$, there was a significant effect of diagnostic group on the number of errors, $F(1,51) = 15.83$, $p < .0005$, partial $\eta^2 = .24$ (shape error > colour error > distractor error). Cohen's *d* (.83) showed a large effect size. There was no significant interaction between condition and diagnostic group, Wilks' $\lambda = .94$, $F(2,49) = 1.86$, $p = .17$, after co-varying for 'performance IQ', which had a significant interaction with condition, Wilks' $\lambda = .86$, $F(2,49) = 4.01$, $p = .03$.

Response Latency for the Delayed Matching to Sample task

Differences in the latency (ms) of the responses on the DMTS task, across groups, were analysed using repeated measures ANOVA. There were no significant effects of condition, Wilks' $\lambda = .86$, $F(3,49) = 2.57$, $p = .07$, or diagnostic group, $F(1,51) = 0.47$, $p = .50$, on speed of response. There was no significant interaction between latency and diagnostic group, Wilks' $\lambda = .86$, $F(3,49) = 2.70$, $p = .06$. However, given the trends towards significance for condition and interaction between latency and diagnostic group, post-hoc t-tests were completed. They revealed that the DD group performed no differently than the healthy control participants at the simultaneous, 0 second delay and 4 second delay conditions, but were faster at the 12 second delay condition [DD: mean=3957ms, S.D.=1375; control: mean=4712ms, S.D.=1306; $t(51)=-2.05$, $p=.05$].

Correlation between Parent and Child Reported Depressive Symptoms, Inattention Symptoms and DMTS Total Accuracy Scores

The DMTS total accuracy score had a large negative correlation with the child-reported depressive symptoms (CDI total score) ($r = -.50$, $p<.0005$), a medium negative correlation with the parent report of child depressive symptoms (CBCL anxiety/depressive subscale score) ($r = -.46$, $p<.0005$), and a medium negative correlation with the parent report of child inattentive symptoms (CBCL inattentive subscale score) ($r = -.48$, $p<.0005$).

Discussion

Children with DD demonstrated significantly impaired visuospatial memory. In the DD group, worse performance was evident both when the exemplars were visible (MTS) and when they had been removed from view (DMTS). Although the pattern of decreased accuracy from the MTS condition to the DMTS conditions was qualitatively similar for both groups, the DD group performed more poorly across all conditions (Figure 1). This suggests an overall impairment in visuospatial memory associated with DD.

Poor performance in the MTS condition suggests deficits in the processes of attending to and/or matching the visual stimuli. Thus, poor performance during the delay conditions of the task may have occurred not because of a deficit in retention and recall but because of an attentional deficit affecting processes implicated in the early stages of task performance, including the initial process of orienting attention to the task and the encoding of visual stimuli. This is consistent with the hypothesis that memory deficits in mood disorders may involve poor encoding arising from deficits in attention [29]. Four additional aspects of our results support this contention.

Firstly, a significant independent association was observed between accuracy of performance on the MTS condition and accuracy of performance on the DMTS conditions. Secondly, the initial significant interaction between condition and diagnostic group did not remain when MTS performance was controlled, suggesting that the accuracy of performance by the DD group did not decrease with an increase in delay. Decreased memory accuracy, as a function of increasing delay [13] is associated with lesions of the medial temporal lobes, amygdala and hippocampal formation [12]. The present findings thus suggest that DD in children is not associated with retention and recall deficits that are mediated by medial temporal lobe-linked neural network dysfunction. Thirdly, between-groups analyses of the types of errors made across all conditions of the DMTS task indicated that the DD group made qualitatively similar and more of each type of error compared to the healthy control group across all conditions. The lack of a significant interaction between the types of errors and diagnostic group suggests that the difference in DMTS task performance is unlikely to be due to the use of different approaches to task completion by each group. Finally, there was no significant between-groups difference in the response times. Taken together, these findings imply that the DD group were motivated to perform on the task according to the task requirements, rather than simply select targets at random. The similar response times also suggest that DD in children is not associated with motor dysfunction.

Overall, the findings suggest that the observed deficit in visuospatial memory reflects impairing levels of inattention, consistent with the impairing cognitive symptoms of inattention clinically observed in children with DD [4,6,7]. This is not consistent with a recent study of a group of children and adolescents (6 to 17 years) with depressive disorders, including MDD and DD, which found verbal memory deficits and no associated deficits in attention [30]. However, this discrepancy may be due to between-study differences in age and developmental-stage sample characteristics, the inclusion of children with MDD in the previous study and the use of a verbal rather than a visuospatial memory task.

However, we have previously demonstrated the association of inattention with poor visuospatial memory encoding performance in children with ADHD-CT [10]. This suggests that the memory deficit observed in the present study may be associated with symptoms of inattention more generally, rather than DD specifically. Indeed, our DD group rated highly on an additional measure of inattention relative to the healthy control group (see Table 1). Furthermore, poor accuracy of performance on the DMTS task was significantly correlated with an increase in the parent report of child inattentive symptoms, as well as an increase in both the parent and child report of child depressive symptoms. This suggests that the examination of visuospatial memory in children with DD and no inattention is required, in order to further investigate whether encoding deficits in visuospatial memory are associated with DD *per se* (see next section).

The findings from the present study are clinically important given that children with DD may display impairments in everyday or academic functioning that appear to be mnemonic in nature, whereas the problem may lie in the ability to attend to and encode stimulus information. Impaired attention has been found to contribute to learning difficulties observed in children with DD [16,31]. The present study provides further evidence that interventions targeting inattention may be helpful. For example, interventions that encourage children to attend to and encode information are likely to be more useful than approaches that emphasise the remembering and retrieval of information (such as memorising lists etc.)

In summary, the present study found that pre-pubertal children with DD displayed impaired performance on a task of visuospatial memory. In particular, dysfunction in the attentional processes of encoding stimulus information was implicated rather than retention and recall processes. Future examination of visuospatial memory performance in larger epidemiologically derived samples of children with DD without inattention is needed, along with investigation of adolescents or adults with DD and patients with DD and co-morbid disorders, especially MDD.

The next study will address the nature of and association of visuospatial working memory with children with DD.

Visuospatial Working Memory

DD is associated with cognitive symptoms of inattention in addition to the core diagnostic symptom of a chronically depressed and/or irritable mood [21]. Symptoms of inattention that have been clinically observed in children with DD include poor attention, difficulty concentrating and difficulty with decision making [4,6-8]. These symptoms of DD are thought to impair cognitive development and functioning in academic domains [16]. In the context of Attention Deficit Hyperactivity Disorder, combined type (ADHD-CT), previous studies have found that inattentive symptoms are associated with impaired performance on neuropsychological measures of visuospatial working memory (VSWM) [9,32]. The interaction between processes of visuospatial attention and VSWM [33,34] is thought to be underpinned by overlap of the neural substrates that subserve these two processes, specifically right hemisphere dominant activation in frontal and parietal brain regions [35].

Importantly, disruption to fronto-striatal neural networks has been found to be related to impairments in attention [9,11,36] and VSWM [12,37]. Given that cognitive symptoms of inattention are associated with DD, fronto-striatal dysfunction that is reflected by impairments to VSWM may also be implicated in DD. The examination of VSWM is further relevant to neuropsychological studies of children, because models of the brain-behaviour relationship between VSWM and the pre-frontal cortex (PFC) are well evidenced by single neuronal firing rates in alert primates [38], studies of behaviour following focal PFC lesions in adult humans [39] and studies of patterns of regional cerebral blood flow in healthy humans performing VSWM tests [40]. In addition, the experimental paradigm can be applied to studies of children and adolescents without modification [9]. Finally, VSWM is largely non-verbal, so that deficits in verbal functioning observed in children with depressive disorders [16] do not confound testing.

The Cambridge Neuropsychological Test Automated Battery (CANTAB) [17] VSWM task allows for an overall measure of VSWM, measured as 'between search error' (BSE) performance, as well as measures of two key components of VSWM: (1) the ability to maintain information 'on line' in a visuospatial sketchpad [41], measured as 'spatial span', and (2) the ability to develop a systematic search strategy during task performance, measured as 'strategy' [37,42-44]. To further analyse VSWM deficits, the CANTAB approach allows examination of the contribution of either or both components of VSWM to observed poor BSE performance [9,37,44]. This approach of deconstructing VSWM has also informed the analysis of the functional neural networks that may subserve the construct of VSWM and its two key components.

VSWM (as defined by BSE or a comparable measure of performance) has been associated with activation of frontal-striatal-parietal neural networks, particularly the PFC and posterior parietal brain regions [45-47]. VSWM is thought to rely on the integrity of the dorsolateral prefrontal cortex (DLPFC) in non-human primates and human beings [48,49]. In one functional imaging study of healthy adult humans, Owen et al. [17] found evidence suggesting that two functionally distinct subdivisions of the lateral frontal cortex may subserve different components of VSWM. They found that during the 'online' maintenance of visuospatial information in working memory, assessed using a task identical to the CANTAB measure of 'spatial span', there was significant activation in the ventrolateral prefrontal cortex (Brodmann Area 47), while the active monitoring and manipulation of spatial information within working memory was specifically associated with significant activation in mid-dorsolateral prefrontal cortical areas 9 and 46.

To date, no known neuropsychological or functional imaging studies have examined the neurocognitive dysfunction underpinning DD in children. Hence, the present study investigated the association of DD with VSWM in pre-pubertal children aged 6 to 12 years by examining the VSWM performance of medication-naive, pre-pubertal children with DD. The CANTAB VSWM task was used to measure overall VSWM ability, as well as the strategy component of VSWM, while the CANTAB Spatial Span (SSP) task allowed a measure of the spatial span component of VSWM. It was hypothesised that (1) VSWM performance would be impaired in the DD group compared to a healthy control group, with additional impairments in the (2) spatial span and (3) strategy components of VSWM in the DD group.

Method

Participants

The characteristics of the DD and healthy control participant groups are the same as those in the Visuospatial memory study.

Measures

Computerised Neuropsychological Tasks

VSWM was assessed through measurement of performance on the Spatial Working Memory and Spatial Span tasks selected from the CANTAB [17]. The computerised tests were presented on a high-resolution IBM monitor with a touch-sensitive screen. All the children reported previous experience with computers and were tested using the same apparatus.

The CANTAB Spatial Span task is a computerised version of the Corsi block tapping test that assesses visuospatial short-memory capacity [50]. This task measures the ability to remember a sequence of squares presented on the screen. After an incorrect attempt at choosing the squares in sequence, the next trial remains at the same difficulty level. A Spatial Span score was calculated as the highest level at which the participant successfully remembered at least one sequence of boxes.

The CANTAB Spatial Working Memory task is a self-ordered search task that measures working memory for spatial stimuli and requires the subject to use mnemonic information to work towards a goal. Participants are required to search through boxes that appear on the screen with the aim of finding the blue tokens hidden inside. The key instruction is that once a token has been taken out of a box, that box will not be used again to hide a token. There were four test trials with each of three, four, six and eight boxes. Returning to an 'empty' box, already opened and a token removed on a previous search, constituted a 'forgetting' or 'Between Search' error (BSE). Performance accuracy was defined as the total number of BSE's (i.e., higher BSE rates indicate lower accuracy of VSWM performance). This was the key functional measure of VSWM. Response latencies, measured in milliseconds (ms), were obtained for each trial. This recorded the time difference between the presentation of boxes on the screen and the end of the trial when all the blue tokens have been found.

A Strategy score was calculated from each participant's performance on the six and eight box levels, to reflect how often a searching sequence was initiated from the same box during a given trial. Higher Strategy scores represent low use of strategy (i.e., many sequences beginning with a different box in a given trial). Lower scores represent efficient use of strategy (i.e., many sequences starting with the same box in a given trial).

Statistical analysis

Performance on the (1) Spatial Working Memory BSE variable, including both the accuracy and response latency variables, and (2) the Strategy and Spatial Span variables was compared between groups using respective (1) repeated-measures and (2) one-way analysis of covariance (ANCOVA), co-varying for the effects of age and PIQ, given the known sensitivity of these VSWM measures to these variables [10,27,28]. To estimate effect sizes, Cohen's d calculation for unequal sample sizes was used to examine differences between group performance on both accuracy and latency measures. To investigate the contribution of Spatial Span and Strategy to overall VSWM, the correlations between BSE and Spatial Span and between BSE and Strategy were computed using the total number of BSE's (across all levels of difficulty). To investigate the association of VSWM with inattentive symptoms, the correlation between the total number of BSE's and inattention symptom scores was computed. Each of these correlations examined the relationships between variables in the combined sample, including healthy control and clinical participants.

Results

Descriptive Statistics

These are presented in the Visuospatial memory study (pages 5,6)

VSWM Task Accuracy (Between-Search Errors)

Differences in accuracy of performance (BSE's) across diagnostic group were analysed using a 2 (group) × 4 (level) repeated measures ANCOVA. Table 2 shows the mean BSE's for each group at each difficulty level on the VSWM task. There was a significant effect of condition (number of boxes), Wilks' $\lambda = 0.50$, $F(3,48) = 16.30$, $p < 0.0005$, and diagnostic group $F(1,50) = 37.78$, $p < 0.0005$, partial $\eta^2 = 0.43$, on the number of BSE's, after co-varying for age, $F(1,50) = 8.64$, $p = 0.005$, partial $\eta^2 = 0.15$, and PIQ, $F(1,50) = 18.98$, $p < 0.0005$, partial $\eta^2 = 0.28$, both of which had a significant independent association with the number of BSE's. The DD group made significantly more errors than the healthy control group (see Figure 2). Cohen's *d* (1.67) showed a large effect size. There was also a significant interaction between condition and group, Wilks' $\lambda = 0.57$, $F(3,48) = 11.98$, $p < 0.0005$, after co-varying for age and PIQ. The difference between the number of BSE's for each group increased with increasing level of task difficulty (Figure 2). Significant independent interactions were also found between condition and age, Wilks' $\lambda = 0.85$, $F(3,48) = 2.84$, $p = 0.048$, and condition and PIQ, Wilks' $\lambda = 0.73$, $F(3,48) = 5.93$, $p = 0.002$.

Differences in the response latency (milliseconds) on the VSWM task across diagnostic group were analysed using a 2 (group) × 4 (level) repeated measures ANCOVA. There was a significant effect of condition, Wilks' $\lambda = 0.72$, $F(3,48) = 6.21$, $p = 0.001$, and diagnostic group, $F(1, 50) = 4.24$, $p = 0.045$, partial $\eta^2 = 0.08$, after co-varying for age, $F(1,50) = 6.095$, $p = 0.017$, partial $\eta^2 = 0.11$, and PIQ, $F(1,50) = 0.74$, $p = 0.39$, partial $\eta^2 = 0.02$. Only age had a significant independent association with response latency. The DD group displayed longer response latencies than the healthy control group (see Figure 3). Cohen's *d* (0.64) showed a medium effect size. There was also a significant interaction between latency and diagnostic group, Wilks' $\lambda = 0.72$, $F(3,48) = 6.38$, $p = 0.001$, after co-varying for age and PIQ. The difference in latency between groups differed with increasing level of difficulty (see Figure 3). No significant interactions were found between latency and PIQ, Wilks' $\lambda = 0.902$, $F(3,48) = 1.73$, $p = 0.17$, nor latency and age, Wilks' $\lambda = 0.899$, $F(3,48) = 1.803$, $p = 0.16$.

Table 2. Group Performance on the Spatial Span Task and the Visuospatial Working Memory Task, including the Between Search Errors (BSE) and the Strategy Components

	DD *(n = 26)* *M (SD)*	Control *(n = 28)* *M (SD)*	*p*
Visuospatial Working Memory			.000*
BSE level 3	0.31 (0.74)	0.00 (0.00)	
BSE level 4	2.81 (2.48)	0.61 (1.13)	
BSE level 6	18.27 (7.00)	8.89 (4.94)	
BSE level 8	35.38 (7.92)	23.61 (10.31)	
Spatial Span	5.08 (1.06)	6.11 (1.34)	.008
Strategy	37.88 (3.66)	33.75 (4.92)	.006

* The significance of the repeated measures ANCOVA across BSE levels of difficulty p<.0005.

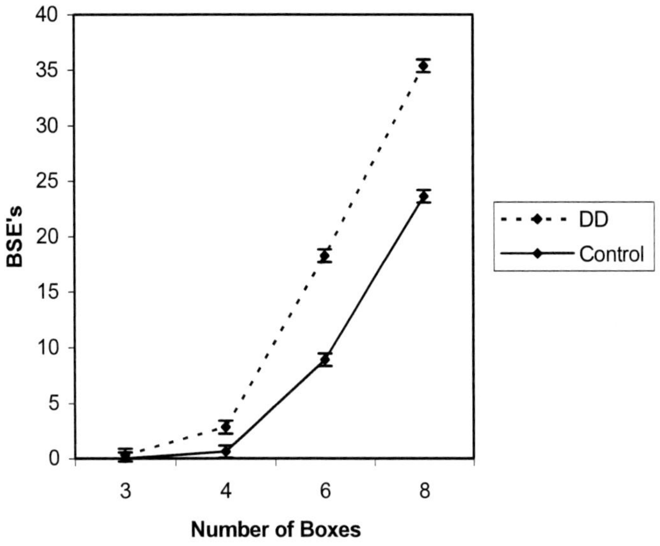

Figure 2. The number of between search errors (BSE's) at each level of difficulty of the Visuospatial Working Memory task, for the healthy control group and DD group (standard error bars included).

VSWM Task Response Latency

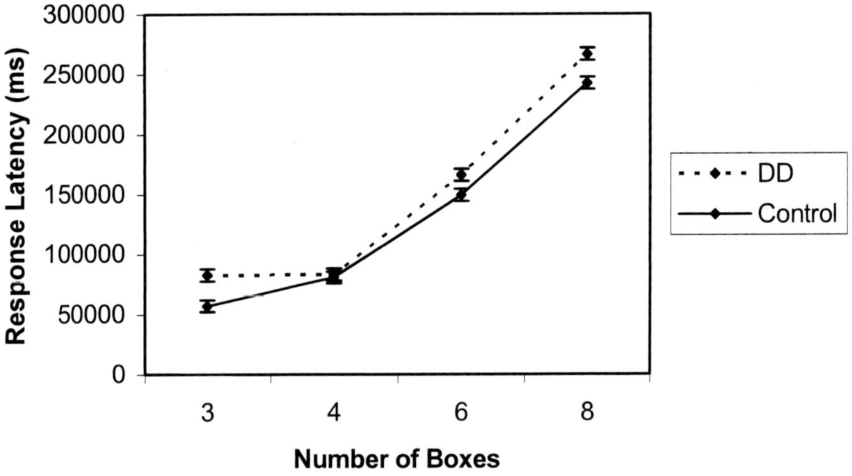

Figure 3. Response latency on the VSWM task at each difficulty level for each group (standard error bars included).

Spatial Span

A univariate analysis of covariance (ANCOVA) was used to analyse the difference between the mean spatial span for each diagnostic group. There was a significant difference between the two diagnostic groups in spatial span performance, $F(1,50) = 7.727$, $p = 0.008$, partial $\eta^2 = 0.13$ (see Table 2), after co-varying for age, $F(1,50) = 9.09$, $p = 0.004$, partial $\eta^2 = 0.15$, and PIQ, $F(1, 50) = 2.17$, $p = 0.15$, partial $\eta^2 = 0.04$. Only age had a significant independent association with spatial span performance. The spatial span for the DD group (M = 5.08, SD = 1.06) was lower than for the healthy control group (M = 6.11, SD = 1.34). Cohen's *d* (0.85) indicated that this was a large effect.

Strategy

Univariate ANCOVA was used to analyse the difference between the mean strategy score for each diagnostic group. There was a significant difference between the two diagnostic groups in search strategy used during the VSWM task, $F(1,50) = 8.27$, $p = 0.006$, partial $\eta^2 = 0.14$ (see Table 2), after co-varying for age, $F(1,50) = 4.02$, $p = 0.05$, partial $\eta^2 = 0.07$, and PIQ, $F(1,50) = 13.45$, $p = 0.001$, partial $\eta^2 = 0.21$. Only PIQ had a significant independent association with search strategy performance. The strategy score for the DD group (M = 37.88, SD = 3.66) was higher, indicating a less efficient search, than for the healthy control group (M = 33.75, SD = 4.92). Cohen's *d* (0.95) again showed a large effect size.

Correlations between VSWM, Span and Strategy

The relationships between VSWM (BSE's) and the spatial span and strategy components of VSWM were assessed in the combined sample. There was a significant negative correlation between total BSE's and spatial span, $r = -0.57$, $p < 0.0005$, and a significant positive correlation between total BSE's and strategy, $r = 0.67$, $p < 0.0005$.

Correlations between Parent and Child Reported Depressive Symptoms, Inattention Symptoms and VSWM

The relationships between problems of inattention, depressive symptoms and VSWM performance in the combined sample, including healthy control and clinical participants, were examined with Pearson product-moment correlation coefficients. The VSWM total accuracy score (as defined by the number of BSE's across all VSWM task levels) had a large positive correlation with the parent report of child inattentive symptoms (CBCL inattentive subscale score) ($r = 0.62$, $p < .0005$), a medium positive correlation with the parent report of child depressive symptoms (CBCL anxiety/depressive subscale score) ($r = 0.49$, $p<.0005$), and a large positive correlation with the child report of depressive symptoms (CDI total score) ($r = 0.51$, $p<.0005$).

Discussion

VSWM deficits (as defined by poor BSE performance) were observed in pre-pubertal children with DD. When performing the VSWM task, children with DD would continually return to search 'boxes' in which a target had already been found. These searches were redundant as a target could only be located once in a box. Analyses revealed that VSWM deficits for the DD group were more evident at levels 6 and 8 of the task. These are the most difficult levels of the task, which suggests that the observed VSWM impairment in DD worsens as the cognitive demands of the task increase. Analyses also showed deficits in both the 'spatial span' and 'strategy' components of VSWM for the DD group. This suggests that children with DD were impaired in their ability to maintain spatial information 'online' in VSWM and in their ability to develop a systematic search strategy during task performance. Correlational analyses showed that, across both diagnostic groups, VSWM deficits (poor BSE performance) were related to poor performance on the 'spatial span' and 'strategy' measures. This suggests that deficits in the maintenance and manipulation of spatial information in VSWM contributed to the impairment in overall VSWM ability displayed by the DD group.

Additional analyses revealed longer response times on the VSWM task for children with DD, evident at levels 3, 6 and 8 of the task. The similar response times between groups on level 4 suggest that motor dysfunction is unlikely to be associated with DD in pre-pubertal children. Further, the longer response times on level 3, but not level 4, may reflect that the DD group took longer to initially orient their attention to the VSWM task. Finally, the longer response times and the lower accuracy of performance on levels 6 and 8 are consistent with the use of less efficient search strategies by the DD group. This further suggests that children with DD had difficulties with manipulating information held 'online' in VSWM.

It is known that dysfunction to fronto-striatal-parietal neural networks is associated with impaired abilities in the manipulation of spatial information in VSWM [12,37,51]. The present findings of deficits in strategy performance and overall VSWM functioning suggest that DD in children is associated with dysfunction to these fronto-striatal-parietal neural networks. Deficits in VSWM 'spatial span' ability suggest there is also dysfunction involving mid-ventrolateral prefrontal and posterior parietal cortical regions in DD [17,52].

Fronto-striatal-parietal dysfunction is also associated with inattention [9]. The present finding that children in the DD group rated highly on a measure of inattention, relative to the healthy control group (see Table 1), further supports the suggestion of dysfunction to these neural networks in DD. More specifically, dorsolateral prefrontal cortex (DLPFC) linked neural networks are involved in higher cognitive processes, or 'executive functions', including working memory [53]. Also, the association of inattentive symptoms with cognitive aspects of executive function, such as working memory, is thought to be underpinned by dysfunction to the DLPFC, anterior cingulate cortex and striatal brain regions [54]. Correlational analyses in the present study found that inattentive symptoms were significantly associated with VSWM impairments. Taken together, these findings suggest there is dysfunction to DLPFC fronto-striatal neural networks in childhood DD. However, the association between VSWM and inattention may suggest that the observed deficits of VSWM are linked to symptoms of inattention in general, rather than DD specifically. Further studies should delineate whether or not VSWM deficits are associated with the neurobiology of DD *per se,* for example by examining VSWM in children with DD and no inattentive symptoms.

The present findings highlight the cognitive and neuropsychological symptoms of DD. Dysfunction to *the interaction between* the DLPFC and other fronto-striatal neural networks may facilitate the spectrum of cognitive, affective and subtle motor symptoms that present in children with DD [4,55,56]. DLPFC fronto-striatal neural networks influence the motor and oculomotor networks [53]. The DLPFC also has connections with orbito-frontal-striatal neural networks, which are associated with motivation for goal directed behaviour [53], as well as medial PFC-linked networks, which have connections to limbic regions and are associated with the expression of emotion [53,57,58]. The 'flow' of affective and cognitive information between the DLPFC, orbital and medial fronto-striatal networks appears to be facilitated by the close proximity of these circuits in the basal ganglia [53,55]. There is need for further research examining whether dysfunction to DLPFC fronto-striatal neural networks, *as well as* their connections with limbic regions, are associated with the cognitive and affective symptoms of DD.

Clinical Implications

Inattentive symptoms may contribute to the learning difficulties and impairments in academic functioning that have been observed in children with DD [16,31]. Interventions targeting inattention may thus be helpful. The observed VSWM deficits also suggest that children with DD have trouble with holding spatial information 'online' in working memory, and manipulating this information. This may have implications for the presentation of information. For example, when children with DD are learning or receiving instructions, they may respond better to smaller, more simple pieces of information that are presented repeatedly, particularly in high stimulus, novel environments like the school classroom. These interventions may also be useful in the home or clinical settings. Further, stimulant medication may be helpful for this group of children who can become severely oppositional and defiant in these contexts [59]. However future randomised controlled trials are needed.

Poor academic performance may exacerbate the symptoms of low self-esteem displayed by children with DD [7]. Low self-esteem is also likely to contribute to the impaired peer relationships, frequently observed during the symptomatic period of DD [60]. Clearly, addressing cognitive, academic and social functioning is important in the treatment of childhood DD.

Study limitations

The levels of the VSWM task were presented in order of increasing cognitive demand, rather than randomised. This may suggest that the poor performance of children with DD on levels 6 and 8 of the task reflects increases in cognitive fatigue, inattention or low motivation as the task progressed. However, the order of presentation was controlled for between the two diagnostic groups. Further, the CANTAB battery has been validated in developmental studies of children and adolescents [61,62], and employed in previous clinical studies of children with psychiatric disorders featuring inattentive symptoms, such as ADHD [9,63-65] and early onset schizophrenia [44]. Thus, the present findings are more likely to reflect actual deficits of VSWM, and the impact of poor spatial span and strategy abilities on VSWM performance. Another limitation is that the present study was a clinical study of children with 'pure' DD. It is not certain whether the findings may be generalised to the wider community or to patients with DD and a further diagnosed co-morbid disorder. Future research should examine the neuropsychological profile of children with DD and key co-morbid disorders, particularly MDD [4].

Conclusion

In summary, the present findings support an association between VSWM and DD in pre-pubertal children. VSWM deficits, including deficits to both the 'spatial span' and strategy components of VSWM, as well as associated symptoms of inattention, taken together, imply dysfunction to dorsolateral and ventrolateral fronto-striatal-parietal neural networks. Further neuropsychological and functional neuroimaging studies are required to extend these findings.

In the next study, a VSWM mental rotation fMRI paradigm will be used to examine fronto-striatal-parietal neural network activation in post-pubertal adolescents and pre-pubertal children with DD compared to a carefully matched healthy control participant group.

Study Two

To date, seminal structural and functional neuroimaging research has been conducted in children and adolescents with ADHD. Decreased volumes of prefrontal cortical, basal ganglia (primarily striatal) and temporal brain regions have been demonstrated [66], while increased volumes in parietal brain regions have been noted [67]. Apart from the significant fMRI response inhibition paradigm studies in ADHD, recent VSWM fMRI paradigm studies have demonstrated decreased activation of right prefrontal cortical, striatal and parietal brain regions in children and adolescents with ADHD [51, 68-70]. In contrast, there is a striking lack of structural and functional neuroimaging research in children and adolescents with DD given its clinical importance. Hence, it is difficult to determine any key research directions based on the extant literature. Steingard et al. [71] have reported decreased frontal lobe volume and increased ventricular size in children and adolescents with DD. Lyoo et al. [72] showed a decreased size of the corpus callosum genu in young adults with 'minor depression' (DD or depressive personality disorder) while Trimble and van Elst [73] demonstrated increased amygdala volumes in adults with DD and temporal lobe epilepsy. Further, Sarikaya et al. [74] reported decreased regional cerebral blood flow (rCBF) in inferior frontal (bilateral), superior frontal (right), posterior temporal (left) and parietal (bilateral) brain regions in adults with DD. However, it remains unclear whether these findings are also evident in children and adolescents with DD. In contrast, there is relatively more evidence implicating the prefrontal cortex, striatal, temporal, and amygdala brain regions in children and adolescents with MDD. Tutus et al. [75] noted decreased rCBF in left anterofrontal and temporal brain regions in adolescents with major depressive disorder while Kowatch et al. [76] reported decreased rCBF in anterior thalamus, left parietal and right caudate brain regions and increased rCBF in mesial, right superior anterior and left inferior lateral temporal brain regions. Thomas et al. [77] reported decreased amygdala activation in depressed adolescents and contrasting increased amygdala activation in anxious adolescents. However, there are also replicated findings of increased amygdala volume and activation in children and adolescents with MDD [78]. In addition, Killgore and Yurgelen-Todd [79], using fMRI, recently demonstrated increased medial orbitofrontal cortex and rostral anterior cingulate cortex activation in healthy adolescents experiencing a sad mood and demonstrating a sad affect. Further they noted that depressed mood correlated positively with left DLPFC and anterior cingulate cortex activity and negatively with right DLPFC activity, consistent with affective lateralisation seen in adulthood [80].

The adult MDD functional neuroimaging literature is much more developed: Decreased activity in the left dorsolateral and dorsomedial prefrontal cortex, and hippocampus along with increased activity in the subgenual prefrontal cortex, bilateral post orbital cortex, left ventrolateral prefrontal cortex and anterior insula are known associations [81-82]. Recently, Grimm et al. [83] have noted the increased activity of the ventromedial prefrontal cortex, pregenual anterior cingulate cortex, posterior cingulate cortex, subgenual cingulate cortex (SGCC) and insula. Further, Wagner et al. [84] have linked increased rostral anterior cingulate cortex activity with decreased orbitofrontal cortex, left dorsolateral and dorsomedial prefrontal cortex and subgenual cingulate cortex volumes. In addition, Liotti et al. [85] have investigated healthy adults in the state of being sad: they demonstrated increased activity in the SGCC and insula associated with decreased activity of the right DLPFC and posterior parietal cortex. Further, this group has hypothesized that direct and indirect connections between the right DLPFC and SGCC may be associated with respective reciprocal deactivation and hyperactivation of these brain regions that in turn subserve diminished attention in a sad mood. Given (1) these same fronto-parietal brain regions subserve VSWM, (2) DD is characterized by chronic sad and/or irritable mood and has a greater than chance association with inattention, and (3) the behavioural neuroscience VSWM data presented earlier in this chapter suggest the inattention in the DD participants is subserved by decreased VSWM performance, Study two aims to examine the robust VSWM mental rotation fMRI probe in (1) post-pubertal adolescents and (2) pre-pubertal children with categorically and dimensionally defined DD. Both DD groups examined have significant inattentive symptoms. Based on our previous work using the same fMRI mental rotation probe in children and adolescents with ADHD, combined type, we hypothesize that (1) the post-pubertal adolescents will activate less the right inferior parietal cortex (BA 40), the right superior parietal (BA 7) and right middle frontal (BA 10) regions; and (2) the pre-pubertal children will activate less the right parieto-occipital areas (cuneus and precuneus, BA 19), the right inferior parietal lobe (BA 40) and the right caudate nucleus. Based on the current DD literature, we were unable to make any systematic predictions.

Method

Participants

Eight male post-pubertal (Tanner stage III-IV [20]) adolescents aged 12 to 17 years [14.6 (1.1) years] and twelve male pre-pubertal (Tanner stage I [20]) children aged 8-12 years [10.1 (1.2) years] were identified with medication naïve DD (DSM-IV, [21]) during their initial clinical evaluation. The cases were recruited from primary health practitioners in respective primary and secondary schools in metropolitan Melbourne. DD was defined through separate semi-structured clinical interviews with parent(s) and child/adolescent [κ>0.8] (A-DISC, [22]). Symptoms of DD were also evaluated dimensionally using parent report (CBCL anxiety depression subscale, [23]) and child/adolescent report (CDI total depression scale, [24]), where clinical level DD symptoms were observed to be greater than 1.5 standard deviations above the mean for a child's/adolescent's age and gender. Patients also exhibited inattentive symptoms [adolescent: 70.88 (9.75); child: 70.68 (9.44)] (CBCL attention subscale, [23]). These eight patients had full scale IQs >80 [adolescents: mean 'performance IQ' = 106.1 (11.9); children: mean 'performance IQ' = 98.9 (9.64)] and no other known medical, neurological or endocrine disorders, MDD, Attention Deficit Hyperactivity Disorder, combined type, Conduct Disorder, Developmental Coordination Disorder or reading/spelling learning disorders (Wide Range Achievement Test, 3rd Edition, [25]).

Eight post-pubertal (Tanner stage III-IV [20]) and twelve pre-pubertal (Tanner stage I [20]) healthy control participants, who did not meet criteria for any psychiatric, neurological or endocrine disorder, were again defined through a semi-structured clinical interview (A-DISC, [22]) with their parent(s) and with each child/adolescent [κ>0.8], and by the parent

(CBCL, anxiety depression subscale, [22]) and child/adolescent (CDI total depression scale, [24]), reports. They did not differ from the DD group in age [adolescents: 14.5 (1.8); children: 10.1 (1.4)]; gender or 'performance IQ' [adolescents: 113.0 (8.3); children: 104.6 (9.9)], as assessed by the perceptual reasoning index from the Wechsler Intelligence Test for Children, 4th edition [26].

Measures

The mental rotation stimuli (3D rotation of complex figures) consisted of Shepard-Metzler-type three-dimensional cube objects. Over a total scan time of 6 minutes and 36 seconds, participants were presented with 18 baseline and 18 mental rotation trials. Each trial comprised one target stimulus and four (adolescents)/two (children) test stimuli and participants were given speed and accuracy instructions by indicating through a button-press which stimulus matched the target. The four/two button response pad was spatially concordant with the display of the test stimuli positions. A single trial consisted of the continuous presentation of a target and four/two test stimuli for 10 seconds, followed by a 1 second inter-stimulus interval. In the mental rotation condition, Shepard-Metzler-type three-dimensional cube objects were used, with each of the target stimuli rotated at a unique three-dimensional angle ranging 45-180° (Figure 4).

In the baseline condition no mental rotation was required, but participants were required to judge which of the four/two test stimuli of Fourier transformed 'noise' patches was most similar to the target (Figure 5). Mental rotation and baseline trials alternated in their presentation and were viewed in groups of three (forming 33 second blocks).

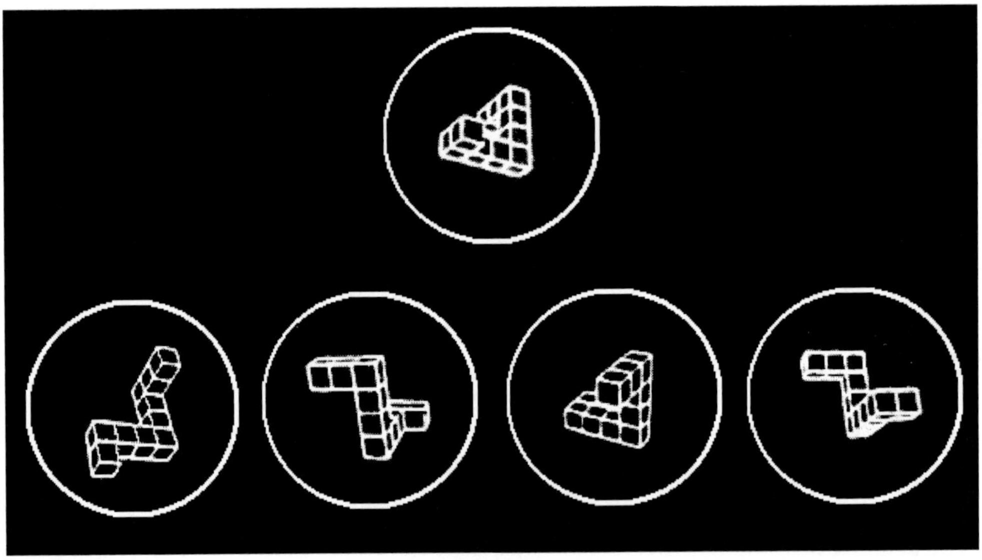

Figure 4. An example of a test stimulus display used in the mental rotation condition (adolescents).

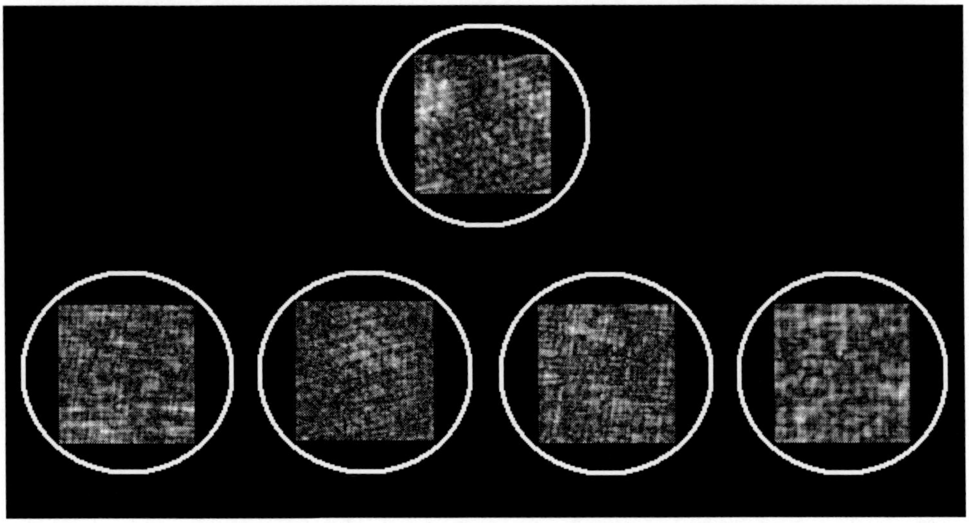

Figure 5. An example of a test stimulus display used in the baseline condition (adolescents)

Procedure

Prior to the fMRI scanning session, all participants and their parents/guardians were invited to an information session with a senior member of the research team. At this time the mental rotation task was practised so that participants were familiar with the stimuli and understood the task. Information about the scanning procedure and aims of the study were also explained at this time and informed consent was obtained from both parent and child. The second session was conducted at the Brain Research Institute (BRI), Austin and Repatriation Medical Centre (adolescents) or Royal Children's Hospital (children). Prior to scanning, all participants were prepared for the experience by use of a Mock scanner which was designed to simulate the experience of being inside the scanner. Assessment for MR risk was completed by standard procedures by the Radiographer at the BRI.

When in the MRI scanner, participants were positioned supine with their head supported in a volume head coil. Participants were instructed to wear loose clothing and blankets were draped over them if they were cold. The bed of the MRI scanner did not enter the bore until each participant was comfortable as they were required to keep their head as still as possible for the entire scanning time.

Stimuli were displayed using E-Prime 1.0 Software and were projected onto a 1.6 x 1.2 metre screen that was positioned at the foot of the MRI scanner bed. The screen was viewed by participants through a mirror that was mounted on the head coil. A CD or DVD of each participant's choice was played to lessen any anxiety during the anatomical scanning. Participants were reminded at all stages that their involvement was voluntary and that they could leave the study if they felt claustrophobic or simply changed their mind. Data was not saved under the name of the participant, but rather participant codes were used.

At the completion of scanning, the radiographer showed each participant and their parent/guardian the scans that were obtained. At the completion of analyses, participants were told that the results of the study and also a picture of their brain would be sent to them.

Imaging Methods

Adolescent Sample

Data were acquired on a 3-Tesla GE Signa MR scanner (GE Medical Systems, USA) at the Brain Research Institute, Austin Health, Melbourne. Participants lay supine with their head supported in a volume coil. For functional imaging, T2*-weighted gradient-echo echo-planar images (EPI) were acquired (TR = 3000 ms, TE = 40 ms, FA = 60°, 128 x 128 matrix at 1.875 x 1.875 mm resolution, 22 axial slices with slice thickness = 4.5 mm + 0.5 mm gap). Whole brain images were therefore acquired every three seconds as participants alternated between performing rotation and baseline tasks. A total of 136 image volumes were acquired per 6 min 36 s scanning session. High resolution T1-weighted structural MRI images were also acquired for each participant (TR = 120 ms, 256 x 256 x 128 matrix, voxel size = 0.9 x 0.9 mm, slice thickness = 1.4mm).

Child Sample

Images were obtained using a 3-Tesla Siemens Magnetom scanner (Siemens, Erlangen, Germany) at the Royal Children's Hospital, Melbourne. Participants lay supine with their head supported in a volume coil. T2*-weighted functional images were acquired using a gradient-echo, echo-planar imaging (EPI) pulse sequence with the following parameters: TR (repetition time) = 2000 ms, TE (echo time) = 30 ms, FA (flip angle) = 90 °, matrix = 128 x 128 at 1.875 x 1.875 mm resolution, FOV (field of view) = 25 cm. Twenty-eight contiguous 3.0 mm transverse slices were taken (in-plane resolution 2.0 x 2.0 mm). The field of view was aligned parallel with the commissural line and included the dorsal-most aspect of the brain. A total of 174 whole-brain volumes were acquired in the rotation condition. High resolution T1-weighted structural MRI images were also recorded for each participant (TR = 190 ms, matrix = 256 x 256 x 128 matrix, voxel size = 0.9 x 0.9 mm, slice thickness = 1.0 mm).

Imaging Analysis

Functional images were converted from the DICOM proprietary scanner format to the NifTI format via MRIcron (Rorden, 2000). The first two images of each EPI series were removed before any pre-processing to allow the MR signal to reach a steady state. The remaining brain volumes for each individual were subjected to pre-statistical processing that was carried out automatically in FSL software (FMRIB, Oxford, UK) as was motion correction (MCFLIRT), spatial filtering, nonlinear highpass filtering and then the FSL time-series statistics were corrected for temporal smoothness with the application of pre-whitening (Woolrich et al., 2001). Images for each participant were then registered to standard space using the MNI152 standard template brain supplied with FSL software so that all participants' functional images approximately conformed to the same standard space (approximate Talairach co-ordinates). Quantitative studies have shown that the use of a standard brain template, although derived from adults, can be used equally for participants from 7-8 years of age with negligible effect on fMRI results. Spatial realignment was conducted to correct for movement of the individual's head during MRI acquisition. Spatial normalisation to standard Talairach space was performed using an EPI image template in order to ensure that all functional images conformed to the same standardized space. This procedure ensured that direct voxel-wise comparisons could be made. Data was smoothed using an 8mm Gaussian kernel (full width at half maximum) to reduce signal changes caused by normal physiological variance in brain size and structure, as well as correcting for motion artefacts.

General Linear Model (GLM) statistical analysis was performed using the fMRI Expert Analysis Tool (FEAT) within FSL using a mixed block and event related design model. The fMRI block design allows the 'state' dependent effects of mental rotation versus baseline (large effect size d >1SD) to be examined within and between the groups. The event related modeling of fMRI activation based on behavioural reaction time data and separated for correct and incorrect trials ensures that mental rotation events for only correct trials can be compared. The realignment parameters, representing the degree of head movement (translation and rotation in x, y, z directions) were also included in the model to account for any residual variance associated with head motion. In the first level analysis, single-sample t-tests were used to identify the areas of significant activation in the two contrast conditions identified within the mental rotation task for each individual in the DD and healthy control participant groups. In the higher order group analysis, between-group random-effects analysis was then performed using independent t-tests, in order to identify areas of activation associated with the mental rotation task that differed significantly between DD and healthy control participant groups. Significant activation was defined as clusters of voxels ($z>2.33$) with cluster-level ($p_{corrected}<0.05$) corrected for multiple comparisons. Voxels within significant clusters with the highest z-score compared to their direct neighbours (within a 10mm sphere) were reported in terms of standard stereotactic (Talairach) coordinates, in the x, y, and z axes, and Brodmann areas (BA). For both within and between-group contrasts obtained from FSL, statistical maps were created using MRIcron by overlaying the mean activation map data onto a standard anatomical template. Areas of activation were described with reference to standard stereotactic (Talaraich) co-ordinates. Areas were labelled in terms of Brodmann areas (BA) using classification from the Talairach Daemon Client 1.1 (Research Imaging Centre, San Antonio, USA). There were no apparent differences in head motion between the DD and control groups and individuals were not excluded from this analysis due to excessive head motion.

Results

Behavioural Performance

The adolescent DD and control groups differed significantly in their accuracy on the mental rotation task [DD: 33.40% (13.88); Control: 56.00% (11.00)]. However response times (sec) did not differ significantly between groups [DD: 5.06 (1.80); Control: 6.40 (0.65)]. In contrast, the child DD and control groups did not differ in their accuracy [DD: 77.82% (7.58); Control: 85.13% (5.86)] or response times (sec) [DD: 2.26 (0.76); Control: 2.35 (0.44)] on the mental rotation task.

fMRI Results

The adolescent DD group activated the left parietal/precuneus region extending into the middle temporal region while the matched healthy control participant group activated the parietal/precuneus and prefrontal cortical regions with greater right versus left hemisphere activation. In particular the right DLPFC, VLPFC, VMPFC and PGCC brain regions were activated while the DLPFC and PGCC were activated on the left. Importantly, the healthy control group activated the right parietal/ precuneus region and the DLPFC and VMPFC regions significantly more than the DD group (Figure 6; Table 3).

The child DD group activated the right occipital region extending into the middle temporal region while the matched healthy control participant group activated the right precuneus, right insula, bilateral inferior temporal, bilateral striatal, right globus pallidus, bilateral DLPFC and right VLPFC and PGCC brain regions with greater right versus left hemisphere activation. Importantly, the healthy control group activated the right precuneus, right insula, bilateral inferior temporal, right posterior cingulate, right striatal and right DLPFC and PGCC brain regions significantly more than the DD group (Figure 7; Table 4).

Discussion

Behavioural Performance

The adolescents with DD performed the 4-choice mental rotation fMRI task significantly worse than the healthy control participants while their reaction times did not differ. This is consistent with the demanding nature of the 4-choice task, evidenced by the relatively low performance accuracy of the healthy control participants. In contrast, the pre-pubertal children with DD and the healthy control children did not differ in either their performance accuracy or the response times for the easier 2-choice mental rotation fMRI task. Further, their accuracy level was clearly higher than that achieved by the adolescent participants. Nevertheless, the adolescent and child DD participants had qualitatively similar differences in brain activation compared to the healthy control participants.

fmri Results: Adolescents

The adolescent DD sample demonstrated deceased activation of the right DLPFC and right parietal/precuneus regions, consistent with Liotto et al.'s [85] findings of deactivation of this brain region in healthy adults in the state of being sad. Interestingly, Wagner et al.'s [84] finding of increased activity in VMPFC (Brodmann area 10) is consistent theoretically with the presented findings because the DD group activated this region less than the healthy control group: Decreased activation may signify an abnormally high basal level of activity in a particular brain region or a failure to induce activation from a normal or decreased basal level of activity [83]. Some caution with these interpretations is warranted because these are the first data published for adolescents with carefully diagnosed DD while Liotti et al.'s [85] and Wagner et al.'s [84] work are based on healthy adults and adults with MDD, respectively. It remains unclear whether their findings relate to children and adolescents who are healthy but sad, have MDD, DD or both conditions.

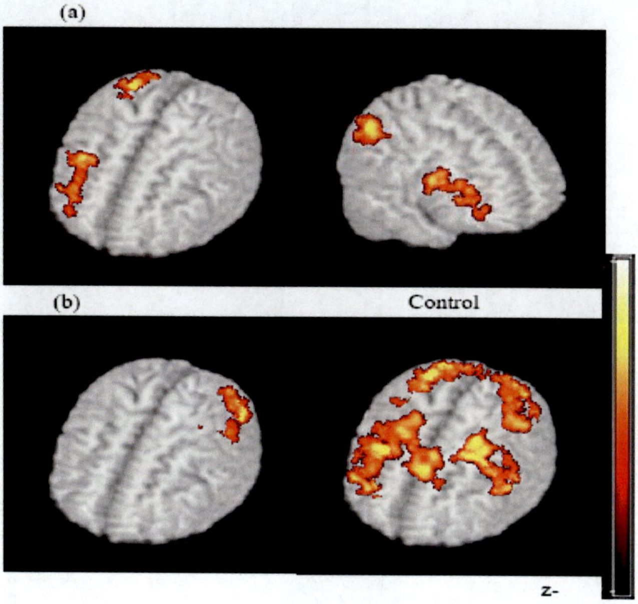

Figure 6. Statistical activation maps showing: (a) regions showing significantly greater activation in the Control group compared with the DD group during mental rotation; and (b) regions of significant activation during the mental rotation task in DD and Control groups separately.

Table 3. Regions showing significantly greater activation in Control compared with DD adolescents. Listed are peak voxels ($P_{uncorrected}$ < 0.005) that are located within significant activation clusters ($P_{corrected}$ < 0.05)

Greater Activation for Control than Dysthymic Disorder				
Region	BA	x	y	z
Right Frontal Lobe				
Inferior Frontal Gyrus	9	42	10	22
Middle Frontal Gyrus	46	44	42	14
Middle Frontal Gyrus	46	40	18	20
Middle Frontal Gyrus	10	34	40	20
Inferior Frontal Gyrus	44	50	14	14
Right Parietal Lobe				
Inferior Parietal Lobule	40	40	-58	44
Superior Parietal Lobule	7	36	-74	44
Inferior Parietal Lobule	39	48	-62	40
Superior Parietal Lobule	7	30	-74	44
Precuneus	19	34	-66	36
Inferior Parietal Lobule	40	42	-44	44

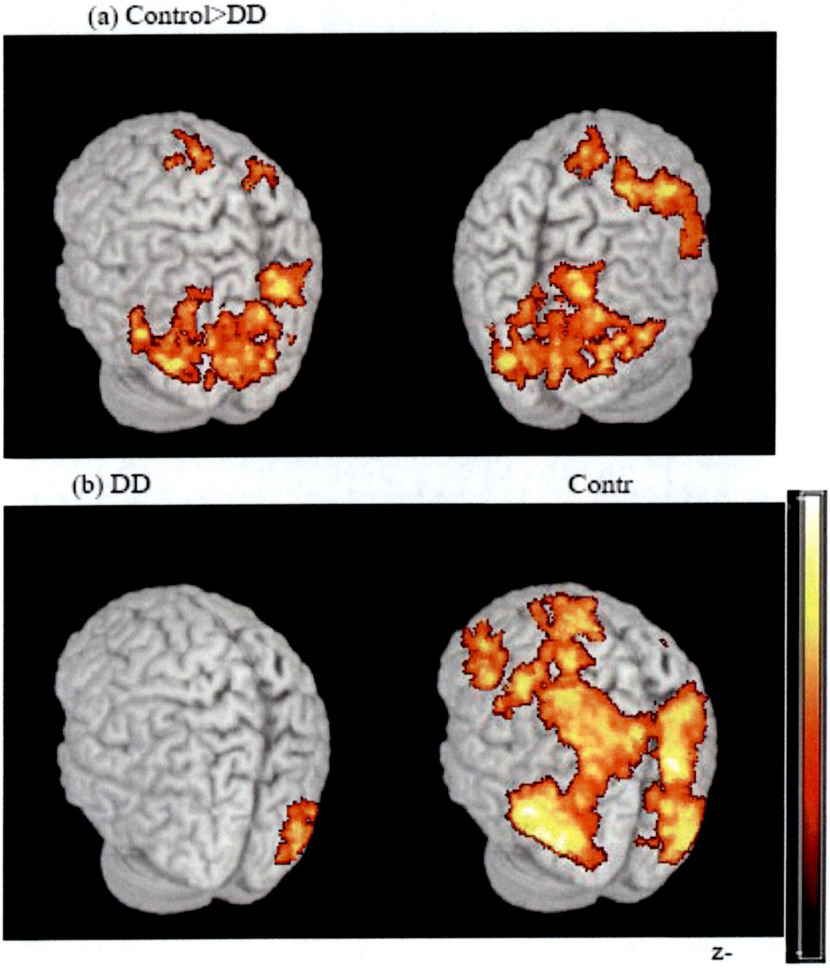

Figure 7. Statistical activation maps showing: (a) regions showing significantly greater activation in the Control group compared with the DD group during mental rotation; and (b) regions of significant activation during the mental rotation task in DD and Control groups separately.

Importantly, the adolescent DD findings are remarkably consistent with our group's previous findings in adolescent ADHD, combined type using the same fMRI mental rotation paradigm [51,86]: Two, albeit interconnected, neural network systems appeared to be activated less in the ADHD-CT group compared to the healthy control subjects; (1) the 'action-attentional' [87] system (including BA 46,39,40) that subserves disengaged, reoriented and maintained attentional focus and inhibition of contextually irrelevant stimuli and (2) the superior parietal (BA 7) and middle frontal (BA 10) areas that are involved in visuospatial manipulation [88]. This most probably reflects the similar high levels of inattention evident in both these disorders, given that inattentive symptoms are part of the core symptom domains of both conditions.

Table 4. Regions showing significantly greater activation in Control compared with DD children. Listed are peak voxels ($P_{uncorrected} < 0.005$) that are located within significant activation clusters ($P_{corrected} < 0.05$)

Greater activation for control than dysthymic disorder group

Region	BA	x	y	z
Bilateral frontal				
R Inferior Frontal Gyrus	9	52	4	34
R Inferior Frontal Gyrus	47	44	18	2
R Inferior Frontal Gyrus	47	46	14	-8
R Middle Frontal Gyrus	6	30	-6	48
R Medial Frontal Gyrus	6	6	12	44
R Superior Frontal Gyrus	8	2	18	50
R Superior Frontal Gyrus	6	6	8	50
R Precentral Gyrus	6	32	-4	36
R Precentral Gyrus	6	40	-6	46
R Precentral Gyrus	6	44	-4	44
L Superior Frontal Gyrus	6	-10	16	48
R Caudate	*	8	0	12
R Putamen	*	26	0	14
R Posterior Cingulate	31	22	-64	16
L Parahippocampal Gyrus	19	-20	-50	-4
L Parahippocampal Gyrus	36	-28	-30	-18
T Thalamus	*	-16	-30	-2
L Cingulate Gyrus	32	0	14	38
Right Temporal				
R Inferior Temporal Gyrus	37	44	-66	-2
L Inferior Temporal Gyrus	19	-46	-56	-4
R Insula	13	42	20	8
Right Parietal				
R Precuneus	7	22	-68	38
R Precuneus	7	20	-72	42
R Precuneus	7	16	-64	44
R Precuneus	7	16	-74	52
R Precuneus	19	28	-80	40
Bilateral occipital				
R Middle Occipital Gyrus	18	29	-82	-6
R Middle Occipital Gyrus	18	26	-82	2
L Inferior Occipital Gyrus	19	-34	-78	-4
R Lingual Gyrus	19	20	-68	-6

* No associated Brodmann area

fmri Results: Children

The child DD sample demonstrated a similar qualitative pattern of deceased activation of the right DLPFC and right parietal/precuneus regions to the adolescent DD group, consistent with Liotto et al.'s [85] findings of deactivation of this brain region in healthy adults in the state of being sad. Interestingly, Grimm et al.'s [83] findings of increased basal activity in posterior cingulate cortex and PGCC (Brodmann areas 31/32) in adults with MDD are theoretically consistent with the presented findings because the DD group activated these regions less than the healthy control group. Further, the decreased activation in the right insula of the DD group is consistent with prior studies suggesting increased basal activity in the insula region in adults with MDD [83] and healthy adults in the state of experiencing a sad mood and observed to have a sad affect [85]. Some caution with these interpretations is warranted because these are the first data published for children with carefully diagnosed DD while Liotti et al.'s [83] and Grimm et al.'s [85] work are based on healthy adults and adults with MDD, respectively. It remains unclear whether their findings relate to children and adolescents who are healthy but in a sad state, have MDD, DD or both conditions.

The decreased activation of the right VLPFC and right inferior temporal region in the children with DD implicates decreased function of the ventral visuospatial pathway involved in object permanence [86]. Further, the right striatal region was activated less in the prepubertal DD participants, consistent with a more widespread inactivation of right frontal-striatal-parietal neural networks known to subserve visuospatial attention and working memory [34,35]. This widespread frontal-striatal-parietal inactivation was again remarkably consistent with our group's previous findings in pre-pubertal ADHD, combined type using the same fMRI mental rotation paradigm [51]: As in these pre-pubertal ADHD, combined type participants, these activation differences occurred despite a lack of behavioural performance difference on the mental rotation task, suggesting that activation differences are not simply due to poorer performance in the DD group. Rather, these activation differences may reflect a dysfunctional use of the same/and or a different strategy that the children with DD use to complete the VSWM fMRI task, aside from the conscious willed approach taken by each child. As in the adolescents with DD, this most probably reflects the similar high levels of inattention evident in both ADHD-CT and DD, given that inattentive symptoms are part of the core symptom domains of both conditions.

In future, (1) regression analyses of the key fronto-striatal-parietal brain regions less active in both disorders and clinical levels of inattentive symptoms are needed to quantify their association, (2) DD without impairing symptoms of inattention, DD with MDD and MDD alone need to be examined with the same fMRI mental rotation probe to see if the same pattern of fronto-parietal decreased activation is evident, and (3) randomized controlled trials of stimulant medication in DD groups with ADHD, inattentive type symptoms need to be conducted to examine and describe the potential benefits in this non-ADHD, combined type group. As always, pre-pubertal child and post-pubertal adolescent samples need to be examined separately if developmental stage specific effects are to be delineated.

Integration and Implications of these Findings

The two studies present data that enhance our understanding of the association between impairing inattentive symptoms and dysthymic disorder. The clinical and research implications for children and adolescents presenting with DD are considered below.

Impairing symptoms of inattention in children and adolescents presenting with dysthymic disorder need to be identified, treated and the psychosocial and/or medication treatment monitored carefully. The behavioural cognitive neuroscience data outlined in this chapter implies that the visuospatial memory and working memory correlates are qualitatively similar to those found in children and adolescents with ADHD, combined type. This contention is further strengthened by the fMRI data demonstrating impaired frontal-striatal-parietal neural networks, known to subserve visuospatial working memory and clinical symptoms of inattention, that seem developmental stage independent.

Future research examination of the following issues are required: (1) DD with and without the three ADHD subtypes, (2) DD with and without MDD and MDD alone, (3) DD with and without key further well known comorbid conditions with a 'greater than chance' association, excluded in these two studies, (4) longitudinal examination of cases pre- and post-puberty, (5) examination using affective cognitive neuroscience behavioural and fMRI working memory paradigms, (5) more specific fMRI paradigms for key brain regions - parietal, basal ganglia and prefrontal cortex, and (6) randomised controlled trials of targeted medication and psychosocial treatments for impairing inattentive symptoms.

References

[1] Vance ALA, Luk ESL. *Heart of the Matter Review*: Attention Deficit Hyperactivity Disorder: Progress and Controversies. *Australian and New Zealand Journal of Psychiatry* 2000; 34: 719-730.

[2] Vance A, Arduca Y, Sanders M. The associations of oppositional defiant behaviour in children with Attention Deficit Hyperactivity Disorder, combined type (ADHD-CT). *Journal of Affective Disorders* 2005; 86: 329-333.

[3] Maughan B, Rowe R, Messer J, Goodman R, Meltzer H. Conduct disorder and oppositional defiant disorder in a national sample: developmental epidemiology. *Journal of Child Psychology and Psychiatry*. 2004; 45: 609-621.

[4] Kovacs M, Akiskal HS, Gatsonis C, Parrone PL. Childhood-onset dysthymic disorder. Clinical features and prospective naturalistic outcome. *Archives of General Psychiatry*. 1994; 51:365-374.

[5] Klein DN, Lewinsohn PM, Seeley JR. Psychosocial characteristics of adolescents with a past history of dysthymic disorder: comparison with adolescents with past histories of major depressive and non-affective disorders, and never mentally ill controls. *Journal of Affective Disorders* 1997; 42: 127-135.

[6] Ferro T, Carlson GA, Grayson P, Klein DN. Depressive disorders: Distinction in children. *Journal of the American Academy of Child and Adolescent Psychiatry* 1994; 33: 664- 670.

[7] Masi G, Favilla L, Mucci M, Poli P, Romano R. Depressive symptoms in children and adolescents with dysthymic disorder. *Psychopathology* 2001; 34: 29-35.

[8] Mitchell J, McCauley E, Burke PM, Moss SJ. Phenomenology of depression in children and adolescents. *Journal of the American Academy of Child and Adolescent Psychiatry* 1988; 27: 12-20.

[9] Barnett R, Maruff P, Vance A, Luk E, Costin J, Wood C, Pantelis C. Abnormal execution function in attention deficit hyperactivity disorder: The effect of stimulant medication and age on spatial working memory. *Psychological Medicine* 2001; 31: 1107-1115.

[10] Barnett R., Maruff, P., and Vance, A. An investigation of visuospatial memory impairment in children with attention deficit hyperactivity disorder (ADHD), combined type. *Psychological Medicine* 2005; 35, 1433-1443.

[11] Lawrence AD, Watkins LHA, Sahakian BJ, Hodges JR, Robbins RW. Visual object and visuospatial cognition in Huntington's disease: implications for information processing in corticostriatal circuits. *Brain* 2000; 123: 1349-1364.

[12] Owen AM, Sahakian BJ, Semple J. Visuo-spatial short-term recognition memory and learning after temporal lobe excisions, frontal lobe excisions or amygdalo-hippocampectomy in man. *Neuropsychologia* 1995; 33: 1-24.

[13] Sahakian BJ, Morris RG, Evenden JL, Heald A, Levy R, Philpot M, Robbins TW. A comparative study of visuospatial memory and learning in Alzheimer-type dementia and Parkinson's disease. *Brain* 1988; 111, 695 – 718.

[14] Lauer RE, Giordani B, Boivin MJ, Halle N, Glasgow B, Alessi NE, Berent S. Effects of depression on memory performance and metamemory in children. *Journal of the American Academy of Child and Adolescent Psychiatry* 1994; 33: 679-685.

[15] Osborn RG, Meador DM. The memory performance of selected depressed and nondepressed nine-to-eleven-year-old male children. *Behavioral Disorders* 1990; 16: 32-38.

[16] Kovacs, M., and Goldston, D. Cognitive and social cognitive development of depressed children and adolescents. *Journal of the American Academy of Child and Adolescent Psychiatry* 1991; 30: 388-392.

[17] Owen AM, Evans AC, Petrides M. Evidence for a two-stage model of spatial working memory processing within the lateral frontal cortex: a positron emission tomography study. *Cerebral Cortex* 1996; 6: 31-38.

[18] Robbins TW, James M, Owen AM, Sahakian BJ, McInnes L, Rabbitt P. Cambridge Neuropsychological Test Automated Battery (CANTAB): A factor analytic study of a large sample of normal elderly volunteers. *Dementia* 1994; 5: 266-281.

[19] Mathes B, Wood SJ, Proffitt TM. Early processing deficits in object working memory in first episode schizophreniform psychosis and established schizophrenia. *Psychological Medicine* 2005; 35: 1053-1062.

[20] Tanner JM. Growth at Adolescence. 2nd ed. New York, NY: Appleton-Century-Crofts, 1966.

[21] American Psychiatric Association. Diagnostic and statistical manual of mental disorders (4th, text revision ed.). Washington: American Psychiatric Association, 2000.

[22] Silverman WK, Albano AM. Anxiety Disorders Interview Schedule for DSM-IV. Texas: Graywind, 1996.

[23] Achenbach TM, Edelbrock CS. Manual for the child behaviour checklist and behaviour profile. Burlington: University of Vermont, 1983.

[24] Kovacs M. The Children's Depression Inventory. New York: Mental Health Systems, 1992.

[25] Wilkinson GS. Wide Range Achievement Tests-Revised. Wilmington, DE: Jastak Assessment Systems, 1993.

[26] Wechsler D. The Wechsler Intelligence Scale for Children (4th Edition). San Antonio, TX: The Psychological Corporation, 2003.

[27] Kravariti E, Morris R, Rabe-Hesketh S, Murray RM, Frangou S. The Maudsley early-onset schizophrenia study: Cognitive function in recent onset schizophrenia. *Schizophrenia Research* 2003a; 61: 137-148.

[28] Kravariti E, Morris R, Rabe-Hesketh S, Murray RM, Frangou S. (2003b). The Maudsley early-onset schizophrenia study: Cognitive function in adolescent-onset schizophrenia. *Schizophrenia Research* 2003b; 61: 95-103.

[29] Sweeney JA, Wetzler S, Stokes P, Kocsis J. Cognitive functioning in depression. *Journal of Clinical Psychology* 1989; 45: 836-842.

[30] Günther T, Holtkamp K, Jolles J, Herpertz-Dahlann B, Konrad K. Verbal memory and aspects of attentional control in children and adolescents with anxiety disorders or depressive disorders. *Journal of Affective Disorders* 2004; 82: 265-269.
[31] Friedman RA, Markowitz JC, Parides M, Kocsis JH. Acute response of social functioning in dysthymic patients with desipramine. *Journal of Affective Disorders* 1995; 34: 84-88.
[32] Kempton S, Vance ALA, Maruff P, Luk SL, Costin J, Pantelis C. Executive Function and Attention Deficit Hyperactivity Disorder: Stimulant Medication and better Executive Function Performance in children. *Psychological Medicine* 1999; 29: 527-538.
[33] Smyth MM. Interference with rehearsal in spatial working memory in the absence of eye movements. *Journal Experimental Psychology* 1996; 49: 940-949.

[34] Awh E, Vogel EK, Oh SH. Interactions between attention and working memory. *Neuroscience* 2006; 139: 201-208.
[35] Awh E, Jonides J. Spatial selective attention and spatial working memory. In: *The attentive brain* (Parasuraman, R., ed.), pp 353-380. Cambridge, MA: MIT Press, 1998.
[36] Lange KW, Robbins TW, Marsden CD, James M, Owen AM, Paul GM. L-Dopa withdrawal in Parkinson's disease selectively impairs cognitive performance in tests sensitive to frontal dysfunction. *Psychopharmacology* 1992; 107: 394-404.
[37] Pantelis C, Barnes TRE, Nelson HE, Tanner S, Weatherley L, Owen AM, Robbins TW. Fronto-striatal cognitive deficits in patients with chronic schizophrenia. *Brain* 1997; 120: 1823-1843.
[38] Goldman-Rakic PS. Circuitry of primate prefrontal cortex and regulation of behavior by representational memory. In F. Plum (Ed.), *Handbook of Physiology, the Nervous System Higher Functions of the Brain* (Vol. V, pp373-417). Bethesda: American Physiological Society, 1987.
[39] Owen AM, Roberts AC, Hodges JR, Summers BA, Polkey CE, Robbins TW. Contrasting mechanisms of attentional set-shifting in patients with frontal lobe damage or Parkinson's disease. *Brain* 1993; 116: 1159-1175.
[40] D'Esposito M, Detre JA, Alsop DC, Shin RK, Atlas S, Grossman M. The neural basis of the central executive system of working memory. *Nature* 1995; 378: 279-281.
[41] Baddeley, A. *Working memory*. New York: Oxford University Press, 1986.
[42] Owen AM, Downes JJ, Sahakian BJ, Polkey CE, Robbins TW. Planning and spatial working memory following frontal lobe lesions in man. *Neuropsychologia* 1990; 28: 1021-1034.
[43] Robbins TW, James M, Owen AM, Sahakian BJ, McInnes L, Rabbitt P. Cambridge Neuropsychological Test Automated Battery (CANTAB): A factor analytic study of a large sample of normal elderly volunteers. *Dementia* 1994; 5: 266-281.
[44] Vance A, Hall N, Bellgrove M, Casey M, Karsz F. Visuospatial working memory deficits in adolescent-onset schizophrenia. *Schizophrenia Research* 2006b; 87: 223-227.
[45] Braver TS, Barch DM, Kelley WM, Buckner RL, Cohen NJ, Miezen FM, Snyder AZ, Ollinger JM, Akbudak E, Conturo TE, Petersen SE. Direct comparison of prefrontal

cortex regions engaged by working and long-term memory tasks. *NeuroImage* 2001; 14: 48-59.

[46] Braver TS, Cohen JD, Nystrom LE, Jonides J, Smith EE, Noll DC. A parametric study of prefrontal cortex involvement in human working memory. *NeuroImage* 1997; 5: 49-62.

[47] Carlson S, Martinkauppi S, Rama P, Salli E, Korvenoja A, Aronen HJ. Distribution of cortical activation during visuosptial n-back tasks as revealed by functional magnetic resonance imaging. *Cerebral Cortex* 1998; 8: 743-752.

[48] Goldman-Rakic PS, Selemon LD. Functional and anatomical aspects of prefrontal pathology in schizophrenia. *Schizophrenia Bulletin* 1997; 23: 437-458.

[49] Cannon TD, Glahn DC, Kim J, Van Erp TGM, Karlsgot K, Cohen MS, Nuechterlein KH, Bava S, Shirinyan D. Dorsolateral prefrontal cortex activity during maintenance and manipulation of information in working memory in patients with schizophrenia. *Archives of General Psychiatry* 2005; 62: 1071-1080.

[50] Milner B. Interhemispheric differences in the localisation of psychological processes in man. *British Medical Bulletin* 1971; 27: 272-277.

[51] Vance A, Silk, T, Casey, M, Rinehart N, Bradshaw J, Bellgrove M, Cunnington R (2007). Right parietal dysfunction in children with Attention Deficit Hyperactivity Disorder, combined type: A functional MRI study. *Molecular Psychiatry* 2007; 12: 826-832.

[52] Smith EE, Jonides J, Koeppe RA. Dissociating verbal and spatial working memory using PET. *Cerebral Cortex* 1996; 96: 11-20.

[53] Haber SH. The primate basal ganglia: Parallel and integrative networks. *Journal of Chemical Neuroanatomy* 2003; 26: 317-330.

[54] Castellanos FX, Sonuga-Barke EJS, Milham MP, Tannock R. Characterizing cognition in ADHD: Beyond executive dysfunction. *Trends in Cognitive Sciences* 2006; 10: 117-123.

[55] Pantelis C, Brewer W. Neurocognitive and neurobehavioral patterns and the syndromes of schizophrenia: Role of fronto-subcortical networks. In C. Pantelis, H. E. Nelson and T. R. E. Barnes (Eds.), *Schizophrenia: A Neuropsychological Perspective* (pp. 317-343). New York: J. Wiley, 1996.

[56] Vance A, Arduca Y, Sanders M, Karamitsios M, Hall N, Hetrick S (2006a). Attention deficit hyperactivity disorder, combined type, dysthymic disorder and anxiety disorders: Differential patterns of neurodevelopmental deficits. *Psychiatry Research* 2006a;143: 213-222.

[57] Carmichael ST, Price JL. Limbic connections of the orbital and medial prefrontal cortex in macaque monkeys. *Journal of Comparative Neurology* 1995; 363: 615-641.

[58] Mayberg HS, Liotti M, Brannan SK, McGinnis S, Mahurin RK, Jerbek PA, Silva JA, Tekell JL, Martin CC, Lancaster JL, Fox PT. Reciprocal limbic-cortical function and negative mood: Converging PET findings in depression and normal sadness. *American Journal of Psychiatry* 1999; 156: 675-682.

[59] Vance A, Arduca Y, Sanders M. The associations of oppositional defiant behaviour in children with Attention Deficit Hyperactivity Disorder, combined type (ADHD-CT). *Journal of Affective Disorders* 2005; 86: 329-333.

[60] Klein DN, Schwartz JE, Rose S, Leader, JB (2000). Five-year course and outcome of dysthymic disorder: A prospective, naturalistic follow-up study. *American Journal of Psychiatry* 2000; 157: 931-939.

[61] Luciana M, Nelson CA. The functional emergence of prefrontally-guided working memory systems in four- to eight-year old children. *Neuropsychologia* 1998; 36: 273-293.

[62] De Luca CR, Wood SJ, Anderson V, Buchanan J, Proffitt TM, Mahony K, Pantelis C. Normative data from the CANTAB. I: Development of executive function over the lifespan. *Journal of Clinical and Experimental Neuropsychology* 2003; 25: 242-254.

[63] Williams D, Stott CM, Goodyer IM, Sahakian BJ. Specific language impairment with or without hyperactivity: Neuropsychological evidence for frontostriatal dysfunction. *Developmental Medicine and Child Neurology* 2000; 42: 368-375.

[64] Cairney S, Maruff P, Vance A, Barnett R, Luk E, Currie J. Contextual abnormalities of saccadic inhibition in children with attention deficit hyperactivity disorder. *Experimental Brain Research* 2001; 141: 507-518.

[65] Vance AL, Maruff P, Barnett R. Attention deficit hyperactivity disorder, combined type: Better executive function performance with longer-term psychostimulant medication. *Australian and New Zealand Journal of Psychiatry* 2003; 37: 570-576.

[66] Castellanos FX, Lee PP, Sharp W. Developmental trajectories of brain volume abnormalities in children and adolescents with ADHD. *Journal American Medical Association* 2002; 288: 1740-1748.

[67] Sowell ER, Thompson PM, Welcome SE. Cortical abnormalities in children and and adolescents with attention deficit hyperactivity disorder. *Lancet* 2003; 362: 1699-1707.

[68] Konrad K, Neufang S, Hanisch C, Fink GR, Herpetz-Dahlmann B. Dysfunctional attentional networks in children with ADHD: Evidence from an event-related fMRI study. *Biological Psychiatry* 2006; 59: 643-651.

[69] Booth JR, Burman DD, Meyer JR, Lei Z, Trommer BL, Davenport ND. Larger deficits in brain networks for response inhibition than for visual selective attention in ADHD. *Journal of Child Psychology and Psychiatry* 2005; 46: 94-111.

[70] Silk T, Vance A, Rinehart N, Egan G, O'Boyle M, Cunnington R. Decreased frontal-striatal-parietal activation in Attention Deficit Hyperactivity Disorder, combined type (ADHD-CT): an fMRI study. *British Journal of Psychiatry* 2005; 187: 282-283.

[71] Steingard RJ, Renshaw PF, Turgelen-Todd D, Lyoo IK, Barnes P. Structural abnormalities in brain magnetic resonance images of depressed children. *Journal of the American Academy of Child and Adolescent Psychiatry* 1996; 35: 307-311.

[72] Lyoo IK, Kwon JS, Lee SJ, Han MH, Chang CG, Seo CS, Lee SI, Renshaw PF. Decrease in genu corpus callosum in medication naïve early onset dysthymia and depressive personality disorder. *Biological Psychiatry* 2002; 52: 1134-1143.

[73] Trimble MR, van Elst LT. The amygdala and psychopathological studies in epilepsy. *Annals of the New York Academy of Sciences* 2003; 985: 461-468.

[74] Sarikaya A, Karaşin E, Cermik TF, Abay E, Berkarda S. Evaluation of dysthymic disorder with technetium-99 brain single-photon emission tomography. *European Journal of Nuclear Medicine* 1999; 26: 260-264.

[75] Tutus A, Simsek A, Sofuoglu S, Nardali M, Kugu N, Karaaslan F, Gönül AS. Changes in regional cerebral blood flow demonstrated by single-photon emission computed tomography. *Psychiatry Research* 1998; 83: 169-177.

[76] Kowatch RA, Devous MD Sr, Harvey DC, Mayes TL, Trivedi MH, Emslie GJ, Weinberg WA. A SPECT HMPAO study of regional cerebral flow in depressed adolescenst and normal controls. *Progress in Neuropsychopharmacology and Biological Psychiatry* 1999; 23: 643-656.

[77] Thomas Thomas KM, Drevets WC, Dahl RE, Ryan ND, Birmaher B, Eccard CH, Axelson D, Whalen PJ, Casey BJ. Amygdala response to fearful faces in depressed and anxious children. *Archives of General Psychiatry* 2001; 58: 1057-1063.

[78] Roberson-Nay R, McClure EB, Monk CS, Nelson EE, Guyer AE, Fromm SJ, Charney DS, Leibenluft E, Blair J, Ernst M, Pine DS. Increased amygdala activity during successful memory encoding in adolescent major depressive disorder: an fMRI study. *Biological Psychiatry* 2006; 60: 966-973.

[79] Killgore WD, Yurgelen-Todd DA. Ventromedial prefrontal activity correlates with depressed mood in adolescent children. *Neuroreport* 2006; 17: 167-171.

[80] Killgore WD, Gruber SA, Yurgelen-Todd DA. Depressed mood and lateralized prefrontal activity during a Stroop task in adolescent children. *Neuroscience Letters* 2007; 416: 43-48.

[81] Dreverts WC. Neuroimaging studies of mood disorders. *Biological Psychiatry* 2000; 48: 813-829.

[82] Liotti M, Mayberg HS. The role of functional neuroimaging in the neuropsychology of depression. *Journal of Clinical and Experimental Neuropsychology* 2001; 23: 121-136.

[83] Grimm S, Boesonger P, Beck J, Schuepbach D, Bermpohl F, Walter M, Ernst J, Hell D, Boeker H, Northoff G. Altered negative BOLD responses in the default-mode network during emotion processing in depressed subjects. *Neuropsychopharmacology* 2008: 1-12.

[84] Wagner G, Koch K, Schachtzabel C, Reichenbach JR, Sauer H, Schlosser RGM. Enhanced rostral anterior cingulate cortex activation during cognitive control is related to orbitofrontal volume reduction in unipolar depression. *Journal of Psychiatry and Neuroscience* 2008; 33: 199-208.

[85] Liotti M, Mayberg HS, Brannan SK, McGinnis S, Jerabek P, Fox PT. Differential limbic-cortical correlates of sadness and anxiety in healthy subjects: implications for affective disorders. *Biological Psychiatry* 2000; 48: 30-42.

[86] Silk T, Vance A, Rinehart N, Egan G, O'Boyle M, Cunnington R. Decreased frontal-striatal-parietal activation in Attention Deficit Hyperactivity Disorder, combined type (ADHD-CT): an fMRI study. *British Journal of Psychiatry* 2005; 187: 282-283.

[87] Mesulam MM. Large-scale neurocognitive networks and distributed processing for attention, language and memory. *Annals of Neurology* 1990; 28: 597-613.

[88] Booth JR, MacWhinney B, Thulborn KR. Developmental and lesion effects in brain activation during sentence comprehension and mental rotation. *Developmental Neuropsychology* 2000; 18: 139-169.

In: Attention Deficit Hyperactivity Disorder (ADHD)
Editors: Stuart M. Gordon and Aileen E. Mitchell
ISBN 978-1-60741-581-7

Chapter 3

Modeling the Mesocortical Variant of ADHD: The Naples High Excitability Rats

Lucia A. Ruocco, Adolfo G. Sadile and Ugo A.Gironi Carnevale
Dept. Exptl Medicine, Second Univ. Naples, Italy

Abstract

Attention-Deficit Hyperactivity Disorder (ADHD) is a developmental problem characterized by hyperactivity, sustained attention problems and impulsivity. Two main variants have been described, i.e. mesocortical (MC), with altered executive functions, and mesolimbic (ML) with delay aversion. The MC and ML variants are associated with altered MC and ML dopamine (DA) branches respectively. The Naples High Excitability rats (NHE) model the MC variant, whereas Spontaneously Hypertensive Rats (SHR) model the ML variant. Here, multiple behavioural, histochemical, pharmacological and molecular biology studies are reviewed as evidence for and against the MC hypothesis for NHE. Behavioural studies have included exposure to spatial novelties, i.e. Làt maze to monitor activity and non selective attention (NSA), and radial maze for NSA and selective spatial attention (SSA). In addition histochemical and molecular biology studies of Tyrosine Hydroxylase (TH), DAT, DA-D1 and DA-D2 receptors, and DA-related phosphoprotein 32 (DARPP32) as functional markers have been carried out in the forebrain. The results indicate that NHE rats feature the main aspects of the MC variant of ADHD, which is associated with hypertrophic and hyperfunctional MC DA branche, as assessed by larger A10 neurons, higher TH activity, and higher DAT and DARPP32 density in the ventral tegmental area. This profile was reverted by subchronic MPH (3 mg/kg). The MPH-induced changes in TH, DAT and DARPP32 in the PFC and striatum are consistent with a drug-induced reduction in MC activity. In addition, HPLC studies revealed high tissue content of excitatory amino acids (EAA) across the NHE forebrain. This, in turn, may lead to neurotoxicity and neurodegeneration in the striatum, as proposed for human ADHD by several fMRI studies. Finally the higher DA and EAA release in forebrain sites of NHE rats is likely to be associated with higher nitric oxide (NO) synthesis. In fact, behavioural studies with acute or subchronic inhibitors of NO synthesis reduced hyperactivity and increased NSA in NHE rats. These data may open new drug/no drug strategies for diagnosis and therapy of ADHD in humans.

Introduction

Attention-Deficit Hyperactivity Disorder (ADHD) is a neurodevelopmental problem that is characterized by hyperactivity, sustained attention problems and impulsivity [1, 45, 81]. It affects 1–3% of the population, most of whom are male, with a high male-to-female ratio (4:1). Seventy percent of cases are of the age 6 to 14 years prepuberal type, and 30% of cases persist as the adult type. There are two main variants of the disorder, i.e. the mesocortical with altered executive functions, and the mesolimbic variant with delay aversion.

The Dopamine (DA) hypothesis of ADHD is based on theoretical, pharmacological, experimental and clinical evidence (for a rev. see e.g. [45, 81]). In particular, different branches of the mesocorticolimbic DA system have been associated with clinical heterogeneity in ADHD. In fact, the mesocortical (MC) variant is associated with alteration of the MC DA branche, whereas the mesolimbic (ML) variant is associated with altered ML DA branches. The neurogenetic approach in animal models has proven to be useful in mice and rats (see e.g. [35]). The most frequently used rats are the Naples High Excitability (NHE) and Spontaneously Hypertensive (SHR) rats. In particular, the NHE rats model the main aspects of the MC variant whereas the SHR model the ML variant. Here, multiple behavioural, pharmacological, histochemical and molecular biology studies are reviewed to provide evidence for and against the MC hypothesis of NHE. Since behavioural arousal to novelty has been associated with the integrity of hippocampal formation [18], these rat lines have been thought to provide a useful tool to study this limbic structure. Moreover, since the hyperactivity of NHE rats appears to be related to spatial novelty, the mesocorticolimbic DA system is involved [94]. Recently NHE rats have been demonstrated to be a suitable animal model for studying neurodevelopmental disorders such as ADHD and autism, in relation to impaired attentive processes [94].

Behavioural Profile

The phenotype of NHE rats has been described in earlier reviews [16, 68, 99]. In essence it is based on a number of spatial-novelty exposures with different complexity levels. In addition learning and memory paradigms have been carried out.

Non Associative Tasks

Spontaneous activity in the home cage – Adult male NHE/NLE rats were kept in activity cages continuously for 3 days. No differences in 24-h activity during the dark or light phase were observed, thus indicating that Naples rat lines do not differ in tonic basal level, but instead in phasic reactivity [71]. In addition NHE rats anticipated the light-on stimulus in the morning by reducing their activity 1 h earlier than NLE rats.

Thresholds for nociceptive stimulation

Nociceptive thresholds were measured with the hot-plate and the tail-flick test, to probe the possibility that NHE/NLE rats could be differentially sensitive to nociceptive stimuli. Data indicate that no differences were found with these two tests.

Animex Box: in a standard box of the Animex type, under a low illumination level, NHE/NLE and NRB rats behaved similarly in photo-beam interrupted cells. In fact, a one-way analysis of variance (ANOVA) revealed no significant differences in activity among lines. Thus, Naples rat lines show normal activity level when challenged with an environment of very low complexity.

Holeboard Test: in this apparatus, described in detail elsewhere [99], NHE and NRB behaved similarly, and both showed higher scores over time of testing in comparison to NLE rats, as well as frequency of horizontal activity (HA), vertical activity (VA) and head-dips (HD).

Làt Maze: these apparatus and testing procedure [99] were used for the Genetic Selection the naples lines. The main behavioural parameters are the frequency of corner crossings (HA), of rearings (VA), the duration of rearing episodes (RD – scanning time) and the number of fecal boluses as emotionality index in Broadhurst's terms [11]. In addition two forms of rearing on hindlimbs were monitored: free rearing and leaning against the wall with one or both forepaws. These behavioural traits are thought to represent two forms of attention: fast orienting and sustained attention towards environmental stimuli (Ruocco et al. in preparation). The activity scores upon first exposure to the Làt-maze ranked NHE> NRB> NLE. All three lines showed a significant time-dependent activity decrement during the single exposure (operationally defined as short-term habituation – STH). Furthermore the activity decrement between exposures as a percent of that during the first exposure (operationally defined as long-term habituation – LTH [17, 69]) was also significant in all three lines but was more pronounced in NHE and NRB rats. The duration of rearing episodes (RD), as an index of non-selective attention (NSA)[2, 3] toward the new environment, differed across lines. In particular NHE had lower scanning times than NLE and NRB rats. In addition, rearing duration was time- and line-dependent as it increased at a lower rate in NHE and steadily increased in NLE and NRB rats. Both NHE/NLE produced higher emotionality scores than NRB rats, consistent with higher plasma corticosterone levels [32].

Radial Maze: an eight arm radial maze was used to test rats at low motivation (LM) or high motivation (HM), as previously described [99]. The rationale for this comes from the observation that ADHD children have attentional problems mainly at low levels of motivation [82]. No differences were found at low or high motivational levels among the three rat lines in terms of working memory, defined as the position of the first repetitive arm entry during non reinforced maze exploration on day 1. When all arms were baited with pieces of chocolate (days 2-13), working memory was similar across rat lines, but NHE rats showed very low or lower chocolate consumption at the low and high motivational level, respectively. When the reinforcement was restricted to a single arm (days 14-23), rats of all three lines showed improved reference memory in finding the single baited arm at the high, rather than at the low, motivational level. Similarly, chocolate consumption increased at high motivational levels in all lines, but NHE rats paid little attention to reinforcement upon visiting the single baited arm at a low motivational level. At a low motivational level, both NHE and NLE rats displayed a more stable reference memory than controls.

Tunnel Maze: the hexagonal tunnel maze described elsewhere [99], was used in the full (Dashiell's maze) or mirror configuration. On days 1-3 total activity was recorded during a 6-min exposure. Testing was run in the dark or light, relying on internal (proprioceptive and olfactory) cues, or external (visual) cues, respectively. In both cases the rat lines ranked NHE >NRB> NLE. However external cues lowered overall activity in NHE and NLE rats, due to light-induced activity inhibition. Exploration efficiency based on the number of photocells interrupted before 18-24-30-36 different ones were scored in raw, revealed that high total activity of NHE rats on days 1-3 was not associated with a higher efficiency, independent of external cues. On days 4-8 in the 6-arm and its mirror configuration (day 8), alley visits (AV) revealed a poor working memory in both NHE/ NLE vs. NRB rats. Similarly, blind alley visits (BAV) over four consecutive days indicated a poor reference memory in both NHE/ NLE rats.

Morris Water Maze: all animals learnt to escape onto the platform during the acquisition phase (days 1-5); latencies decreased over days [99]. On the last acquisition day with the hidden platform (day 5), NHE /NLE rats showed an impaired reference memory vs. NRB controls. All rats were allowed to search for the hidden platform. Both NHE and NLE rats spent more time in the opposite quadrant (SW), whereas NRB rats spent more time where the platform had been hidden before (NE).

Elevated Plus Maze: two experiments were run in NHE/NLE with NRB as controls. Our aim was to assess whether genetic differences were present in emotionality levels in the Naples lines. Testing was carried out in an elevated plus maze (experiment 1) or in the non elevated plus configuration of a radial maze (experiment 2)[28]. NHE did not differ from NRB in either experiment, and only NLE rats spent significantly longer time in the open arms. These data are consistent with a behavioural profile where the emotional dimension does not overlap with the reactivity dimension. In fact, the hyperactivity of NHE rats is not correlated with increased emotionality. In contrast the hypoactivity of NLE rats can be explained only partially by elevated emotionality.

Associative Tasks

Two-Way, Active Avoidance: The apparatus and procedure have been described elsewhere [14]. During the acquisition phase (learning), NHE and NLE rats did not significantly differ in the number of trials necessary to reach serial consecutive conditioned responses (from 1 to 4). In the retention phase, while NHE rats were heterogeneous with high inter-individual variability, NLE rats showed a significantly impaired performance, thus revealing a shift in coping strategy from avoidance to freezing.

Conditioned Taste Aversion: A two-bottle water–0.1% saccharin (test choice; CTA) paradigm was used, as described by Garcia [30], on NHE and NLE rat lines: they did not differ in this viscero-gustatory conditioning. Further, during forced extinction, NHE rats were consistent in avoiding saccharin intake that had been paired with the LiCl-induced malaise whereas NLE showed an extinction of this avoidance response.

Selective Breeding

The Naples High (NHE) and Naples Low Excitability (NLE) rat lines have been bidirectionally selected since 1976 over 122 generations from a Sprague-Dawley population [35, 99]. The selection trait has been the reactivity to spatial novelty (Lát-maze), as indexed by the frequency of corner crossings (horizontal activity: HA) and rearing on hindlimbs (vertical activity: VA). The latter includes free rearing and leaning against the wall with one or both forepaws. This selection has produced behavioural divergence with high activity scores for NHE and low scores for NLE respectively [35, 99]. As described earlier, this behavioural divergence has been reproduced in other novel situations and found to be dependent upon the complexity of the spatial novelty [99]; this is probably associated with the limbic rather than motor systems [94]. Along with selective breeding, a control stock, referred to as Naples Random Bred (NRB), has been replicated as a reference parental line. As a result, two strategies have been followed either with all three lines or with NHE and NRB as controls.

Our initial approach has been to directly relate genetics to behaviour in NHE and NLE rat lines. We found that the neurobehavioural phenotypic differences are based on strong genetic determinants [35] and epigenetic influences [29, 65, 70]. The relative weight of genetic contribution has been defined in a quantitative study based on phenotypic expression in the hybrids obtained from a classical Mendelian cross-breeding [35]. The behavioural traits considered are the same used to select the lines, i.e. total activity (HVA) in the Lát-maze and its HA and VA components. These activity parameters are considered to have cognitive and non-cognitive meaning respectively [34] [21] and have been associated with different genes in mice [87] and rats [74]. First of all, we observed the continuous distribution of the main behavioural trait in the hybrids, thus revealing the quantitative nature of the phenotype. Then, by repeating Mendelian cross-breeding with different parental gender, the sex-linkage of the trait was excluded. However, a generally higher activity level was found in females, probably due to the oestrogen level [58] [85]. The fact that females have a smaller body size than males should also be taken into consideration, as they may cover relatively longer travelling distance than males with the same HA score.

The heritability index (h^2) of a trait, evaluated by offspring/parents regression, was very high (82.4% – Fig. 1), thus confirming the strong genetic basis of the divergent behaviour. Finally an estimation of the possible heritability models was made using two different quantitative analysis approaches: the joint-scaling test according to the simplified model proposed by M. Lynch and B. Walsh [47] and a regression study between experimental and estimated values of trait expression. Both approaches confirmed a polygenic model with epistatic control for the main trait, i.e. total activity (HVA), and its HA component. In addition a simpler model was defined for the VA component.

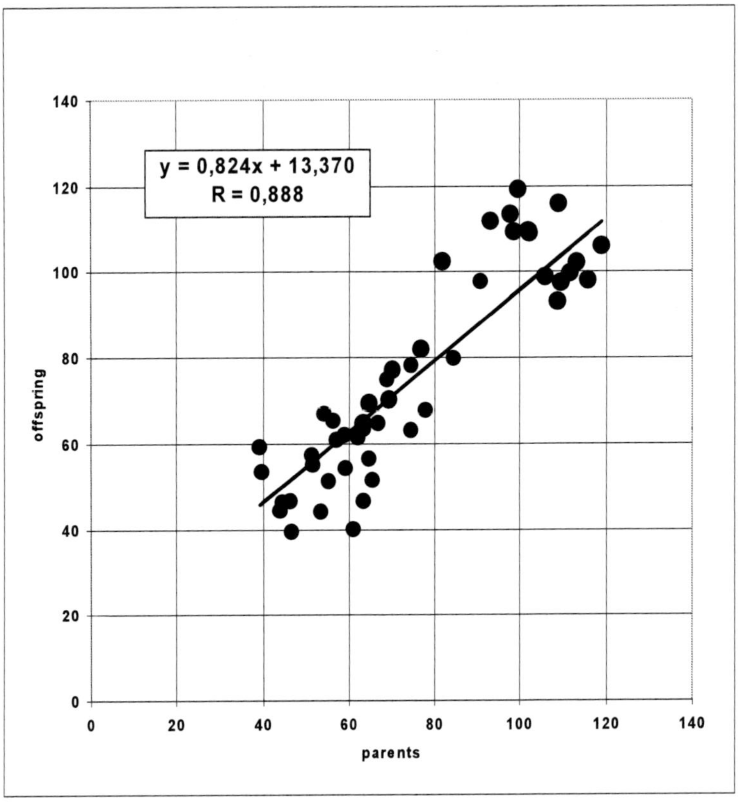

Figure 1. Offspring–parents regression. Total activity scores for offspring are plotted against those for parents over 20 generations of selection. The box shows the equation of the regression line (used to calculate the heritability index) and the regression coefficient (R). Modified from [35].

The existence of a more complex model for HA than VA would confirm differential genetic control of the two behavioural components and their different biological meaning [87] [74] [34] [21].

Differential Functional State of Da Branches in Naples Lines

1. HISTOCHEMICAL AND MOLECULAR BIOLOGY –

Histochemical and neurochemical studies on the brain of NHE rats, as reviewed in [97] [96], reveal a different functional architecture of DA brain systems, as neural substrate of behavioural differences in the Naples lines. In essence, a hypertrophic mesocortical DA system has been identified in the ventral tegmental area (VTA) based on i) the higher volume of A10 mesencephalic neurons (30%) [95], ii) the higher density of tyrosine hydroxylase (TH) positive fibres, iii) the higher expression of TH protein by western blot, and iv) the over-expression of DA-related phosphoprotein (DARP32). In addition the prefrontal cortex (PFC) shows i) a higher density of axonal varicosity, ii) a higher density of dopamine transporter (DAT), and iii) a lower density of DA D1 and D2 receptors. These findings suggest an elevated functional state of the mesocortical DA branch in NHE rats. In fact, repeated injections of the psychostimulant drug methylphenidate (MPH 3 mg/Kg for 14 days), a DAT-blocker, increase DA D1 and D2 receptors in the PFC. This may indicate the reduced release of DA with "up-regulation" of DA D1 and D2 receptors. Moreover, MPH also reduces the higher basal density of DAT binding sites in the PFC. Furthermore, in the mesencephalon this drug reduces the expression of DARP32, a multifunctional transduction protein that is controlled by DA D1 and D2 receptors and is involved in a multi-step activation system for receptor, channel and exchanger membrane proteins [53].

On the other hand, an in vivo microdialysis study of the ventral striatum in both NHE and NLE rats demonstrated that both rat lines show lower basal DA levels than the control in the nucleus accumbens core but not in the shell. In the same region a single injection of morphine sulphate (1 mg/Kg) increases DA to a higher level in NLE rats [64]. This in vivo evaluation of DA release strongly suggests that the mesolimbic DA branch does not discriminate NHE and NLE rats.

2. Morpho-Functional Analysis Of Dopamine Systems –

The DA systems were initially characterized at the nuclei of origin in the VTA and Substantia Nigra pars compacta (SN-PC) by TH ICC and CO histochemistry [72, 90] in NHE rats with NRB as controls. Morphometric analysis was carried out by PC-assisted image analysis (MCID-M2; Imaging Res. Inc. Canada), measuring neuronal size and number and intensity of staining by optical density measurements (relative optical density, ROD). The data indicated larger DA neurons in the VTA, but not in the SN-PC, in NHE rats. Moreover, in the VTA the neuropile was also more intensely stained by TH ICC [72, 90]. The ventral striatum and the medial PFC represent the main targets of the VTA, whereas the SN-PC project mainly to the dorsal striatum or Caudate Putamen. The ventral striatum is composed of the Nucleus Accumbens (divided into the pole, core and shell) and the olfactory tubercle. Analysis of the TH-immunoreactive (IR) terminals in these regions showed a slight increase in optical density in NHE rats. However, the number of Parvalbumin (PV)-IR interneurons, Calcium-Calmodulin-dependent-protein-kinase-II (CAMK II) (the main component of postsynaptic density), and AChE histochemical activity in the striatum did not differ significantly from the control. Therefore, the dorsal striatum did not show significant alterations, as expected based on the SN-PC integrity. Nor did the ventral striatum show any significant changes. This is in agreement with previous studies on basal metabolic activity [36] and NMDA-glutamate binding sites [59], which showed no change in NHE rats in this region. Therefore, further analyses of the mesocortical DA system were performed. DA-containing fibres are present in the frontal cortex, extending from the rostral pole to the retrosplenial cortex. Most of the DA fibres are within the prefrontal subareas, i.e. in the medial precentral, anterior cingulate, and prelimbic areas. The DA terminals in the rodent PFC are subdivided into anteromedial, suprarhinal and supragenual systems [8, 88]. These fibres are characterized by TH-IR (TH + intervaricose segments and irregularly spaced varicosities [88]. The number of varicosities is a useful index of DA innervation in the same region [27]. The deep layers of medial PFC primarily receive TH + DA fibres from VTA neurons. In fact, two different DA populations in the VTA project separately to the PFC or the ventral striatum. The more superficial layers and the lateral PFC receive TH + fibres, mainly of norepinephrine (NE) origin from the locus coeruleus. Therefore, a quantification of TH + varicosities in the deep medial and lateral PFC can give insight into the DA/NE innervation of this region. The number of TH + varicosities/mm^2 of deep layers of medial PFC was higher in NHE than NRB control rats [99]. Axonal varicosities in NHE also appeared to be smaller than in NRB rats. Moreover, these varicosities were mainly localized in deep layers of the medial PFC, but not in more superficial layers and the lateral PFC [99]. In agreement with these findings, the staining for DAT, a specific marker for DA terminals, was higher in NHE than NRB rats [99]. This specific alteration in the mesocortical pathway did not modify the basal metabolic activity of this region, as assessed by cytochrome oxidase histochemistry. However, previous studies showed a lower number of NMDA-glutamate binding sites in deep layers of the frontal cortex [59]. Furthermore, analysis of the perisynaptic environment revealed a lower number of perisynaptic WFA-positive chondroitinsulphates (CHS). The detection of N-acetyl galactosamine-containing binding sites in CNS was performed by histochemistry with the lectin Wisteria Floribunda agglutinin (WFA; [41, 89, 91]). In the nervous system N-acetylgalactosamine is mainly found on extracellular CHS at perisynaptic sites. The reaction was revealed by the ABC system (Vector), using diaminobenzidine (DAB)/hydrogen peroxide as substrates. NHE rats showed a marked decrease in the number of perisynaptic CHS. Cells with perisynaptic staining on their soma revealed normal amounts of CHS, as assessed by densitometry on target sites. Moreover, the amount of CHS in the region was not diminished, revealing that the CHS did not aggregate around neuronal bodies. This was consistent with the normal amount of PV-IR interneurons in the same region, these being the main cells covered by CHS in the cerebral cortex [89, 91]. It is interesting to note that WFA binding sites are complementary to TH-IR areas, and a direct negative interaction between CHS deposition and catecholamine innervation is likely to be present. In fact, the altered deposition of CHS is likely to be a local phenomenon, because in other regions, such as the red nucleus, deposition of CHS in NHE rats is not significantly different from controls.

3. Pharmacological Studies

Molecular biology studies have revealed a lower expression of DA D1 receptors in the PFC of NHE rats that is likely to be due to down-regulation [99]. To analyze the effects of pharmacological changes in DA level under different basal DA conditions, a behavioural pharmacology study was carried out using a D-1 receptor agonist and antagonist. The DA system was probed using i) low doses of a selective DA D1-receptor antagonist, SCH23390 (0 (saline), 0.01 and 0.1 mg/kg), and ii) a low dose of a specific D1 DA agonist SKF 81297 (0 and 0.1 mg/kg). All drugs were dissolved in saline. The animals were randomly distributed among the treatment and control groups, and the behavioural analysis was conducted in blind conditions. Animals were tested in the Lat maze, 30 min after injection: rats were allowed to explore the resulting corridor, and their locomotor activity (travelled distance, assessed by the number of `corner crossings'), orienting frequency (number of rearings) and scanning times (non-selective attention assessed as duration of rearing episodes) were studied for 30 min. Low doses (0.01 mg/kg) of DA antagonist SCH 23390 significantly increased locomotor activity in NHE rats (128 ± 7% of basal activity; p, 0.05), mainly in the middle part of the test, but not in NRB rats (94 ± 11% of basal activity). The orienting frequency and scanning times were not modified by this dose of D1 antagonist in either NHE rats or NRB rats. Higher doses of SCH 23390 (0.1 mg/kg) totally abolished locomotor activity and rearing episodes in both NHE and NRB rats. Low doses (0.1 mg/kg) of DA agonist SKF 81297 did not modify locomotor activity in NHE or NRB rats (72 ± 19 and 75.7 ± 12% of basal activity, respectively). In contrast, SKF 81297 reduced orienting frequency (63 ± 11% of basal state), but increased the scanning duration (130 ± 11% of basal state) in NHE rats only, mainly in the first test period. In summary, 0.1 mg/kg of D1 antagonist drastically reduced activity in both lines. However, low doses of D1 agonist/antagonist paradoxically decreased/increased, respectively, the exploratory activity in NHE rats, with a non-significant effect in NRB rats. Thus, the increased efficacy and the paradoxical effects of low doses of D1 modulators reveal an unbalance of the network asset in this animal model of ADHD.

Response of Dopamine to Drug Treatment

Dopamine (DA) is a neurotransmitter that is present in many brain control systems. Attention, reward, motor activity and hormonal secretion are directly or indirectly influenced by DA action [7, 50]. Several diseases, such as Parkinson's, are linked to diffused alterations of DA neuronal circuits, and other neuropsychiatric problems, such as Attention-Deficit Hyperactivity Disorder (ADHD)[24, 77], have been correlated with altered brain DA levels [25]. Therapy involves modification of DA brain levels by external and internal mechanisms [55, 60, 80]. Neuronal DA level is mainly regulated by a passive diffusion and an active reuptake system, i.e. the DA membrane transporter (DAT) (for a rev. see e.g. [98]). Reuptake can be modified by Methylphenidate (MPH), which acts on the specific transporter (DAT). On the other hand, brain DA is increased by administration of its precursor L-DOPA, which enters the CNS via the amino acid transporter (system L) [49], crossing the blood–brain barrier (BBB).

NHE rats show histochemical and neurochemical evidence of a different functional architecture of DA brain systems (see above).

1- Galactosilated DA (Galda), Activity and Attention

We attempted to modify this typical DA asset by administration of a galactosylated form of DA (GAL-DA) [66] that can cross the BBB [10, 20, 61] using the carrier-mediated transport (Glut-1) that is located on the membrane of endothelial cells [52, 56]. The aim of this study was to investigate the effects of brain GAL-DA entry on the hyperactivity and inattention that NHE rats typically showed vs. NRB rats. Our hypothesis was that GAL-DA could block the NHE hyperfunctioning of the mesocortical branch of the mesocorticolimbic system by mesencephalic D2-DA autoreceptors [37]. Using two extreme doses, i.e. 10 and 100 mg/kg, and two vehicles as controls, we verified the effects of DA released by GAL-DA on high and low affinity target sites.

Histochemical analyses confirmed that GAL-DA crosses the BBB and increases DA neuronal levels. In fact we found an increment of brain galactose residues by lectin histochemistry and we directly measured DA-succinate and DA-galactose in brain extracts by the capillary depletion method. In addition altered mesolimbic DA covariation was found by HPLC-EC. The histochemical analyses revealed the DA peaks in the brain three hours after treatment. The active plasma level, as shown in previous studies on drug stability, was achieved only after 90–120 min [9]. This latency is probably due to the crossing of the BBB and to enzymatic cleavage at target sites.

On the behavioural side, the higher dose of GAL-DA, i.c. 100 mg/kg, reduced hyperactivity in NHE, as demonstrated by a 25% decrement of horizontal activity in the first part of the test period in the Làt maze, and ameliorated non specific attention (NSA), increasing the rearing duration in the second part of the test period. These behavioural effects were not related to any peripheral actions of GAL-DA, as very few effects on the main physiological parameters, i.e. heart rate and blood pressure, have been reported after intravenous administration of this compound [9].

GAL-DA produced differential effects on DA level in the mesocorticolimbic system of NHE and NRB rats, i.e. the target sites. We found increased DA levels in the neostriatum and prefrontal cortex of NHE, but decreased levels in NRB rats. This increment in GAL-DA-treated NHE rats may be linked to insufficient DAT functioning induced by GAL-DA itself. Conversely, the NRB decrease could be related to the blockade of mesocorticolimbic neurons by D2 autoreceptors, which decreases DA release [31], increases the activity of the DA transporter [13, 75, 76, 101], regulates potassium channels [46, 86], and also normalizes DAT functioning.

By extracting the information content of within group variability, we also observed subtle covariations in DA level between the mesencephalon and neostriatum. In fact, a high negative covariation of DA content between the origin and the terminal fields of the mesostriatal and mesolimbic systems was found in NRB under basal conditions. Conversely in the NHE rats the covariation was positive. In both cases GAL-DA administration disrupted this association.

2. Intranasal Dopamine, Activity and Selective Attention

Based on the findings of a profound action of intranasally applied dopamine (DA) on dopamine release in the striatum, it was considered a possibility that intranasal application of DA (IN-DA) would modify indices of attention and activity in juvenile male NHE rats [62]. To this end, NHE rats received daily IN-DA (0.0, 0.075, 0.15, 0.3 mg/kg) for 15 days. On day 14, rats were tested in the Làt maze one hour after treatment, and one day later, in the radial maze. *Activity in the Làt maze*: The highest dose of DA (0.3 mg/kg) decreased horizontal (HA) and vertical (VA) activity during the first 10 min of the test. No effect was found for duration of scanning (RD), which indexes non-selective attention (NSA). *Activity in the radial maze:* No treatment effects were found for HA and VA components, or for RD. *Attention indices:* The intermediate dose of DA (0.15 mg/kg) significantly improved the position of the first repetitive arm entry in the radial maze, an index of selective spatial attention (SSA). Thus, intranasal application of DA at the highest dose reduced hyperactivity, whereas the intermediate dose improved attention in an animal model of ADHD. These results suggest the potential of employing intranasal DA for therapeutic purposes.

3. Involvement of Endocannabinoids in Activity and Attention

Several pieces of evidence suggest that endocannabinoids (EK) exert a neurotrophic effect on developing mesencephalic dopamine neurons. In addition, EK have been shown to modulate neurotransmitter release in DA, glutamate, GABA and other systems through vanilloid receptors [5].

A series of studies were carried out in prenatal, juvenile and adult NHE rats to verify the possible role of EK in activity and attention. The rationale was based on an earlier observation that AM404, an inhibitor of anandamide reuptake into terminals, reduces hyperactivity and increases NSA in the SHR model of ADHD, in comparison to WKY controls [6].

These results were confirmed in adult NHE rats, using NRB as controls [38]. We then attempted to interfere in the prenatal development of the DA neuron phenotype. To this end, pregnant NHE and NRB females received a subcutaneous injection of AM-404 (1 mg/kg) or vehicle daily from E11 until E20 [93]. Young adult male offspring were exposed to a spatial novelty (Lat maze) for 30 min and their behaviour was videotaped and analyzed. Then, morphological analysis of the brains was carried out using tyrosine hydroxylase as a marker of the dopamine systems. Prenatal AM-404 reduced activity (by about 20%) throughout the test period, and reduced scanning times in the first part only in NHE rats. In addition, image analysis revealed increased DA innervation of the dorsal striatum in AM-404-treated NHE rats. Thus, the unbalance between mesostriatal and mesocorticolimbic systems in favour of the latter appears to be corrected through mesostriatal hyperinnervation, leading eventually to reduced hyperactivity and non selective attention in this animal model of ADHD.

Excitatory Amino Acid Distribution in NHE Forebrain

L-glutamate (L-Glu) and L-aspartate (L-Asp) are the most diffuse amino acid neurotransmitters in the nervous system of invertebrates and vertebrates (for a rev. see[19]). L-glutamate mediates the cross-talk between the prefrontal cortex and striatum, which operates through AMPA and NMDA receptors. In particular, prefrontal cortex axon terminals synapse upon dendrites of medium-spiny GABA projection neurons of the dorsal and ventral striatum [12]. Axon terminals release L-glutamate, but L-aspartate and its stereoisomer D-aspartate are also found. These excitatory amino acids can play a role in synaptic transmission, neural plasticity and information processing (for a rev. see [23]). The proposed involvement of D-aspartate has multiple biological bases [63, 65, 67] . Briefly D-Asp can be converted into the L-Asp isomer by the racemase enzyme, into N-methyl D-Asp by NMDA synthetase, and can be inactivated by the D-Asp oxidase. Moreover, D-asp can interact with glutamate receptors of the AMPA subtype, whereas the methylated form of D-Asp i.e. NMDA, can bind and stimulate glutamate receptors of the NMDA subtype. In addition, NMDA receptors are modulated by Dopamine (DA) and Serotonin (5HT). With the above premises, since DA modulates EAA neurotransmission, an increased DA functional state (see above) would imply a parallel increase in EAA synthesis and release. With this in mind, we have recently addressed three questions concerning the possible involvement of EAA neurotransmission in the forebrain of NHE rats.

1.1 Are Forebrain Level Of L-Glu And D- / L-ASP Different in Prepuberal Rats of NHE and NRB Control Line?

The NHE rats were used as they have been shown to model the mesocortical variant of ADHD [82, 84]; NHE rats are characterized by altered executive functions involving the fronto-striato-pallido-thalamo-cortical pathway (see e.g. [22, 33]).

The rationale was multiple: i) Làt et al. (unpublished data) had previously shown in the early 1980s a high level of L-glutamate and γ-aminobutyric acid (GABA) in the whole brain of rats behaviourally selected for high scores in horizontal and vertical activity in a spatial novelty. This construct was defined as the "non-specific excitability" level (NEL) [43], ii) DA is known to "modulate" L-Glu transmission in the frontostriatal pathway through AMPA and NMDA receptors [51] (see Introduction), and iii) a high level of L-Glu is likely to be associated with the elevated activity of the mesocortical DA branch [97].

The results indicated a higher level of L-Glu in the forebrain of NHE rats associated with hyperactivity in two spatial contexts, and impaired selective spatial attention in the radial maze [67].

The increment in EAA level accounted for about 50% of NRB controls across the forebrain.

The nature of this increment remains to be ascertained, given the heterogeneity of glutamate pools. In fact, L-Glu is distributed in three compartments: a very large metabolic one (10 mM) of neuron-glial origin, a smaller vesicular one and an even smaller extra-synaptic one (for a rev. see [100]). Our aim was not to determine the specific weight of each compartment. However, our findings refer mainly to the metabolic pool, as it overwhelms the others with its 10 mM size. Moreover, the three pools are not independent, as the neurotransmitter L-Glu is stored in the glial compartment, is transferred to the neuron as glutamine, then is reconverted to L-Glu and packed into vesicles to be secreted into the synaptic cleft. Therefore, the higher level of L-Glu should be proportionally distributed among the three pools. Interestingly, in this study the forebrain level of L-Glu and D/L-Asp was region- and amino acid-dependent. In fact, for L-Glu the NHE-NRB divergence pertained to STR, HPC and HYP but not to PFC. In contrast, for L-Asp the divergence was restricted to PFC and HPC, whereas for D-Asp it included HYP as well. Thus the three amino acids act independently, because i) L-Glu and L-Asp may bind to different receptors [48, 57],

ii) the role of D-Asp as a neurotransmitter/neuromodulator remains controversial (see above), and iii) the three amino acids may interact with different modulators in the various neural systems e.g. in the mesocortical DA system their release is affected not only by DA and 5-HT, but also by norepinephrine (NE), for instance in the medial PFC (see e.g. [92]). Conversely NE is not involved in the target of the mesostriatal DA system, i.e. STR. Thus there appears to be heterogeneity within the three amino acids studied here, as no overlap exists.

1.2 Can Differential, Prepuberal Handling Modify L-GLU, D and L-Asp Across The Forebrain?

Recent studies indicated that daily stimulation decreased and sensory deprivation increased the forebrain level of L-Glu, D and L-Asp [65].

In particular i) in the Làt maze, no-postnatally stimulated (NO-PS) NHE rats were more active than postnatally stimulated (PS) rats, but only for HA, ii) in the radial maze NO-PS rats of both lines showed shorter rearing durations than PS rats, iii) the EAA level was higher in NHE than in NRB rats, and iv) NO-PS vs. PS treatment increased the EAA level across the forebrain in both rat lines. In contrast L-Glu decreased in the HYP of NHE NO-PS rats and L-Asp decreased in the HPC of NHE NO-PS rats. In conclusion, postnatal stimulation in prepuberal rats significantly affects forebrain EAA and behaviour in the NHE line. Thus EAA appears to be modulated by genetic determinants and environmental (epigenetic) factors.

1.3. Can Prepuberal Subcronic D-Asp Modify L-GLU, D and L-ASP Across the Forebrain?

The free form of D-Asp and its diethyl ester pro-drug exerted a differential effect on forebrain amino acids, activity and attention [63] . Subchronic treatment with D-Asp or DEE i) reduced EAA levels in the NHE and increased it in the random-bred control (NRB) rats, ii) D-Asp increased horizontal activity in NHE but DEE decreased it in NRB rats in the Làt-maze, iii) D-Asp and DEE decreased vertical activity in NHE and NRB rats respectively in the Olton maze, iv) D-Asp impaired attention only in NRB, decreasing the number of arms visited before the first repetition. Therefore, the data demonstrate the differential effects of prepuberal subchronic D-Asp and DEE, which may be related to different basal EAA levels in NHE and NRB rats. In particular, the L-Glu level was significantly affected by D-Asp treatment. All together, these findings demonstrate that D- and L-Asp can modify L-Glu and may support the hypothesis that the L-Glu level across the forebrain is plastic, as it appears to be sensitive to environmental manipulation.

Forebrain amino acids and animal models – The issue of amino acid release in the brain of animal models has already been examined in the rat. In fact variations in L-Glu and GABA have been associated in the hippocampus and amygdala of rats that are genetically susceptible to absence epilepsy [79] or kindling seizures [78] respectively.

A study on L Glu, D and L-Asp in NHE rats may be of particular interest in relation to ADHD in children. In fact, high L-Glu release during development may be associated with neurotoxicity and neurodegeneration (see e.g. [4]). Since the pioneer work by Filipek et al. [26], several FMRI studies have confirmed a degeneration-induced atrophy in the fronto-striatal system in the right hemisphere (see e.g. [44]). However, to confirm the validity of this working hypothesis, the determination of L-Glu in the vesicular pool (see above) remains to be ascertained. Interestingly, the choice of the prepuberal period in the postnatal development of the rat has been appropriate, as it corresponds in humans to the school age (6–14 years) of children affected by ADHD [45, 82, 83]. In fact, this period is very sensitive to interference by drug and no drug treatment (see e.g. [42]).

This neurogenetic approach in a rat model of ADHD confirms the involvement of amino acid neurotransmission in the forebrain associated with behavioural hyperactivity and impaired selective spatial attention. This, in turn, may lead eventually to the understanding of the basic mechanism in the etiopathogenesis, prevention and treatment of ADHD in humans.

Involvement of Nitric Oxide

Nitric oxide (NO) is involved in phenomena such as neurotransmission, neural plasticity and degeneration. Since increased NO release is associated with increased DA and EAA release, our aim was to verify whether blockade of NO synthesis could reduce or revert the hyperactivity and attention deficit of NHE rats. As a matter of fact the pioneer work of Aspide et al. [3] demonstrated that acute inhibition of NO synthesis by L- nitro-arginine-methylester (L-NAME) at 10 mg/kg ameliorated the behaviour of NHE as well as Spontaneously Hypertensive Rats (SHR). In fact, NO inhibition decreased hyperactivity and increased non-selective attention in both animal models of ADHD.

In addition, to assess whether NO inhibition was of neuronal origin, a series of experiments have been carried out using more specific NO inhibitors such as 7-Nitroindazole (7-NINA) [39]. Adult male NHE rats were given a single injection of 7-NINA (1 mg/kg – acute experiment) or repeated injections (14 days – subchronic experiment). The acute experiment involved a fast or slow release rate whereas the subchronic experiment involved a slow rate only. The results showed a significant differential effect of the drug that was dependent on the release rate: fast release yielded an increased NSA whereas both the single and repeated slow rate exerted the opposite effect. Thus, selective inhibition of n-NOS by an allosteric inhibitor that increases arginine availability without displacing the inhibitor from n-NOS, strengthens the hypothesized role of NO in NSA and possibly in ADHD.

Conclusion

The rationale for this review was to update the multidisciplinary evidence gathered on the NHE rats and to discuss this in relation to the proposed hypothesis for the MC variant of ADHD.

From the behavioural point of view, the review has confirmed that NHE rats differ from NLE/NRB rats in reactivity to spatial novelty rather than in basal activity in the home cage and that the divergence depends on the complexity of the environment. Furthermore, this divergence is not associated with novelty-induced analgesia, as is the case for NLE rats [73]. It is worth mentioning that a factor analysis of the Naples lines has shown that they differ in two dimensions, a cognitive and emotional one, with the former discriminating and explaining most of the between-line variance [15].

In addition, the Mendelian cross-breeding study has yielded putative models for the genetic control of HA and VA traits. This, in turn, may eventually lead to the isolation of genes and/or polymorphisms associated with behavioural hyperactivity and/or attention deficit.

The series of studies carried out in our laboratory has been carried out within the theoretical framework of the so-called DA hypothesis (see Introduction). Coherent with this, all studies appear to support the hypothesis of a high functional DA state for the MC DA branch. This has largely been confirmed by molecular biology studies under basal conditions and following MPH subchronic treatment. Moreover, the high functional DA state has also been demonstrated by its reduction through DA-D2 autoreceptor stimulations in the mesencephalon induced by low doses of MPH, by galactosylated DA[66], by IN-DA [62] and by AM404-induced anandamide-elevations [40]. The high functional DA state is restricted to the MC branch, as demonstrated by TH activity and dihydroxyphenyl acetic (DOPAC) level [71] as well as by in-vivo microdialysis studies showing that the basal DA tone in the nucleus accumbens of NHE rats did not differ from NRB control rats [64]. On the other hand, the involvement of the MC is also supported by behavioural studies with subchronic DAT inhibition by MPH or NET inhibition by atomoxetine (ATX). In fact, both treatments improved SSA, without reducing NSA and/or activity. While MPH and ATX are expected to reduce activity in the ML-origin, delay-aversion ADHD variant (modelled by SHR), they do not affect activity in the MC-origin, executive-function ADHD variant (modelled by NHE).

Consistent with these drug effects, long-term modifications in the expression of TH, DAT, DA-D1/D2 receptors and DARP32 have been observed in the mesencephali of NHE rats following subchronic drug treatment [54, 96].

Since DA modulates the cross-talk between prefrontal cortex and striatal medium-spiny neurons, the elevated tissue content of EAA across the NHE forebrain is additional evidence for this hypothesis.

Together, these findings are interesting from the theoretical point of view, as they may open up new strategies for the diagnosis and therapy of ADHD in humans. As a matter of fact, the elevated EAA release may be a point of attack in the chain of events leading to neurotoxicity and neurodegeneration proposed for the right fronto-striatal systems (see Introduction). Another point of attack may be the reduction of the high functional DA state. This may be achieved by reducing the firing rate of mesencephalic DA neurons, by presynaptic inhibition of DA release or by interfering in the coupling of DA release with activation of the NR1 subunit of the NMDA receptors on prefrontal cortex pyramidal neuron dendrites [57].

Acknowledgments

Supported by a MIUR 2005-2007 grant to AGS and by a Young-Investigator project, coordinated by Walter Adriani as PI, to LAR .

References

[1] American Psychiatric Association. Diagnostic and Statistical Manual of Mental Health, Fourth Edition. Washington, DC: 1994.

[2] Aspide R, Fresiello A, De Filippis G, Gironi Carnevale UA, Sadile AG. Non selective attention in a rat model of hyperactivity and attention deficit: subchronic methylphenidate and nitric oxide synthesis inhibitor treatment. *Neurosci. Biobehav. Rev.*, 2000;24: 59-71.

[3] Aspide R, Gironi Carnevale UA, Sergeant JA, Sadile AG. Non-selective attention and nitric oxide in putative animal models of Attention-Deficit Hyperactivity Disorder. *Behav. Brain Res.*, 1998;95: 123-33.

[4] Atlante A, Calissano P, Bobba A, Giannattasio S, Marra E, Passarella S. Glutamate neurotoxicity, oxidative stress and mitochondria. *FEBS Lett*, 2001;497: 1-5.

[5] Beltramo M, Piomelli D. Anandamide transport inhibition by the vanilloid agonist olvanil. *Eur. J. Pharmacol.*, 1999;364: 75-8.

[6] Beltramo M, Rodriguez de Fonseca FR, Navarro M, Calignano A, Gorriti MA, Grammatikopoulos G, Sadile AG, Giuffrida AM, Piomelli D. Reversal of dopamine D_2-receptor responses by an anandamide trasport inhibitor. *J. Neurosci.*, 2000;20: 3401-7.

[7] Bentivoglio M, Morelli M. The organization and circuits of mesencephalic dopaminergic neurons and the distribution of dopamine receptors in the brain. In: Dunnett SB, Bentivoglio M, Bjorklund A, Hokfelt T, editors. *Handbook of chemical neuroanatomy Elsevier,* 2005. p 1-107.

[8] Bjorklund A, Lindvall O. Dopamine containing systems in the CNS. In: Bjorklund A, Hokfelt T, editors. Handbook of chemical neuroanatomy, 55 Edition. Amsterdam: *Elsevier,* 1984. p 55-122.

[9] Bonina F, Puglia C, Rimoli MG, Melisi D, Boatto G, Nieddu M, Calignano A, La Rana G, De Caprariis P. Glycosyl derivatives of dopamine and L-dopa as anti-Parkinson prodrugs: synthesis, pharmacological activity and in vitro stability studies. *J. Drug Target*, 2003;11: 25-36.

[10] Bonina FP, Arenare L, Palagiano F, Saija A, Nava F, Trombetta D, De Caprariis P. Synthesis, stability, and pharmacological evaluation of nipecotic acid prodrugs. *J. Pharm. Sci.* 1999;88: 561-7.

[11] Broadhurst PL. Experiments in psychogenetics: application of biometrical genetics to the inheritance of behaviour. In: Eysenck HJ, editor. Experiments in personality. Vol. I. Psychogenetics and Psychopharmacology. London: Routledge, Regan Paul, 1960. p 1-102.

[12] Broman J, Rinvik E, Sassoe Pognetto M, Khalkhali Shandiz H, Ottersen OP. Glutamate. In: Paxinos G, editor. *The rat nervous system Elsevier,* 2004. p 1269-80.

[13] Cass WA, Gerhardt GA. Direct in vivo evidence that D2 dopamine receptors can modulate dopamine uptake. *Neurosci Lett*, 1994;176: 259-63.
[14] Cerbone A, Grimaldi A, Lamberti C, Manzi G, Sadile AG. Task and genotype-dependent associative and non associative behavioural modifications in the albino rat. *Behav. Brain Res.*, 1985;16: 196.
[15] Cerbone A, Patacchioli FR, Sadile AG. A neurogenetic and morphogenetic approach to hippocampal functions based on individual differences and neurobehavioural covariations. *Behav. Brain Res.*, 1993;55: 1-16.
[16] Cerbone A, Pellicano MP, Sadile AG. Evidence for and against the Naples high- and low-excitability rats as genetic model to study hippocampal functions. *Neurosci. Biobehav. Rev.*, 1993;17: 295-303.
[17] Cerbone A, Sadile AG. Behavioural habituation to spatial novelty: interference and noninterference studies. *Neurosci. Biobehav. Rev.*, 1994;18(4): 497-518.
[18] Chozick BS. The behavioural effects of lesions of the hippocampus: a review. *Int. J. Neurosci.*, 1983;22: 63-80.
[19] D'Aniello A. D-Aspartic acid: an endogenous amino acid with an important neuroendocrine role. *Brain Res. Rev.*, 2007;53: 215-34.
[20] Dalpiaz A, Filosa R, De Caprariis P, Conte G, Bortolotti F, Biondi C, Scatturin A, Prasad PD, Pavan B. Molecular mechanism involved in the transport of a prodrug dopamine glycosyl conjugate. *Int. J. Pharm.*, 2007;336: 133-9.
[21] Damasio AR. Descartes'error - Emotion, reason, and human brain. Putnam Publishing, 1994.
[22] Doya K. Modulators of decision making. *Nat. Neurosci.*, 2008;11: 410-6.
[23] Errico F, Rossi S, Napolitano F, Catuogno V, Topo E, Fisone G, D'Aniello A, Centonze D, Usiello A. D-aspartate prevents corticostriatal long-term depression and attenuates schizophrenia-like symptoms induced by amphetamine and MK-801. *J. Neurosci.*, 2008;28: 10404-14.
[24] Faraone SV, Sergeant J, Gillberg C, Biederman J. The worldwide prevalence of ADHD: is it an American condition? *World Psychiatry*, 2003;2: 104-13.
[25] Fernandez-Espejo E. Pathogenesis of Parkinson's disease: prospects of neuroprotective and restorative therapies. *Mol. Neurobiol.*, 2004;29: 15-30.
[26] Filipek PA, Semrud-Clikeman M, Steingard RJ, Renshaw PF, Kennedy DN, Blederman J. Volumetric MRI analysis comparing attention-deficit hyperactivity disorder and normal controls. *Neurology*, 1997;48: 589-601.
[27] Finkelstein DI, Stanic D, Parish CL, Tomas D, Dickson K, Horne MK. Axonal sprouting following lesions of the rat substantia nigra. *Neuroscience*, 2000;97: 99-112.
[28] Fresiello A. DFGaSAG. The behavioural profile of the naples high excitability and low-excitability rat lines in the elevated plus-maze. *Soc. Neurosci. Abstr.*, 1998;24, 1428.
[29] Fresiello A, Grammatikopolus G, Pignatelli M, Sadile AG. Enviromental factors during post natal period modify activity and non selective attention in the Naples high excitability rat. *Behavioural Brain Research,* 2002;130 : 111-5.
[30] Garcia J, Ervin FR. Gustatory-visceral and telereceptor-cutaneous conditioning: Adaptation in internal and external milieus. *Commun. Behav. Biol.*, 1968;1: 389-415.

[31] Garris PA, Ciolkowski EL, Pastore P, Wightman RM. Efflux of dopamine from the synaptic cleft in the nucleus accumbens of the rat brain. *J. Neurosci.*, 1994;14: 6084-93.

[32] Gentsch C, Lichtensteiner M, Feer H. Locomotor activity, defecation score and corticosterone levels during an open-field exposure: a comparison among individually and group-housed rats, and genetically selected rat lines. *Physiol. Behav.*, 1981;27: 183-6.

[33] Gerfen CR. The basal ganglia. In: Paxinos G, editor. The rat nervous system Elsevier, 2004. p 458-97.

[34] Gironi Carnevale UA, Vitullo E, Sadile AG. Post-trial NMDA receptor allosteric blockade differentially influences habituation of behavioural responses to novelty in the rat. *Behav. Brain Res.*, 1990;39(2): 187-95.

[35] Gironi Carnevale UA, Vitullo E, Varriale B, Ruocco LA, Sadile AG. A classical Mendelian cross-breeding study of the Naples high and low excitability rat lines. *Behav. Brain. Res.*, 2007;183: 130-40.

[36] Gonzalez-Lima F, Sadile AG. Network Operations Revealed by Brain Metabolic Mapping in a Genetic Model of hyperactivity and attention deficit: the Naples High and Low-Excitability Rats. *Neurosci .Biobehav. Rev.*, 2000;24: 157-60.

[37] Grace AA, Bunnney BS, Moore H, Todd CL. Dopamine-cell depolarization block as a model for the therapeutic actions of antipsychotic drugs. *Trends Neurosci.*, 1997;20: 31-7.

[38] Grammatikopolus G, Pignatelli M, Sadile AG. Endocannabinoids modulate activity and non-selective attention in two animal models of ADHD. *Soc. Neurosci .Abstr.*, 2000;26 (part.2): 1540.

[39] Grammatikopoulos G, Pignatelli M, D'Amico F, Fiorillo C, Sadile A. Selective inhibition of neuronal nitric oxide synthesis reduces hyperactivity and increases non-selective attention in the Naples high excitability rats. *Behav. Brain. Res.*, 2002;130 : 127-32.

[40] Grammatikopoulos G, Pignatelli M, Giuliano A, Ruocco LA, Scamardella M, Sadile AG. Blockade of the CB1 endocannabinoid receptor modulates activity and non-selective attention in the naples high exitabililyty rat. *Soc. Neurosci. Abstr.* part II, 2001;27: 2629.

[41] Hartig W, Brauer K, Bruckner G. Wisteria floribunda agglutinin-labelled nets surround parvalbumin-containing neurons. *Neurorep*, 1992;3: 869-72.

[42] Holmes A, le Guisquet AM, Vogel E, Millstein RA, Leman S, Belzung C. Early life genetic, epigenetic and environmental factors shaping emotionality in rodents. *Neurosci. Biobehav. Rev.*, 2005;29: 1335-46.

[43] Irmis F, Làt J, Radil-Weiss T. Individual differences in hippocampal EEG during romboencephalic sleep and arousal. *Physiol. Behav.*, 1971;7: 117-9.

[44] Kelly AM, Margulies DS, Castellanos FX. Recent advances in structural and functional brain imaging studies of attention-deficit/hyperactivity disorder. *Curr. Psychiatry Rep.*, 2007;9: 401-7.

[45] Kieling C, Goncalves RR, Tannock R, Castellanos FX. Neurobiology of attention deficit hyperactivity disorder. *Child Adolesc. Psychiatr Clin. N. Am.*, 2008;17: 285-307, viii.

[46] Lacey MG, Mercuri NB, North RA. On the potassium conductance increase activated by GABAB and dopamine D2 receptors in rat substantia nigra neurones. *J. Physiol.*, 1988;401: 437-53.

[47] Lynch M, Walsh B. Genetics and analysis of quantitative traits. Sinauer Associates Inc. ed. Sunderland (USA): Sinauer Associates Inc., 1998.

[48] Mayer ML, Armstrong N. Structure and function of glutamate receptor ion channels. *Annu. Rev. Physiol.*, 2004;66: 161-81.

[49] Mercuri NB, Bernardi G. The 'magic' of L-dopa: why is it the gold standard Parkinson's disease therapy? *Trends Pharmacol. Sci.*, 2005;26: 341-4.

[50] Missale C, Nash SR, Robinson SW, Jaber M, Caron MG. Dopamine receptors: from structure to function. *Physiol. Rev.*, 1998;78: 189-225.

[51] Moyer JT, Wolf JA, Finkel LH. Effects of dopaminergic modulation on the integrative properties of the ventral striatal medium spiny neuron. *J. Neurophysiol.*, 2007;98: 3731-48.

[52] Mueckler M. Facilitative glucose transporters. *Eur. J. Biochem.*, 1994;219: 713-25.

[53] Nairn AC, Svenningsson P, Nishi A, Fisone G, Girault JA, Greengard P. The role of DARPP-32 in the actions of drugs of abuse. *Neuropharmacology*, 2004;47 Suppl 1: 14-23.

[54] Oades RD, Sadile AG, Sagvolden T, Viggiano D, Zuddas A, Devoto P, Aase H, Johansen EB, Ruocco LA, Russell VA. The control of responsiveness in ADHD by catecholamines: evidence for dopaminergic, noradrenergic and interactive roles. *Dev. Sci.*, 2005;8: 122-31.

[55] Olanow CW, Agid Y, Mizuno Y, Albanese A, Bonuccelli U, Damier P, De Yebenes J, Gershanik O, Guttman M, Grandas F, Hallett M, Hornykiewicz O, Jenner P, Katzenschlager R, Langston WJ, LeWitt P, Melamed E, Mena MA, Michel PP, Mytilineou C, Obeso JA, Poewe W, Quinn N, Raisman-Vozari R, Rajput AH, Rascol O, Sampaio C, Stocchi F. Levodopa in the treatment of Parkinson's disease: current controversies. *Mov. Disord*,. 2004;19: 997-1005.

[56] Oldendorf WH. Brain uptake of radiolabeled amino acids, amines, and hexoses after arterial injection. *Am. J. Physiol.*, 1971;221: 1629-39.

[57] Paoletti P, Neyton J. NMDA receptor subunits: function and pharmacology. *Curr. Opin. Pharmacol.*, 2007;7: 39-47.

[58] Papalexi E, Antoniou K, Kitraki E. Estrogens influence behavioural responses in a kainic acid model of neurotoxicity. *Horm Behav.,* 2005;48: 291-302.

[59] Pellicano MP, Sadile AG. An autoradiographic study of 3H-L-glutamate binding sites in the brain of the Naples High and Low-Excitability rats. *Neurosci. Lett.*, 1992;Suppl.43: S86.

[60] Pisani A, Centonze D, Bernardi G, Calabresi P. Striatal synaptic plasticity: implications for motor learning and Parkinson's disease. *Mov. Disord.,* 2005;20: 395-402.

[61] Polt R, Porreca F, Szabo LZ, Bilsky EJ, Davis P, Abbruscato TJ, Davis TP, Harvath R, Yamamura HI, Hruby VJ. Glycopeptide enkephalin analogues produce analgesia in

mice: evidence for penetration of the blood-brain barrier. *Proc. Natl. Acad. Sci. U S A,* 1994;91: 7114-8.

[62] Ruocco L.A., de Souza Silva M.A., Topic B, Mattern C, Huston JP, Sadile A.G. Intranasal Application of Dopamine Reduces Activity and Improves Attention in Naples High Excitability Rats that Feature the Mesocortical Variant of ADHD. *European Neuropsycopharmacology,* 2009;in press.

[63] Ruocco L.A., Di Pizzo A., Gironi Carnevale U.A., Murolo M., Sadile A.G., Arra C., Topo E., D'Aniello A., Curcio A., Melisi D., Rimoli M.G. Excitatory amino acids in the forebrain of the naples high-excitability rats: neurochemical and behavioural effects of subchronic d-aspartate and its diethyl ester prodrug. *Behav. Brain Res.,* 2008;In press.

[64] Ruocco L.A., Gironi Carnevale U.A., Sadile A., Valentini V., Di Chiara G. Differential Opioid Mediated DA Release in the N. Accumbens Core and Shell of the Naples Rat Lines: a Behavioural and Microdialysis Study. Monitoring Molecules In Neuroscience - 11th International Conference on In Vivo Methods - May 19-22 2006, 2006.

[65] Ruocco L.A., Gironi Carnevale U.A., Sica A., Arra C., Topo E., Di Maio A., Di Giovanni M., D' Aniello A., Sadile A.G. Differential prepuberal handling modifies behaviour and excitatory amino acids in the forebrain of the naples high-excitability rats. *Behav Brain. Res*, 2008;in press.

[66] Ruocco L.A., Viggiano D, Viggiano A, Abignente E., Rimoli M.G., Melisi D, Curcio A., Nieddu M, Boatto G, Carboni E, Gironi Carnevale U.A., Sadile A.G. Galactosilated dopamine enters into the brain, blocks mesocorticolimbic system and modulates activity and scanning time in Naples High Excitability Rats. *Neuroscience*, 2008;152: 234-44.

[67] Ruocco LA, Gironi Carnevale UA, Sica A, Arra C, Topo E, Di MA, D'Aniello A, Sadile AG. Elevated forebrain excitatory l-glutamate, l-aspartate and d-aspartate in the Naples high-excitability rats. *Behav. Brain Res.*, 2008.

[68] Sadile AG. What can genetic models tell us about behavioural plasticity? *Rev. Neurosci.*, 1993;4: 287-303.

[69] Sadile AG. Long-term habituation of theta-related activity components of albino rats in the Làt-maze. In: Sanberg PR, Ossenkopp KP, Kavaliers M, editors. Motor activity and movement disorders: measurement and analysis. New York: Humana Press, 1996. p 1-54.

[70] Sadile AG, Cerbone A, Grimaldi A, Manzi G, Cioffi LA. Postnatal brain growth and behaviour: evaluation of environmental factors. *Bibl. Nutr. Diet.*, 1986;38: 194-205.

[71] Sadile AG, Lamberti C, Siegfried B, Welzl H. Circadian activity, nociceptive thresholds, nigrostriatal and mesolimbic dopaminergic activity in the Naples High- and Low-Excitability rat lines. *Behav. Brain Res.*, 1993;55: 17-27.

[72] Sadile AG, Viggiano D. Incresed number of varicosities of mesocorticolimbic terminals in the frontal cortex in the naples high exitability rats. *Soc. Neurosci. Abstr.*, 2001;27: 2628.

[73] Sadile, A. G., Welzl, H., and Siegfried, B. Novelty-induced analgesia in the Naples High- and Naples Low-Excitable rat lines [abstract]. In: Anonymous. 1989. p 850.

[74] Sanders DC. The Bethlem lines: genetic selection for high and low rearing activity in rats. *Behav. Genet,* 1981;11: 491-503.

[75] Schmitz Y, Lee CJ, Schmauss C, Gonon F, Sulzer D. Amphetamine distorts stimulation-dependent dopamine overflow: effects on D2 autoreceptors, transporters, and synaptic vesicle stores. *J. Neurosci.*, 2001;21: 5916-24.

[76] Schmitz Y, Schmauss C, Sulzer D. Altered dopamine release and uptake kinetics in mice lacking D2 receptors. *J. Neurosci.*, 2002;22: 8002-9.

[77] Sergeant JA, Geurts H, Huijbregts S, Scheres A, Oosterlaan J. The top and the bottom of ADHD: a neuropsychological perspective. *Neurosci. Biobehav. Rev.*, 2003;27: 583-92.

[78] Shin RS, Anisman H, Merali Z, McIntyre DC. Changes in extracellular levels of amygdala amino acids in genetically fast and slow kindling rat strains. *Brain Res.*, 2002;946: 31-42.

[79] Sirvanci S, Meshul CK, Onat F, San T. Immunocytochemical analysis of glutamate and GABA in hippocampus of genetic absence epilepsy rats (GAERS). Brain Res, 2003;988: 180-8.

[80] Solanto MV. Neuropsychopharmacological mechanisms of stimulant drug action in attention-deficit hypractivity disorder:a review and integration. *Behavioural Brain Research*, 1998;94: 127-52.

[81] Solanto MV. Dopamine dysfunction in AD/HD: integrating clinical and basic neuroscience research. *Behav. Brain Res.*, 2002;130: 65-71.

[82] Sonuga-Barke EJ, Sergeant JA, Nigg J, Willcutt E. Executive dysfunction and delay aversion in attention deficit hyperactivity disorder: nosologic and diagnostic implications. *Child Adolesc. Psychiatr. Clin. N. Am.*, 2008;17: 367-84, ix.

[83] Spencer TJ, Biederman J, Mick E. Attention-deficit/hyperactivity disorder: diagnosis, lifespan, comorbidities, and neurobiology. *J. Pediatr. Psychol.*, 2007;32: 631-42.

[84] Stevenson J, Asherson P, Hay D, Levy F, Swanson J, Thapar A, Willcutt E. Characterizing the ADHD phenotype for genetic studies. *Dev. Sci.*, 2005;8: 115-21.

[85] Tropp J, Figueiredo CM, Markus EJ. Stability of hippocampal place cell activity across the rat estrous cycle. *Hippocampus*, 2005;15: 154-65.

[86] Uchimura N, Higashi H, Nishi S. Hyperpolarizing and depolarizing actions of dopamine via D-1 and D-2 receptors on nucleus accumbens neurons. *Brain. Res.*, 1986;375: 368-72.

[87] Van Abeelen JHF. Genetics of rearing behaviour in mice. *Behav. Genet*, 1970;1: 71-6.

[88] Van Eden CG, Hoorneman EM, Buijs RM, Matthijssen MA, Geffard M, Uylings HB. Immunocytochemical localization of dopamine in the prefrontal cortex of the rat at the light and electron microscopical level. *Neuroscience*, 1987;22: 849-62.

[89] Viggiano D. The two faces of perineuronal nets. *Neurorep.*, 2000;11: 1-4.

[90] Viggiano D, Grammatikopoulos G, Sadile AG. A morphometric evidence for a hyperfunctioning mesolimbic system in an animal model of ADHD. *Behav. Brain. Res.*, 2002;130: 181-9.

[91] Viggiano D, Ibrahim M, Celio MR. Relationship between glia and the perineuronal nets of extracellular matrix in the rat cerebral cortex: importance for volume trasmission in the brain. *Prog. Brain Res.*, 2000;125: 193-7.

[92] Viggiano D, Ruocco LA, Arcieri S, Sadile AG. Involvement of norepinephrine in the control of activity and attentive processes in animal models of Attention Deficit Hyperactivity Disorder. *Neural. Plast*, 2004;11: this issue.

[93] Viggiano D, Ruocco LA, Pignatelli M, Grammatikopoulos G, Sadile AG. Prenatal elevation of endocannabinois corrects the unbalance between dopamine systems and reduces activity in the Naples High Excitability rats. *Neurosci. Biobehav. Rev.*, 2003;27: 129-39.

[94] Viggiano D, Ruocco LA, Sadile AG. Dopamine phenotype and behaviour in animal models: in relation to attention deficit hyperactivity disorder. *Neurosci. Biobehav. Rev.*, 2003;27: 623-37.

[95] Viggiano D, Sadile AG. Hypertrophic A10 dopamine neurons in a rat model of Attention-Deficit Hyperactivity Disorder (ADHD). *Neurorep.*, 2000;11: 3677-80.

[96] Viggiano D, Vallone D, Ruocco L.A., Carboni E, Gironi Carnevale U.A., Sadile A.G. Naples High Excitability and Spontaneously Hypertensive model different variants of Attention-Deficit Hyperactivity Disorder. *Soc. Neurosci. Abstr.*, 2007.

[97] Viggiano D, Vallone D, Ruocco LA, Sadile AG. Behavioural, pharmacological, morpho-functional molecular studies reveal a hyperfunctioning mesocortical dopamine system in an animal model of attention deficit and hyperactivity disorder. *Neurosci. Biobehav. Rev.*, 2003;27: 683-9.

[98] Viggiano D, Vallone D, Sadile AG. Dysfunctions in the dopamine systems and ADHD: evidences from animals and modeling. *Neural .Plast*, 2004;11: 93-116.

[99] Viggiano D, Vallone D, Welzl H, Sadile AG. The Naples high-and low excitability rats: selective breeding, behavioural profile, morphometry and molecular biology of the mesocortical dopamine system. *Behav. Genet,* 2002;32: 315-33.

[100] Waagepetersen HS, Sonnewald U, Schousboe A. Glutamine, glutamate and GABA: metabolic aspects. Handbook of Neurochemistry and Molecular Neurobiology. Amino Acid and Peptides in the Nervous System., Abel Lajtha (ed). Edition 2007. p 1-22.

[101] Wu Q, Reith ME, Walker QD, Kuhn CM, Carroll FI, Garris PA. Concurrent autoreceptor-mediated control of dopamine release and uptake during neurotransmission: an in vivo voltammetric study. *J. Neurosci,*. 2002;22: 6272-81.

In: Attention Deficit Hyperactivity Disorder (ADHD)
Editors: Stuart M. Gordon and Aileen E. Mitchell
ISBN 978-1-60741-581-7

Chapter 4

Major Candidate Gene Study on Eastern Indian Indo-Caucasoid Attention Deficit Hyperactivity Disorder Probands

K Mukhopadhyay*[*], *N Bhaduri*[†], *M Das, K Sarkar and S Sinha
Manovikas Biomedical Research and Diagnostic Centre,
Manovikas Kendra Rehabilitation and Research Institute for the Handicapped

Abstract

Attention deficit hyperactivity disorder (ADHD) is one of the most common childhood onset neurobehavioral disorders characterized by a combination of developmentally inappropriate attention, hyperactivity, and impulsivity. A strong genetic basis for ADHD has been documented by family, twin, and adoption studies. Dopamine (DA), a neurotransmitter, has been implicated to play an important role in ADHD since the most frequently prescribed drugs for ADHD are targeted at the dopaminergic system. For the same reason, dopaminergic system genes have long been considered as candidates for study. Two most widely explored dopaminergic genes are the DA transporter (*DAT1*) and DA receptor (*DRD4*) and it is hypothesized that specific alleles of these genes may alter DA transmission. For example, the 10-repeat allele of the *DAT1* gene is believed to be associated with faster re-uptake of DA while the 7-repeat allele of *DRD4* gene was found to generate a post-synaptic receptor with reduced binding affinity for DA. However, association studies between an allele and the disorder have yielded conflicting reports in different ethnic groups. Moreover, some of the ADHD patients failed to respond to the drugs targeted at the dopaminergic system and therefore others, like norepinephric, serotonergic systems etc., known to control the cognitive functions were also studied for association with the disorder. In the present investigation, we have looked into five candidate genes (*DAT1*, *DRD4*, *DBH*, *MAOA*, *SNAP25*) in nuclear

[*] 482, Madudah, Plot-I-24, Sector-J, EM Bypass, Kolkata- 700 107., India. Ph. 033-4001-9179; Fax:033-2442-8275.
[†] Present address: Research Associate, Crystallography and Molecular Biology Division, Saha Institute of Nuclear Physics, 1/AF Bidhannagar, Kolkata 700064, India. Ph. 033-2343-5979.

families with ADHD probands belonging to the Indo-Caucasoid ethnicity. Genomic DNA isolated from leukocytes / buccal cells, donated by volunteers giving informed written consent, was used to study genetic polymorphisms. Data obtained were analyzed for family-based as well as population-based association tests to determine the risk of ADHD in this population. Analysis of five candidate genes revealed transmission of specific haplotypes to Indian ADHD cases from the parents, an information which could be useful while prescribing remedial medication to an ADHD proband.

Introduction

The concept of deficiency in sustained attention as a clinical entity without noted physical impairments [1] first gave rise to the identification of Attention deficit hyperactivity disorder (ADHD), one of the most common childhood onset neurobehavioral disorders. Throughout the world, a large number of school-going children and adolescents with attention problem are referred to pediatricians, neurologists and psychologists [2]. The disorder is diagnosed more often in boys as compared to girls, with a ratio of 3-4:1 [2,3] and a prevalence of 4-12% [4,5]. Although hyperactivity symptoms tend to diminish with age, it persists till adulthood in 30-50% cases [6,7] and long term follow up indicate that about 40% may develop personality disorder, substance abuse and/or criminality during adulthood [8-10].

On the basis of the presenting symptom thresholds three subtypes of ADHD have been described in the most widely accepted diagnostic system, Diagnostic and Statistical Manual for Mental Disorders –IV [2]: predominantly inattentive (I), predominantly hyperactive-impulsive (HI) and combined (C). However, other psychiatric disorders are also detected in ADHD patients [2] and review of literature showed oppositional defiant disorder (33%), conduct disorder (25%), anxiety disorders (25%), depressive disorders (20%) and learning disabilities (22%) as common co-morbid conditions [4,11]. Increased risk for cigarette smoking and substance abuse was detected in juveniles with ADHD and risk for early onset of abuse was found in those with bipolar or conduct disorder [12].

In India, only few systematic studies were carried out on ADHD [13-17]. The first organized study, in north Indian subjects, revealed an occurrence rate of 8.1% with a M/F ratio of 5:1 and mean IQ of 85 (range of 72-109); combined subtype was reported to be the most impaired group [18]. However, among eastern Indian pediatric outpatients, prevalence was reported to be higher (15.5%) with inattentive subtype being predominant (7.1%) [19]. On the contrary, amongst psychiatric clinic referrals belonging to the same ethnic group, the combined subtype (69%) was found to be more prevalent as compared to the inattentive (11%) and hyperactive-impulsive groups (20%) [Unpublished data, K. Mukhopadhyay].

Although laboratory measures are usually not very helpful in diagnosing ADHD subjects, recent observations proved that molecular genetic testing and functional magnetic resonance imaging (fMRI) may aid in the diagnosis. Significantly smaller area in the inferior portions of dorsal prefrontal cortices and anterior temporal cortices of the brain was noticed bilaterally by MRI and this reduction in size of specific brain regions was emphasized as a characteristic feature unique for ADHD [20]. In addition, a prominent increase in the grey matter has been recorded in large portions of the posterior temporal and inferior parietal cortices bilaterally.

An early non-progressive 'lesion' with characteristically smaller total brain volume (4%) and striking decrease in the posterior inferior cerebellar vernal volume (15%), which controls selected dopamine (DA) circuits and did not show any change with aging, was also reported [21]. Parts of the brain, such as substantia nigra and striatum, that revealed changes are regions rich in dopaminergic innervations [22,23].

Therefore, while studying the pathophysiology of ADHD, catecholamine deregulation received prime importance [24,25]. Dysfunction of the dopaminergic system seems to play a major role while norepinephrine (NE) possibly has an indirect effect; this stems from the fact that pharmacological agents that act primarily on the dopaminergic systems appear more effective in treating ADHD [26] whereas medicines targeting the norepinephric system provide relief to only a subset of ADHD patients. Additionally, interface of the cholinergic and catecholaminergic-dopaminergic systems also seems fascinating since ADHD patients are prone to nicotine abuse [27], a compound that stimulates dopaminergic neurotransmission [28]. ADHD being a heterogeneous disorder with multiple behavioral dimensions, it is often hypothesized that a relative balance between different neurotransmitter systems actually control the symptoms manifested in an individual. Role of serotonergic neurotransmission in controlling the behavior is also well studied and a role for 5-HT in ADHD has been hypothesized long back [29].

Strong genetic component in association with ADHD has been proposed since family, twin and adoption studies showed a mean heritability estimate of 76% [30]. Although studies on various ethnic groups worldwide have revealed conflicting results, till date, candidate gene search for ADHD has been focused on the DA receptor D4 (*DRD4*) [31-36], DA receptor D5 (*DRD5*) [37,38], DA transporter (*DAT1*) [39,40], DA metabolizing enzymes such as dopamine beta hydroxylase (*DBH*) [37,41,42], monoamine oxidase (*MAO*) [43-45] and catechol-O-methyl transferase (*COMT*) [46].

In the present investigation, we are summarizing our observations on the eastern Indian Indo-Caucasoid ADHD probands. Both familial transmission patterns as well as population-based analyses of polymorphisms in five candidate genes, namely the *DRD4*, *DAT1*, *DBH*, *MAOA* and *SNAP25*, have been carried out to find out the risk of association with ADHD in this population.

DRD4 receptor is widely distributed in the limbic system, frontal cortex, and other areas of the brain and is known to modulate post-synaptic higher brain functions like affection and personality [47]. With a large number of expressed polymorphisms distributed in its four exons, it has been the primary suspect for ADHD for long [48-53].

The DA transporter, DAT directs re-uptake of DA from the synapse back into the pre-synaptic neuron. The gene encoding the transporter *DAT1*, mapped at chromosome 5p15.3 [39], has also been studied worldwide for its association with ADHD as this is the main target of methylphenidate, the most commonly prescribed medicine for ADHD [54].

Since higher cortical functions including attention, alertness, vigilance and executive functions are under the control of norepinephric system, NE also drew attention while studying genetics of ADHD. Conversion of DA to NE is mediated by the enzyme dopamine β-hydroxylase (DβH) which is readily detectable in the plasma and cerebrospinal fluid [55,56]. The structural gene encoding DβH (*DBH*) is inherited in a autosomal co-dominant manner and is a major locus influencing plasma DβH activity [57,58]. Molecular genetic studies on different ethnic groups have indicated that *DBH* has a possible role in the etiology of ADHD [37,41,42].

Monoamine oxidase (MAO), which catalyzes metabolism of catecholamines, exists in two principal forms, MAOA and MAOB. These enzymes are expected to be directly involved with metabolism of 5-HT, NE and DA. Efficacy of MAOA inhibitors in the treatment of depression of neurobehavioral patients including ADHD gives a hint towards involvement of MAOA in the etiology [43]

It has been speculated that in addition to inefficient receptor-binding and reuptake, abnormal DA availability could be mediated through disorganized release and lead to the analysis of Synaptosomal-Associated Protein 25 (SNAP-25) which is a neuron-specific protein controlling exocytotic neurotransmitter release. Eight genetic polymorphisms have been investigated by different investigators which yielded conflicting results. However, a single nucleotide polymorphism (SNP) at the 3′ end of *SNAP25* (T1065G) showed significant evidence for association with ADHD [59].

Materials and Methods

Subjects

Ninety-eight ADHD probands, 84 complete parent-offspring trios and 14 duos (one parent absent), were selected from the out-patient department of Manovikas Kendra Rehabilitation and Research Institute for the Handicapped, Kolkata. Families were interviewed by mental health professionals (child psychiatrist and clinical psychologist) using a behavioral questionnaire modeled after DSM-IV-TR [2]. Psychological evaluation was carried out by a clinical psychologist through – The Conners' Parents and Teachers Rating Scale [60] for inattention-hyperactivity level and Wechsler Intelligence Scale for children >5 yrs [61] and Developmental Screening Test [62] for children <5 yrs for IQ status. Subjects suffering from any other neuropsychiatric disorders, pervasive developmental disorder, mental retardation (IQ<70) including Down syndrome and Fragile-X syndrome were excluded from the study.

Control individuals evaluated by the same psychometric procedure were included for population based analysis. Informed written consent was obtained from all the individuals /parents of ADHD children for their participation in the study.

ADHD cases and controls belonged to the Indo-Caucasoid ethnic category. The mean age of ADHD probands was 7.5 years (± 2.9 SD), with ~ 10:1 male to female sex ratio. The mean age of controls was 35 years (± 8.2 SD) with ~ 1:2 male to female ratio. Amongst the ADHD cases, 11 probands belonged to the Inattentive subtype, 19 probands belonged to Hyperactive/Impulsive subtype; the rest of the 68 probands belonged to combined subtype of ADHD. The most common comorbid conditions were learning and conduct disorder; 33% suffered from some form of specific learning disorder, while 10% suffered from conduct disorder. Rarely, obsessive compulsive disorder, tic disorder, communication and mood disorder were also observed (<0.01%)

Fifteen polymorphic alleles in five different genes, *DAT1*, *DRD4*, *DBH*, *MAOA*, and *SNAP25* were analyzed (Table 1). Throughout the remaining sections, the polymorphisms are denoted by their rs numbers (where present) available from the SNP database (dbSNP: http://www.ncbi.nlm.nih.gov/SNP/). Primer sequences, details regarding amplification protocols and restriction fragment length polymorphism (RFLP) analyses will be available on request.

Genotyping

Table 1

Gene	Polymorphism	rs number
DRD4	-521 C→T	rs1800955
	-1200 120bp duplication	rs4646984
	Exon 1 12bp duplication	rs4646983
	DRD4 Exon 3 VNTR	--
DAT1	3'UTR VNTR	--
	Intron 8 VNTR	--
DBH	-1021C→T	rs1611115
	Exon 2 G→A	rs1108580
	Intron 5 A→G	rs2519152
MAOA	Promoter VNTR	--
	Exon 8 T→G	rs6323
SNAP25	Intron 7 A→G	rs362988
	3′ UTR T→G	rs3746544
	3′ UTR T→C	rs1051312
	3′ UTR C→T	rs8636

Peripheral blood was collected from ADHD probands, their parents, and control individuals. Genomic DNA was prepared from leukocytes using the high-salt precipitation protocol [63]. Wild-type allele of the SNPs has been designated A1 and the derived allele as A2.

Statistical Analyses

Population-based analysis was carried out to compare allelic association between the case and control groups using the program COCAPHASE, which is part of a suite of programs UNPHASED [64]. Haplotype comparisons were also done with the same software. Family-based association studies were performed using Transmission Disequilibrium Test (TDT) [65] to ascertain association between disease and transmission of genetic polymorphisms; the program TDTPHASE, which is also a part of UNPHASED, was utilized to perform the test. Transmission pattern of haplotypes formed by the polymorphisms was also acquired using TDTPHASE.

Pair-wise linkage disequilibrium (LD) between the studied polymorphisms was investigated for ADHD cases, their parents and control individuals by studying the D' and r2 values obtained using HAPLOVIEW program (version 3.2)[66]. Genetic Power Calculator (Available at: http://pngu.mgh.harvard.edu/~purcell/gpc/) was used to evaluate the power of the association tests at 5% significance level, using 'Additive' model for assessing genotype relative risk for the 'high risk' allele [67].

Results

DRD4

Association Studies

For rs1800955, both case-control and family-based analyses showed no significant bias in either presence or transmission of an allele (Tables 2A and 2B). The single repeat allele of rs4646984 showed a trend towards over-representation in ADHD cases, deviation reaching near statistical significance (P=0.06). At 5% significance level, the power for this association test was 48%. Frequency of single repeat allele of rs4646983 was also higher in cases, though not statistically significant. TDT for both the repeat polymorphisms failed to show any preferential transmission (Tables 2A and 2B).

Table 2A. Case-Control analysis of *DRD4* allele frequencies

Polymorphism	Case		Control		χ^2	P-value
	*Allele (N)**	*Frequency*	*Allele (N)**	*Frequency*		

Polymorphism	Case		Control		χ^2	P-value
	*Allele (N)**	*Frequency*	*Allele (N)**	*Frequency*		
rs1800955	T (110)	0.60	T (100)	0.52	2.9	0.09
	C (74)	0.40	C (92)	0.48		
rs4646984	1 repeat (65)	0.34	1 repeat (59)	0.25	3.6	0.06
	2 repeats (127)	0.66	2 repeats (173)	0.75		
rs4646983	1 repeat (24)	0.13	1 repeat (19)	0.08	2.0	0.16
	2 repeats (168)	0.87	2 repeats (209)	0.92		
Exon 3 VNTR	2R (15)	0.08	2R (17)	0.09	0.3	0.56
	3R (1)	0.005	3R (0)	0	1.4	0.24
	4R (165)	0.85	4R (165)	0.86	0.3	0.59
	5R (0)	0	5R (1)	0.005	1.4	0.24
	6R (10)	0.05	6R (4)	0.02	4.0	0.04
	7R (4)	0.02	7R (4)	0.02	0	1

*N = No. of alleles.

Table 2B. Family-based TDT of DRD4 polymorphisms

Polymorphism	Transmission	Allele	Transmitted	Not-transmitted	χ^2	P-value
rs1800955	Overall	T	32	29	0.15	0.7
		C	29	32		

Table 2B. (Continued)

	Paternal	T	19	13	1.1	0.29
		C	13	19		
	Maternal	T	13	16	0.3	0.58
		C	16	13		
rs4646984	Overall	1R	30	25	0.5	0.50
		2R	25	30		
	Paternal	1R	18	11	1.7	0.19
		2R	11	18		
	Maternal	1R	12	14	0.2	0.69
		2R	14	12		
rs4646983	Overall	1R	17	21	0.4	0.51
		2R	21	17		
	Paternal	1R	9	11	0.2	0.65
		2R	11	9		
	Maternal	1R	8	10	0.2	0.64
		2R	10	8		
Exon 3 VNTR	Overall	2R	10	11	0.0 5	0.83
		3R	1	0	1.4	0.24
		4R	13	21	1.9	0.17
		5R	0	1	1.4	0.24
		6R	9	4	2.0	0.16
		7R	4	0	5.6	0.02
	Paternal	2R	3	5	0.5	0.48
		4R	6	10	1.0	0.32

Polymorphism	Transmission	Allele	Transmitted	Not-transmitted	χ^2	P-value
		6R	5	2	1.3	0.25
		7R	3	0	4.2	0.04
		2R	7	6	0.08	0.78
		3R	1	0	1.4	0.24
	Maternal	4R	7	11	0.9	0.34
		5R	0	1	1.4	0.24
		6R	4	2	0.7	0.41
		7R	1	0	1.4	0.24

Sequence analysis of *DRD4* exon 3 variable number of tandem repeats (VNTR) helped in identifying the following variants in the present study groups: 2R-379bp, 3R-427bp, 4R-475bp, 5R-523bp, 6R-571bp and 7R-619bp. Frequency of the '6R' allele was significantly higher in cases as compared to controls (P=0.04) (Tables 2A and 2B). The '4R' allele was most common variant (86.46%) in the population. Family-based study revealed statistically significant preferential transmission of the 7R allele from parents to ADHD probands (*P*=0.02), which was primarily of paternal origin (P=0.04).

Linkage Disequilibrium and Haplotype Analyses

The repeat polymorphisms were found to be in strong LD in ADHD cases and control group, but only a moderate strength was observed in parents of ADHD probands (Table 3). A haplotype comprising of 'T' of rs1800955, single repeat allele of rs4646984, two-repeat allele of rs4646983 and the common four repeat variant of the VNTR was significantly overrepresented in ADHD cases (Table 4), though the number of observations for this haplotype was only 2. On the other hand, none of the haplotypes formed from the four *DRD4* polymorphisms were transmitted significantly to the probands.

DATI

Association Studies

Five different alleles were observed in the *DAT1* 3′-untranslated region (UTR) VNTR with repeat units varying between 6 and 11 (8R absent). Sizes of repeat were: 6R-324bp, 7R-364bp, 9R-444bp, 10R-484bp and 11R-524bp. Case-control analysis (Table 5A) revealed significantly lower frequency of the 10R allele in ADHD cases as compared to controls (P=0.01). On the other hand, frequency of the 9R allele was higher in cases than in controls but the difference was statistically not significant. Family-based association analysis (Table 5B) revealed significant (P=0.04) preferential transmission of the 9R allele to ADHD cases. Conversely, the 10R allele was preferentially under transmitted.

In case of intron 8 VNTR, five alleles were detected in our population; 4R-380bp, 5R-410bp, 6R-440bp, 9R-530bp, 10R-560bp, 11R-590bp. Case-control analysis (Table 5A) revealed significantly higher frequency of the 5R allele in cases as compared to controls (P=0.004) while the controls had significantly higher percentage of the 6R allele than in cases (P=0.001). However, family-based analysis TDT (Table 5B) revealed no significant bias in transmission of any of the alleles.

Table 3. Pair-wise linkage disequilibrium analysis of *DRD4* polymorphisms

Polymorphism pairs	Parameters	ADHD cases	Parents of cases	Controls
rs1800955 and rs4646984	D'	0.1	0.07	0.09
	r^2	0.003	0.003	0.003
rs1800955 and rs4646983	D'	0.59	0.33	0.043
	r^2	0.036	0.013	0
rs1800955 and Exon 3 VNTR	D'	0.28	0.66	0.42
	r^2	0.004	0.017	0.008
rs4646984 and rs4646983	D'	0.83	0.47	0.89
	r^2	0.19	0.078	0.2
rs4646984 and Exon 3 VNTR	D'	0.47	0.13	1
	r^2	0.031	0.002	0.015
rs4646983 and Exon 3 VNTR	D'	1	1	0.11
	r^2	0.01	0.01	0.007

Table 4. Haplotype comparison for DRD4 polymorphisms between ADHD cases and control group

Haplotype	Frequency in cases (N)*	Frequency in controls (N)*	$\chi2$	P-value
1-1-1-3	0.04 (1)	0	1.6	0.2
1-1-2-3	0.08 (2)	0	3.3	0.07
1-2-2-3	0.46 (11)	0.67 (20)	2.4	0.12
2-1-2-3	0.04 (1)	0	1.6	0.2
2-2-2-3	0.38 (9)	0.33 (10)	0.1	0.75

*N = No. of individuals.

Table 5A. Case-Control analysis of *DATI* allele frequencies

Polymorphism	Case		Control		χ^2	P-value
	Allele (N)*	Frequency	Allele (N)*	Frequency		
3′-UTR 40bp VNTR	11R (4)	0.02	11R (1)	0.005	1.1	0.30
	10R (151)	0.77	10R (172)	0.87	7.1	0.01
Intron 8 30bp VNTR	9R (37)	0.19	9R (25)	0.13	3.4	0.07
	7R (6)	0.03	7R (0)	0	7.1	0.01
	9R (6)	0.03	9R (4)	0.02	0.5	0.48
	6R (122)	0.64	6R (156)	0.79	10.9	0.001
	5R (55)	0.29	5R (33)	0.17	8.3	0.004

*N = No. of alleles.

Table 5B. Family-based association test for *DAT1* polymorphisms

Polymorphism	Transmission	Allele	Transmitted	Not-transmitted	χ^2	P-value (df=1)
3′-UTR VNTR	Overall	11R	3	3	0	1
		10R	14	29	5.34	0.02
		9R	23	11	4.33	0.04
		8R	0	1	1.39	0.24
		7R	5	1	2.91	0.09
	Paternal	11R	1	3	1.0	0.31
		10R	7	15	3.0	0.08
		9R	13	5	3.7	0.05
		8R	0	1	1.4	0.24
		7R	3	0	4.2	0.04
	Maternal	11R	2	0	2.8	0.09
		10R	7	14	2.4	0.12
		9R	10	6	1.0	0.31
		7R	2	1	0.3	0.56
intron 8 VNTR	Overall	10R	4	6	0.40	0.53
		9R	6	3	1.02	0.31
		6R	25	35	1.67	0.20
		5R	32	22	1.86	0.17
		4R	0	1	1.39	0.24
	Paternal	10R	2	5	1.3	0.25
		9R	2	2	0	1
		6R	16	16	0	1

	5R	15	12	0.3	0.56
	10R	2	1	0.3	0.56
	9R	4	1	1.9	0.17
Maternal	6R	9	19	3.6	0.06
	5R	17	10	1.8	0.18
	4R	0	1	1.4	0.24

Table 6A. Haplotype analysis of *DAT1* gene polymorphisms in cases and controls

Haplotype	Case (N)*	Control (N)*	χ^2	P value
11R-6R	0.01 (2)	0.005 (1)	0.4	0.53
11R-9R	0.005 (1)	0	1.4	0.23
10R-5R	0.16 (31)	0.13 (25)	1.4	0.24
10R-6R	0.54 (102)	0.71 (140)	12.0	0.001
10R-9R	0.03 (5)	0.02 (3)	0.2	0.69
10R-10R	0.04 (7)	0.02 (3)	1.7	0.19
10R-11R	0	0.005 (1)	1.4	0.25
9R-5R	0.11 (22)	0.05 (9)	6.4	0.01
9R-6R	0.08 (16)	0.08 (15)	0.02	0.88
9R-9R	0	0.003 (1)	0.3	0.61
9R-10R	0	0	0.2	0.62
7R-5R	0.02 (4)	0	5.6	0.02
7R-6R	0.005 (1)	0	1.6	0.21
7R-10R	0	0	0.9	0.36

*N = No. of observations.

Table 6B. Haplotype transmission of *DAT1* gene polymorphisms

Haplotype	Transmitted	Not transmitted	χ^2	P value
11R-5R	1	1	0	1
11R-6R	2	1	0.34	0.56
10R-5R	22	18	0.40	0.53
10R-6R	24	40	4.04	0.04
10R-9R	6	3	1.02	0.31
10R-10R	4	6	0.40	0.53
9R-4R	0	1	1.39	0.24
9R-5R	12	4	4.19	0.04
9R-6R	9	9	0	1
8R-5R	0	1	1.39	0.24
7R-5R	3	1	1.05	0.31
7R-6R	2	0	2.77	0.10

Linkage Disequilibrium and Haplotype Analyses

The two studied *DAT1* VNTRs showed lack of LD. Case-control analysis of different haplotypes revealed that the frequency of 9R-5R haplotype was significantly higher in cases than in controls (P=0.01) (Table 6A). On the other hand, 10R-6R combination was significantly over represented in controls (P=0.001). Transmission pattern of the different haplotypes showed preferential transmission of the 9R-5R haplotype (P=0.04) and under transmission of the 10R-6R haplotype from parents to ADHD cases (Table 6B).

DBH

Association Studies

Case-Control study for all three polymorphisms showed no significant difference between ADHD cases and controls (Table 7A). For rs1611115 and rs1108580, family-based association analysis revealed no significant preferential transmission of either allele from parents to probands (Table 7B). However, for rs2519152 a statistically significant over-transmission of 'G' was observed from father to the probands. At 5% significance level the power for this association test was 43.5%.

Linkage Disequilibrium and Haplotype Analyses

Pair-wise LD was analyzed for the *DBH* polymorphisms in ADHD cases, their parents and the control group (Table 8). rs1108580 and rs2519152 showed strong LD with each other in ADHD cases and their parents; the strength, however, decreased in the control group. rs1611115 was found to be in significant LD with rs1108580 and rs2519152, particularly in cases and parent group where disequilibria measure D' reached 'absolute' value (= 1). However, the r2 values were low.

Haplotype comparison between ADHD cases and controls (Table 9A) revealed that a haplotype, comprised of rs1611115 'C' allele, rs1108580 'G' allele and rs2519152 'A' allele, was significantly over-represented in the control group (P=0.03). In family-based transmission study, a near significant over transmission of a haplotype comprising of 'C' of rs1611115, 'G' of rs1108580 and 'G' of rs2519152 was noticed (P=0.07) (Table 9B).

Table 7A. *DBH* allele frequency comparison between ADHD cases and control

Polymorphism	Case		Control		χ^2	P-value
	Allele (N)*	Frequency	Allele (N)*	Frequency		
rs1611115	C (146)	0.78	C (196)	0.80	0.2	0.64
	T (40)	0.22	T (48)	0.20		
rs1108580	G (56)	0.29	G (80)	0.32	0.5	0.5
	A (136)	0.71	A (168)	0.68		
rs2519152	A (135)	0.72	A (171)	0.70	0.3	0.60
	G (53)	0.28	G (75)	0.30		

*N = No. of alleles.

MAOA

Association Studies

Four variants of MAOA-u VNTR were identified in the studied population: 2.5R (294bp), 3.5R (324bp), 4.5R (354bp) and 5.5R (384bp). Case-control analysis of the variants (Table 10A) revealed an increased frequency of the 3.5R allele in cases as compared to controls (P=0.09). TDT showed over transmission of the 3.5R allele and under transmission of the 4.5R allele from parents to ADHD probands (Table 10B); however, this bias in transmission did not reach statistical significance.

In case of rs6323, no significant difference in allele frequencies between cases and controls was noticed. Family-based study, too, did not reveal any variation in transmission of any allele (Tables 10A and B).

Table 7B: Family-based TDT of *DBH* polymorphisms

Polymorphism	Transmission	Allele	Transmitted	Not-transmitted	χ^2	P-value (df=1)
rs1611115	Overall	C	19	18	0.03	0.87
		T	18	19		
	Paternal	C	6	9	0.6	0.44
		T	9	6		
	Maternal	C	13	9	0.7	0.39
		T	9	13		
rs1108580	Overall	G	29	20	1.7	0.20
		A	20	29		
	Paternal	G	15	9	1.5	0.22
		A	9	15		
	Maternal	G	14	11	0.4	0.55
		A	11	14		
rs2519152	Overall	A	17	28	2.7	0.10
		G	28	17		
	Paternal	A	5	19	8.7	0.003
		G	19	5		
	Maternal	A	12	9	0.4	0.51
		G	9	12		

Table 8. Pair-wise linkage disequilibrium analysis of *DBH* polymorphisms

Polymorphism pairs	Parameters	ADHD cases	Parents of cases	Controls
rs1611115 and	D'	1.0	1.0	0.79
rs1108580	r2	0.12	0.09	0.07
rs1611115 and	D'	1.0	1.0	0.85
rs2519152	r2	0.11	0.09	0.08
rs1108580 and rs2519152	D'	0.89	0.85	0.69
	r2	0.77	0.71	0.43

Table 9A. Haplotype comparison for rs1611115, rs1108580 and rs2519152 between ADHD cases and control group

Haplotype	Frequency in cases (N)*	Frequency in controls (N)*	χ^2	P-value
C-G-A	0.02 (4)	0.08 (20)	4.9	0.03
C-G-G	0.26 (48)	0.24 (57)	0.1	0.7
C-A-A	0.48 (87)	0.42 (103)	0.9	0.33
C-A-G	0.02 (4)	0.06 (15)	3.4	0.06
T-G-A	0.008 (2)	0	0.4	0.5
T-A-A	0.21 (37)	0.19 (45)	0.4	0.5
T-A-G	0	0.009 (2)	1.0	0.31

*N = No. of observations.

Table 9B. Haplotype transmission of rs1611115, rs1108580 and rs2519152 from parents to ADHD probands

Haplotype	Transmitted	Not-transmitted	χ^2	P-value
C-G-A	2	5	1.4	0.24
C-G-G	28	17	3.4	0.07

Table 9B (Continued)

C-A-A	65	70	0.4	0.51
C-A-G	2	5	1.4	0.24
T-G-A	0	1	1.4	0.24
T-A-A	20	19	0.03	0.86

Linkage Disequilibrium and Haplotype Analyses

rs6323 and the VNTR were found to be in strong LD with each other. (Cases: D'=0.94, r2=0.66; Controls: D'=0.89, r2=0.77). Analysis to examine the combined effect of the two *MAOA* polymorphisms on ADHD revealed that haplotypes containing the 3.5R allele of the VNTR was present in higher frequency in cases as compared to controls, though the difference did not reach statistical significance (Table 11A). Haplotype transmission showed significant preferential transmission of the 3.5R-T haplotype from parents to ADHD cases (P=0.01) (Table 11B).

SNAP25

Association Studies

Table 10A. MAOA Allele frequency comparison between ADHD cases and controls

Polymorphism	Case		Control		χ^2	P-value
	Allele (N)*	Frequency	Allele (N)*	Frequency		
u VNTR	3.5R (80)	0.75	3.5R (110)	0.66	2.9	0.09
	4.5R (26)	0.25	4.5R (56)	0.34	2.5	0.11
	5.5R (0)	0	5.5R (1)	0.006	1.0	0.32
rs6323	T (30)	0.29	T (58)	0.35	1.02	0.31
	G (74)	0.71	G (109)	0.65		

*N = No. of alleles.

Frequency of the 'G' allele of rs362988 was significantly higher in ADHD cases (P=0.05) as compared to controls (Table 12A). None of the other polymorphisms showed any statistically significant deviation in allele frequencies between the two study groups.

TDT were carried out independently for the four polymorphisms. 'T' allele of rs3746544 was found to be preferentially transmitted from parents to ADHD probands (Table 12B, $P<0.05$). This over-transmission was primarily of maternal origin, as was evident from the statistically significant association between transmissions of 'T' from mothers to probands.

Table 10B. Family-based association test for MAOA polymorphisms

Polymorphism	Transmission	Allele	Transmitted	Not-transmitted	χ^2	P-value (df=1)
u VNTR	Overall	2.5R	0	2	2.77	0.09
		3.5R	19	12	1.59	0.21
		4.5R	14	19	0.76	0.38
	Male probands	2.5R	0	2	2.77	0.10
		3.5R	19	11	2.16	0.14
		4.5R	13	19	1.13	0.29
rs6323	Overall	T	17	16	0.03	0.86
		G	16	17		

Table 11A. Case control analysis of haplotypes of *MAOA* gene polymorphisms

Haplotype	Frequency in cases (N)*	Frequency in controls (N)*	χ^2	P-value
3.5R-G	0.70 (73)	0.62 (105)	1.6	0.21
3.5R-T	0.07 (7)	0.03 (5)	2.0	0.16
4.5R-G	0.01 (1)	0.03 (4)	0.9	0.35
4.5R-T	0.22 (23)	0.31 (52)	2.6	0.11
5.5R-T	0	0.006 (1)	1.0	0.32

*N = No. of observations.

Table 11B. Haplotype transmission analysis of MAOA gene polymorphisms

Haplotype	Transmitte	Not- transmitted	χ2	P value
2.5R-G	0	2	2.77	0.10
3.5R-G	18	15	0.27	0.60
3.5R-T	5	0	6.93	0.01
4.5R-G	0	2	2.77	0.10
4.5R-T	13	17	0.53	0.46

Table 12A. Case-Control analysis for SNAP25 polymorphisms

Polymorphism	Case		Control		χ^2	P-value
	Allele (N)*	Frequency	Allele (N)*	Frequency		
rs362988	A (110)	0.56	A (143)	0.65	3.8	0.05
	G (86)	0.44	G (77)	0.35		
rs3746544	T (150)	0.76	T (147)	0.68	1.7	0.19
	G (48)	0.24	G (69)	0.32		
rs1051312	T (176)	0.89	T (188)	0.87	0.64	0.42
	C (22)	0.11	C (28)	0.13		
rs8636	C (149)	0.75	C (163)	0.72	0.41	0.5
	T (49)	0.25	T (63)	0.28		

*N = No. of alleles.

Table 12B. TDT of SNAP25 polymorphisms

SNP	Transmission	Allele	Transmitted	Not-transmitted	χ^2	P value (df=1)
rs362988	Overall	A	28	36	1.00	0.32
		G	36	28		

SNP	Transmission	Allele	Transmitted	Not-transmitted	χ^2	P value (df=1)
	Paternal	A	14	21	1.41	0.24
		G	21	14		
	Maternal	A	14	15	0.03	0.85
		G	15	14		
rs3746544	Overall	T	34	16	6.63	0.01
		G	16	34		
	Paternal	T	15	9	1.52	0.22
		G	9	15		
	Maternal	T	19	7	5.75	0.02
		G	7	19		
rs1051312	Overall	T	21	14	1.41	0.24
		C	14	21		
	Paternal	T	9	8	0.06	0.81
		C	8	9		
	Maternal	T	12	6	2.04	0.15
		C	6	12		
rs8636	Overall	C	33	22	2.21	0.14
		T	22	33		
	Paternal	C	16	9	1.99	0.16
		T	9	16		
	Maternal	C	17	13	0.53	0.46
		T	13	17		

At 5% significance level, power for this association test was 42%. The other SNPs did not reveal any significant transmission of either allele.

Linkage Disequilibrium and Haplotype Analyses

rs3746544 and rs1051312 were found to be in moderately strong LD with each other, D' reaching an absolute value (=1) in the control group (Table 13). None of the haplotypes formed from the four SNPs was over represented or over transmitted in ADHD cases (Tables 14A and B).

Gene-Gene Interaction

Individual association studies revealed that exon 3 VNTR of *DRD4*, 3′-UTR VNTR of *DAT1*, rs2519152 of *DBH*, and rs3746544 of *SNAP25* were positively correlated with ADHD in our study population. The genotypes of these four polymorphisms were combined to identify possible haplotypes that are associated with the disease (Table 15 A and B). A haplotype comprising of the common 4R variant of *DRD4* VNTR, 9R variant of *DAT1* 3′ VNTR, ‘G’ allele of rs2519152 and ‘T’ of rs3746544 was significantly transmitted to ADHD probands. Interestingly, in this haplotype the 9R of *DAT1*, ‘G’ of rs2519152 and ‘T’ of rs3746544 showed individual positive association with ADHD. Again, 9R of *DAT1* and ‘T’ of rs3746544 was part of another haplotype (4R-9R-A-T) that was also significantly associated with the disorder.

Discussion

Majority of referrals to child and adolescent clinics comprise of patients suffering from ADHD and its co-morbid disorders. Therefore, extensive investigations on ADHD have been carried out in different parts of the world, with special emphasis on the molecular genetic anomalies, to characterize the disorder for better management.

Table 13. Pair wise linkage disequilibrium analysis of SNAP25 polymorphisms

Polymorphism pairs	Parameters	ADHD cases	Parents of cases	Controls
rs362988 and rs3746544	D'	0.61	0.49	0.31
	r^2	0.15	0.13	0.09
rs362988 and rs1051312	D'	0.34	0.61	1
	r^2	0.01	0.03	0.08
rs362988 and rs8636	D'	0.53	0.44	0.52
	r^2	0.12	0.11	0.20

rs3746544 and	D'	0.59	0.72	1
rs1051312	r^2	0.01	0.03	0.07
rs3746544 and	D'	0.6	0.74	0.64
rs8636	r^2	0.32	0.5	0.36
rs1051312 and	D'	1	1	1
rs8636	r^2	0.04	0.05	0.06

Table 14A. Haplotype comparison for rs362988, rs3746544, rs1051312, and rs8636 between ADHD cases and control group

Haplotype	Frequency in cases (N)*	Frequency in controls (N)*	χ^2	P value
1-1-1-1	0.57 (12)	0.62 (13)	0.1	0.75
1-2-1-1	0	0.05 (1)	1.4	0.25
1-2-1-2	0.05 (1)	0.05 (1)	0	1
2-1-1-1	0.24 (5)	0.14 (3)	0.6	0.43
2-1-1-2	0	0.05 (1)	1.4	0.25
2-2-1-2	0.14 (3)	0.1 (2)	0.2	0.63

*N = No. of observations.

Table 14B. Haplotype transmissions of rs362988, rs3746544, rs1051312, and rs8636 from parents to ADHD probands

Haplotype	Transmitted	Not-transmitted	χ^2	P value
1-1-1-1	25	20	0.6	0.46
1-1-1-2	4	3	0.1	0.70
1-1-2-1	9	10	0.05	0.82
1-2-1-1	2	4	0.7	0.41

Table 14B (Continued)

1-2-1-2	2	7	2.9	0.09
1-2-2-1	0	1	1.4	0.24
2-1-1-1	16	8	2.7	0.1
2-1-1-2	1	2	0.3	0.56
2-1-2-1	2	5	1.3	0.25
2-2-1-1	3	4	0.1	0.71
2-2-1-2	13	12	0.04	0.84
2-2-2-1	0	1	1.4	0.24

Table 15A. Combined haplotypes of significant DRD4, DAT1, DBH and SNAP25 polymorphisms; comparison between cases and controls

Haplotyp e	Frequency in cases (N)*	Frequency in controls (N)*	χ^2	P value
3-2-1-1	0.11 (2)	0.2 (3)	0.5	0.48
3-2-2-1	0.83 (15)	0.73 (11)	0.5	0.48
3-2-2-2	0.06 (1)	0.07 (1)	0.02	0.89

*N = No. of observations.

Table 15B. Combined haplotype transmission of significant polymorphisms of *DRD4* (exon 3 VNTR), *DAT1* (3′-UTR VNTR), *DBH* (rs2519152) and *SNAP25* (rs3746544) from parents to ADHD probands

Table 15B.	*Table 15B.*	*Table 15B.*	*Table 15B.*	*Table 15B.*
2R-10R-G-T	1	0	1.4	0.24
2R-10R-G-G	0	1	1.4	0.24
2R-10R-A-T	4	3	0.1	0.70
2R-10R-A-G	1	0	1.4	0.24
2R-9R-G-T	0	1	1.4	0.24

2R-7R-G-G	0	1	1.4	0.24
3R-9R-G-T	1	0	1.4	0.24
4R-11R-G-T	0	1	1.4	0.24
4R-11R-A-T	2	1	0.34	0.56
4R-11R-A-G	1	0	1.4	0.24
4R-10R-G-T	13	8	1.2	0.27
4R-10R-G-G	1	5	2.9	0.09
4R-10R-A-T	17	26	1.9	0.17
4R-10R-A-G	10	19	2.8	0.09
4R-9R-G-T	5	0	6.9	0.008
4R-9R-A-T	11	4	3.4	0.065
4R-9R-A-G	3	4	0.1	0.70
4R-8R-A-G	0	1	1.4	0.24
4R-7R-A-T	2	0	2.8	0.10
5R-9R-A-T	0	1	1.4	0.24
6R-10R-G-T	3	1	1.1	0.31
6R-10R-A-T	0	2	2.8	0.10
6R-10R-A-G	1	1	0	1
6R-9R-G-T	1	0	1.4	0.24
7R-10R-G-G	1	0	1.4	0.24
7R-10R-A-T	1	0	1.4	0.24
7R-9R-A-T	1	0	1.4	0.24

Advances in neuroimaging, particularly functional MRI and positron emission tomography studies helped in understanding the regions of the brain that are affected in an ADHD proband [20-25]. To further the rationale, studies on neurogenetics have been put forward to categorize the defect in an individual.

DRD4

Role of the rs1800955 (-521 C>T), located in the CpG island of *DRD4* promoter [68], has been investigated in association with novelty seeking [70], schizophrenia [69,71,72], attachment disorganization [73,74] and the findings are contradictory. Investigation has revealed that the T allele displays ~40% reduced transcriptional efficiency as compared to the C allele in human retinoblastoma cell line [69]; however, another group of investigators have reported identical promoter activity conferred by the two alleles [75]. In the present study, no significant bias in transmission was noticed for this polymorphism.

The *DRD4* 120bp tandem duplication (rs4646984) [76], located approximately 1.2 kb upstream of the initiation codon, is speculated to contain consensus binding sequences for several transcription factors [31]. Both positive and negative association with ADHD was reported [51, 52, 77]. In eastern Indian ADHD cases, case-control analysis revealed a higher frequency of the short single repeat allele as compared to the controls (P=0.06).

In the coding region of *DRD4* exon 1, another 12bp tandem repeat (rs4646983) has been reported [78] which results in duplication of four amino acids (GASA) near the extracellular domain and first transmembrane domain junction of the receptor, which possibly alters agonist binding and signal transduction [35]. The rarer allele (1 repeat) was found to be significantly associated with Italian delusional disorder patients [79]. However, lack of association was noticed between ADHD and transmission of the 1-repeat allele in Canadian population [80]. On the other hand, case-control analysis in the current investigation showed a higher frequency of the single repeat allele (P=0.16) in ADHD cases, while, family-based studies revealed no positive association between the single repeat allele and ADHD. These two repeat polymorphisms of *DRD4* were found to be in strong LD; both in cases and controls, an observation reported for the first time from our lab [81]. The observed higher occurrence of the single repeat alleles of both the polymorphisms in ADHD cases as compared to controls, which showed no transmission bias in familial studies, along with strong LD may indicate that in Indian ADHD subjects, these two polymorphisms may be segregating together as risk haplotypes for ADHD and possibly contributing to the disease etiology.

A VNTR in the exon 3 of *DRD4* has been documented in several different populations [32, 82, 83]. The repeat numbers vary between 2 and 11 and include over 67 different haplotypes [84,85].The exon 3 encodes a proline rich domain in the third inter-cytoplasmic loop of the protein [80] and the 7R variant of the VNTR has been found to have altered pharmacological properties as compared to variants with 2 or 4 repeats [86]. Significant association between ADHD and transmission of the *DRD4*-7R allele have been reported in American children [49,84,87,88] and a possible risk conferred by the 7R variant in the etiology has been suggested [84]. However, lack of any apparent association between the disorder and the higher repeat alleles was reported from Ireland, Israel, UK and New Zealand [49,50]. In eastern Indian ADHD subjects, we have earlier reported an association of the higher repeats of the *DRD4* exon 3 (6- and 7-R) VNTR [81]. In the present investigation, using an extended number of samples, we have noticed a significantly higher frequency of the 6R allele in cases and the 7R allele showed statistically significant preferential transmission from father to ADHD probands, indicating that the higher repeat alleles of the

VNTR may have an important role to play in the etiology of ADHD in the eastern Indian population.

Haplotype analysis for *DRD4* previously showed that a haplotype of markers containing the –521 C allele may confer susceptibility to ADHD [89]. rs1800955 has also been reported to be in LD with the exon 3 VNTR in novelty seeking subjects [90]. Nevertheless, a study on a sample of ADHD children of mixed European Caucasian and non-Caucasian descent, found no bias in transmission of any of the alleles of this polymorphism and found no evidence of LD between the VNTR and the SNP [69,91]. In ADHD children of Irish descent also no statistically significant excess transmission of T allele was observed and lack of LD was noticed between the VNTR and the SNP [92]. Later, the same group extended their work on relation between Sustained Attention to Response Test (SART) in ADHD and *DRD4* variants of the exon 3 VNTR, -521 and –616 SNP and found that 7R allele on VNTR was associated with better performance while the –521 T allele was associated with poorer performance in SART [93].

DAT1

In the 3′ UTR of *DAT*1, a polymorphic 40bp repeat, with repeat numbers ranging between 3 and 11, was identified [94]. Since the 3′UTR is believed to control protein transcription, it was hypothesized that "the 10 repeat (10R) allele may generate a dopamine transporter that is abnormally efficient at the reuptake process, which in turn may produce reduced activity in the DA pathways – both mesolimbic and nigrostriatal" [95]. Measurement of brain tissue and lymphocyte DAT mRNA revealed positive correlation between presence of 10R allele and expression of DAT [96]. Heritability for the trait toward ADHD was estimated at 75% with higher correlation for twins than for other siblings. While working with eastern Indian ADHD probands, we have observed lack of association with the 10R allele of the VNTR [97]. In the present investigation, with increased sample size, significant preferential transmission of the 9R allele to ADHD probands was noticed which supports our previous observation.

The intron 8 VNTR of *DAT1* comprises of a 30bp sequence, repeated 4-12 times; the most common being 5R and 6R alleles. Functional analysis demonstrated statistically significant baseline increase in reporter gene expression by the 'protective' 5R allele as compared to 6R 'risk' allele [98]. Association analysis revealed that the 6R allele and a haplotype comprising of 6R allele of intron 8 VNTR and 10R allele of 3′-UTR VNTR were preferentially transmitted to ADHD cases both in Taiwanese and British subjects [99]. Frequency of the 5R allele was significantly higher in cases and a haplotype comprising of this 5R allele and the 9R allele of the 3′ UTR VNTR was not only significantly over-represented in ADHD cases but also significantly over-transmitted from their parents. This suggests that both the polymorphisms may have a vital function to play in the disease etiology.

DBH

Individuals with a Taq1 RFLP in the intron 5 of *DBH* (rs2519152) were frequently found to be susceptible to ADHD [37,42]. Two polymorphic sites in the *DBH* gene, viz. (a) *DBH* simple tandem repeat (STR) containing a GT repeat sequence and (b) *DBH* * 444 g/a, a single nucleotide polymorphism (SNP) at the 3′ end of *DBH* exon 2, have been found to be in LD. They were found to be associated with CSF and plasma DβH activity prompting the authors to infer that *DBH* is a quantitative trait loci (QTL) influencing both plasma and CSF DβH activity [57].

A novel polymorphism (-1021 C→ T, rs1611115) in the 5′ flanking region of the *DBH* was also reported where homozygosity for the T allele was found to be associated with very low DβH activity and accounting for 35-52% variability observed in the plasma DβH activity [58], implementing rs1611115 as a major genetic marker for plasma DβH activity.

Previously we have reported lack of association between the intron 5 Taq1 RFLP (rs2519152) as well as a trend towards association of the exon 2 444g/a polymorphism (rs1108580) with Indian ADHD subjects [100]. However, in the present study with extended samples, a highly significant paternal over-transmission of 'G' allele of the RFLP was observed (P=0.003), suggesting that the 'G' allele of rs2519152 could be associated with ADHD in the Indian population. This observation is in concordance with a case-control Milwaukee Longitudinal Study in the US, where this allele was significantly associated with ADHD [101]. Again, a notably high LD was observed between rs2519152 and *DBH* * 444 g/a (rs1108580) in ADHD cases and their parents as compared to controls. This indicates higher chances for the two polymorphisms to be transmitted together in families with ADHD probands, implying that this region of the gene may be close to the true polymorphism that is responsible for susceptibility to ADHD. The other SNP studied, rs1611115, showed lack of association between ADHD and the eastern Indian population.

MAOA

Among numerous different genetic polymorphisms explored for association with neurobehavioral disorders, the most functionally significant in the MAOA gene is a 30bp VNTR, known as *MAOA*-upstream (*MAOA*-u) VNTR [102]. It is located approximately 1.2 kb upstream of the coding region and both the 5′ and 3′ flanking regions of the VNTR contain a number of transcription factor binding sites believed to affect transcriptional activity of the *MAOA* promoter [102,103]; transcriptional efficiency being directly proportional to the number of repeats [103]. In a population-based study, short allele (2 and 3 repeats) with low enzyme activity was found to be associated with impulsivity and aggression [104] and association of this VNTR with ADHD have also been reported [45]. In Indian ADHD probands, we have previously reported probable association of the short 3.5 repeat allele [105], which was further supported from the present investigation; both case-control and family-based studies showed that the short repeat allele had a strong tendency towards association with ADHD.

The second functional polymorphism studied is a silent T/G SNP (rs6323) located at exon 8 of *MAOA* gene; the T and G alleles, in spite of being silent transition, have been reported to be associated significantly with low and high MAOA activity respectively [106]. This polymorphism has been studied in association with bipolar disorder [107] and ADHD [108,109]. In British Caucasian ADHD children no significant association was observed between this SNP and the disorder [108]. However, the high activity G allele and a haplotype containing the short repeat allele of the *MAOA*-u VNTR and G allele was reported to be preferentially transmitted to Irish ADHD children [44].

In Indo-Caucasoid ADHD children, the rs6323 SNP did not reveal any transmission bias. Haplotype analysis showed significant preferential transmission of 3.5R-T haplotype with a transmission percentage of 100 from parents to ADHD cases. It is also noteworthy that another haplotype containing the 3.5R of the VNTR, the 3.5R-G haplotype, was more often transmitted (18 times) than not transmitted (15 times) to ADHD cases. Moreover, under transmission of haplotypes containing the 4.5R allele of the VNTR was also noticed. Since these two polymorphisms were found to be in strong LD in both the case and control groups, we may conclude that a haplotype formed between these polymorphisms has a higher chance of being transmitted as a haplotype block and the shorter 3.5R allele of the MAOA VNTR confers a risk of ADHD in this population.

SNAP25

Synaptosomal-Associated Protein 25 (SNAP-25) is a neuron-specific protein that controls exocytotic neurotransmitter release and eight genetic polymorphisms have been investigated by different investigators. Significant evidence for association with ADHD was reported for rs3746544 [59]. In Han Chinese population, case-control analysis of rs362988 showed significant association (P=0.033) with inattentive subtype of ADHD [109]. In the present investigation, three SNPs, rs362988, rs3746544 and rs1051312 were studied. Case-control analysis of rs362988 in eastern Indian population revealed significant over-representation of the 'G' allele in ADHD cases; however, no correlation was observed between genetic polymorphism and ADHD subtypes.

Functional importance of rs3746544 and rs1051312 are not known till today. However, In Canadian ADHD subjects, significant association with a haplotype comprising of 'T' allele of rs3746544 and 'C' allele of rs1051312 (P=0.03) was reported [79]. An over-transmission (P=0.027) of this haplotype from father to ADHD probands belonging to Caucasian ethnicity was also observed [110]. Screening of twelve *SNAP25* polymorphisms (including rs3746544 / T1065G and rs1051312 / T1069C) in Canadian and southern Californian families revealed significant association with four markers in the Canadian sample but not in the Californian samples [111]; difference in observation was attributed to discrepancy in sample selection, ethnicity and response to medication.

In the present investigation on Indo-Caucasoid population, family-based transmission analyses showed significant overtransmission of the 'T' allele of rs3746544, particularly from mothers to probands (P=0.05). Earlier in Irish ADHD subjects, preferential transmission of paternal alleles of several candidate genes, including *DRD4*, *DRD5*, and *DAT* was reported;

the 'T' allele of rs3746544 showed a trend towards paternal overtransmission (P=0.18) [112]. This observed difference in transmission bias between the two study groups could be due to marked population distinction.

Gene-Gene Interactions

For neurobehavioral disorders like ADHD, schizophrenia, and bipolar disorder, exploration for disease-causing genes is very difficult. Susceptibility towards these disorders is caused by multiple genes of relatively small effect or by a combination of genetic and environmental factors, thus presenting substantial challenges for the genetic inquest. Hence, molecular geneticists worldwide have tried to identify chromosomal regions that confer susceptibility to the disorder with an idea of recognizing the contribution of these genes in the etiology of the disorder, which may open avenues for exploring pharmacogenetic interactions for better therapeutic intercession.

In an attempt to reach this target, the present study took into account fifteen polymorphisms in five different genes in the dopaminergic pathway with an aim to identify variations that are possibly leading to susceptibility towards ADHD in the eastern Indian population. We have noticed that several polymorphisms were positively associated with the disorder independently. In order to find out whether their individual small effects are combining together to produce gene-gene interaction, the genotypes of those polymorphisms were combined to identify possible haplotypes that are associated with the disorder. The study led to the identification of a "risk haplotype", comprising of the 4R variant of *DRD4* VNTR, 9R variant of *DAT1* 3′ VNTR, 'G' allele of rs2519152 and 'T' of rs3746544, which showed higher chances of transmission to ADHD probands.

Although the functions of TaqI RFLP (rs2519152) of *DBH* and 3′-UTR T→G (rs3746544) of *SNAP25* are not yet clear, we are aware that the lower repeat variant of *DAT1* 3′ VNTR may produce a transporter protein with normal reuptake of DA from the synapse [96], and the lower repeat variants (4R) of the *DRD4* is associated with a receptor with normal binding affinity [86]. Further, our analysis showed higher transmission of the short 3.5R allele of the MAOA upstream VNTR that confers reduced enzymatic activity [102, 103] (this site was not considered for gene-gene interaction due to localization in the sex chromosome). Hence, we may conclude from the present finding that the "haplotype" that showed preferential transmission in the Indo-Caucasoid ADHD children is different from that so far being reported in other populations [113,114]. The main draw back of the present study is the limited number of ADHD samples used and further analysis, including some other ethnic groups, would be necessary for validation of the data.

Inference

A complicated disorder like ADHD deserve multifaceted attention and in the post-genomic era, with rapidly advancing field of information and treatment strategies, we should be capable of using the knowledge of genomics together with these advancements. The comparatively new field referring to the spectrum of genes that determine drug response is pharmacogenomics [115]. ADHD with a high heritability [116] has received extensive attention for both candidate gene studies and genome wide approaches since ethnic heterogeneity is an important factor while conducting genetic association studies. The highly complicated nature of the disorder have also necessitated studies on pharmacogenomics and individualized response to medication, a topic which has been recently very critically reviewed [117]. Categorization of patients who could be poor responder to a certain group of drugs and therefore are at increased risk for treatment failure could be spared. Alternatively, they could be provided with "tailored medication" for better management of the problem. In-depth analysis employing increased number of samples and different ethnic populations is warranted to avoid interpretation bias. Impact of gene-environment interactions, as have been reviewed recently [118], also deserves consideration in outlining management strategies for ADHD patients.

References

[1] Still GF. (1902) Some abnormal physical condition in children. *Lancet* 1: 1008-1012.

[2] American Psychiatric Association. (2000) Diagnostic and Statistical Manual for Mental Disorders-IV-Text Revised version. Washington, DC: American Psychiatric Association.

[3] Swanson JM, Sergeant JA, Taylor E, et al. (1998) Attention-deficit hyperactivity disorder and hyperkinetic disorder. *Lancet* 351: 429-433.

[4] Berkeley RA, Fisher M, Smallish L, Fletcher K. (2002) The persistence of attention-deficit/hyperactivity disorder into young adulthood as a function of reporting source and definition of disorder. *J Abnorm Psychol* 111: 279-289.

[5] Faraone SV, Sergeant J, Gillberg C, Biederman J. (2003) The worldwide prevalence of ADHD: Is it an American condition? *World Psychiatry* 2: 104-113.

[6] Weiss G, Hetchman L. (1993) Hyperactive children grown up. New York, NY: Guilford Press.

[7] Wolraich ML, Hannah JN, Pinnock TY, et al. (1996) Comparison of diagnostic criteria for attention-deficit hyperactivity disorder in a country-wide sample. *J Am Acad Child Adolesc Psychiatry* 35: 319-324.

[8] Fischer M, Barkley RA, Fletcher KE, Smallish L. (1993) The adolescent outcome of hyperactive children: predictors of psychiatric, academic, social, and emotional adjustment. *J Am Acad Child Adolesc Psychiatry* 32: 324-332.

[9] Mannuza S, Klein RG, Bessler A, et al. (1993) Adult outcome of hyperactive boys: Educational achievement, occupational rank and psychiatric status. *Arch Gen Psychiatry* 50: 565-576.

[10] Weiss G, Hechtman L, Milroy T, Perlman T. (1985) Psychiatric status of hyperactives as adults: a controlled prospective 15-year follow-up of 63 hyperactive children. *J Am Acad Child Psychiatry* 24:211-220.

[11] Biederman J, Newcorn J, Sprich S. (1991) Comorbidity of attention deficit hyperactivity disorder with conduct, depressive, anxiety, and other disorders. *Am J Psychiatry* 148: 564-577.

[12] Wilens TE, Biederman J, Mick E, et al. (1997) Attention deficit hyperactivity disorder (ADHD) is associated with early onset substance use disorders. *J Nerv Ment Dis* 185: 475-482.

[13] Chawla PL, Shashi G, Sunderam KR, Mehta M. (1981) A study of prevalence pattern of hyperactive structural syndrome in primary school children. *Ind J Psychiatry* 24: 443-455.

[14] Prakash S. (2002) Patterns of child and adolescent psychiatric disorders in India. In Ramachandran V, Palaniappan V, Shah LP (eds): Continuing Medical Education Programme. Bangalore, India, Ind Psychiatric Society.

[15] Gada M. (1987) A study of prevalence and pattern of attention deficit disorder with hyperactivity in primary school children. *Ind J Psychiatry* 29: 113-118.

[16] Singhal PK, Bhatia MS, Dhar BMK, et al. (1988) Psychiatric morbidity. *Ind J Pediatrics* 55: 575-579.

[17] Bhatia MS, Choudhary S, Sidana A. (1999) Attention deficit hyperactivity disorder among psychiatric outpatients. *J Child Psychol Psychiatry* 36: 583-587.

[18] Malhi P, Singhi P. (2000) Spectrum of attention-deficit hyperactivity disorders in children among referrals to psychology services. *Ind Pediatrics* 37: 1256-1260.

[19] Mukhopadhyay M, Misra S, Mitra T, Niyogi P. (2003) Attention deficit hyperactivity disorder. *Ind J Pediatrics* 70: 789-792.

[20] Sowell ER, Thompson PM, Welcome SE, et al. (2003) Cortical abnormalities in children and adolescents with attention-deficit hyperactivity disorder. *Lancet* 362: 1699-1707.

[21] Rapoport JL, Castellanos FX, Gogate N, et al. (2001) Imaging normal and abnormal brain development: new perspectives for child psychiatry. *Aust N Z J Psychiatry* 35: 272-281.

[22] Durston S. (2008) Converging methods in studying attention-deficit/ hyperactivity disorder: What can we learn from neuroimaging and genetics? *Development and Psychopathology* 20: 1133–1143.

[23] Krause KL, Dresel SH, Krause J, et al. (2000) Increased striatal dopamine transporter in adult patients with attention deficit hyperactivity disorder: effects of methylphenidate as measured by single photon emission computed tomography. *Neurosci Letters* 285: 107-110.

[24] Barkley RA. (1997) Behavioral inhibition, sustained attention, and executive functions: constructing a unifying theory of ADHD. *Psychol Bull* 121: 65-94.

[25] Zametkin A, Liotta W. (1998) The neurobiology of attention-deficit/hyperactivity disorder. *J Clin Psychiatry* 59: 17-23.

[26] Spencer T, Biederman J, Wilens T, et al. (1996) Pharmacotherapy of attention deficit disorder across the life cycle. *J Am Acad Child Adolesc Psychiatry* 35: 409-432.

[27] Levin E. (1992) Nicotinic systems and cognitive function. *Psychopharmacology* 108: 417-431.

[28] Westfal T, Grant H, Perry H. (1983) Release of dopamine and 5-hydroxytryptamine from rat striatal slices following activation of nicotinic cholinergic receptors. *Gen Pharmacol* 14: 321-325.

[29] Spivak B, Vered Y, Yoran-Hegesh R, et al. (1999) Circulatory levels of catecholamines, serotonin and lipids in attention deficit hyperactivity disorder. *Acta Psychiatry Scand* 99: 300-304.

[30] Faraone SV, Perlis RH, Doyle AE, et al. (2005) Advancing the neuroscience of ADHD: Molecular genetics of attention-deficit/hyperactivity disorder. *Biol Psychiatry* 57: 1313-1323.

[31] Seaman MI, Fisher JB, Chang FM, Kidd KK. (1999) Tandem duplication polymorphism upstream of the dopamine D4 receptor gene (DRD4). *Am J Med Genet* 88B: 705-709.

[32] Litcher JB, Barr CL, Kennedy JL, et al. (1993) A hypervariable segment in the human dopamine receptor D4 (DRD4) gene. *Human Mol Genet* 2: 767-773.

[33] Cichon S, Nothen MM, Catalano M, et al. (1995) Identification of two novel polymorphisms and a rare deletion variant in the human dopamine D4 receptor gene. *Psychiatric Genet* 5: 97-103.

[34] Nothen MM, Cichon S, Hemmer S, et al. (1994) Human dopamine D4 receptor gene : frequent occurrence of a null allele and observation of homozygosity. *Human Mol Genet* 3: 2207-2212.

[35] Seeman P, Ulpian C, Chouinard G, et al. (1994) Dopamine D4 receptor variant D4GLYCINE194, in Africans, but not in Caucassians: no association with schizophrenia. *Am J Med Genet* 54B: 384-390.

[36] Schoots O, Sanyal S, Guan H-C, et al. (1996) Cryptic inhibition at the human D4 receptor reveals a functional role for the amino terminus. *Biochemistry* 35: 3614-3618.

[37] Daly G, Hawi Z, Fitzgerald M, Gill M. (1999) Mapping susceptibility loci in attention-deficit hyperactivity disorder: preferential transmission of parental alleles at DAT1, DBH and DRD5 to affected children. *Mol Psychiatry* 4: 192-196.

[38] Barr CL, Wigg KG, Feng Y, et al. (2000) Attention-deficit hyperactivity disorder and the gene for the dopamine D5 receptor. *Mol Psychiatry* 5: 548-551.

[39] Vandenbergh DJ, Persico AM, Hawkins AL, et al. (1992) Human dopamine transporter gene (DAT1) maps to chromosome 5p15.3 and displays a VNTR. *Genomics* 14: 1104-1106.

[40] Barr CL, Xu C, Kroft J, et al. (2001) Haplotype study of three polymorphisms at the dopamine transporter locus confirms linkage to attention-deficit/hyperactivity disorder. *Biol Psychiatry* 49: 333-339.

[41] Roman T, Schmitz M, Polanczyk GV, et al. (2002) Further evidence for the association between attention-deficit/ hyperactivity disorder and the dopamine B-hydroxylase gene. *Am J Med Genet* 114: 154-158.

[42] Hawi Z, Lowe N, Kirley A, et al. (2003) Linkage disequilibrium mapping at DAT1, DRD5 and DBH narrows the search for ADHD susceptibility alleles at these loci. *Mol Psychiatry* 8: 299-308.

[43] Nolen WA, Hoencamp E, Bouvy PF, Haffmans PM. (1993) Reversible monoamine oxidase-A inhibitors in resistant major depression. *Clin Neuropharmacol* 16: S69-S76.

[44] Domschke K, Sheehan K, Lowe N, et al. (2005) Association analysis of the monoamine oxidase A and B genes with attention deficit hyperactivity disorder (ADHD) in an Irish sample: preferential transmission of the MAO-A 941G allele to affected children. *Am J Med Genet* 134B: 110-114.

[45] Manor I, Tyano S, Mel E, et al. (2002) Family-based and association studies of monoamine oxidase A and attention deficit hyperactivity disorder (ADHD): preferential transmission of the long promoter-region repeat and its association with impaired performance on a continuous performance test (TOVA). *Mol Psychiatry* 7: 626-632.

[46] Eisenberg J, Mei-Tal G, Steinberg A, et al. (1999) Haplotype relative risk study of catechol-O-methyltransferase (COMT) and attention deficit hyperactivity disorder (ADHD): association of the high enzyme activity Val allele with ADHD impulsive-hyperactive phenotype. *Am J Med Genet* 88:497-502.

[47] Civelli O, Bunzow JR, Grandy DK, et al. (1991) Molecular biology of the dopamine receptors. *Eur J Pharmacol (Mol Pharmacol Section)* 207: 277-286.

[48] Swanson JM, Sunohara GA, Kennedy JL, et al. (1998) Association of the dopamine receptor D4 (DRD4) gene with a refined phenotype of attention deficit hyperactivity disorder (ADHD): a family-based approach. *Mol Psychiatry* 3:38-41.

[49] Hawi Z, McCarron M, Kirley A, et al. (2000) No association of the dopamine D4 receptor (DRD4) gene polymorphism with attention deficit hyperactivity disorder (ADHD) in the Irish population. *Am J Med Genet* 96B: 268-272.

[50] Holmes J, Payton A, Barrett JH, et al. (2000) A family-based and case-control association study of the dopamine D4 receptor gene and dopamine transporter gene in attention-deficit hyperactivity disorder. *Mol Psychiatry* 5: 523-530.

[51] McCracken JT, Smalley SL, McGough JJ, et al. (2000) Evidence for linkage of a tandem duplication polymorphism upstream of the dopamine D4 receptor gene (DRD4) with attention deficit hyperactivity disorder (ADHD). *Mol Psychiatry* 5: 531-536.

[52] Kustanovich V, Ishii J, Crawford L, et al. (2004) Transmission disequilibrium testing of 11 dopamine-related candidate gene polymorphisms in ADHD: confirmation of association of ADHD with DRD4 and DRD5. *Mol Psychiatry* 9: 711-717.

[53] Leung PW, Lee CC, Hung SF, et al. (2005) Dopamine receptor D4 (DRD4) gene in Han Chinese children with attention-deficit/hyperactivity disorder (ADHD): Increased prevalence of the 2-repeat allele. *Am J Med Genet* 133B: 54-56.

[54] Wolraich ML, Greenhill LL, Pelham W, et al. (2001) Randomized, controlled trials of oral methylphenidate once a day in children with attention-deficit/hyperactivity disorder. *Pediatrics* 108: 883-892.

[55] O'Connor DT, Cervenka JH, Stone RA, et al. (1994) Dopamine beta-hydroxylase immunoreactivity in human cerebrospinal fluid: properties, relationship to central noradrenergic neuronal activity and variation in Parkinson's disease and congenital dopamine beta-hydroxylase deficiency. *Clin Sci (Lond)* 86:149-158.

[56] Biaggioni I, Goldstein DS, Atkinson T, Robertson D. (1990) Dopamine-beta-hydroxylase deficiency in humans. *Neurology* 40: 370-373.

[57] Cubells JF, van Kammen DP, Kelley ME, et al. (1998) Dopamine beta-hydroxylase: two polymorphisms in linkage disequilibrium at the structural gene DBH associate with biochemical phenotypic variation. *Human Genet* 102: 533-540.
[58] Kim CH, Zabetian CP, Cubells JF, et al. (2002) Mutations in the dopamine beta-hydroxylase gene are associated with human norepinephrine deficiency. *Am J Med Genet* 108: 140-147.
[59] Mill J, Richards S, Knight J, et al. (2004) Haplotype analysis of SNAP-25 suggests a role in the etiology of ADHD. *Mol Psychiatry* 9: 801-810.
[60] Conners CK. (1997) Conners' Rating Scales – Revised. Multi-Health Systems: Toronto, Canada.
[61] Wechsler D. (1991) Wechsler Intelligence Scale for Children-Third Edition: Manual. San Antonio, TX: Psychological Corporation.
[62] Bharat Raj J. (1971) AIISH norms on SFB with Indian children. *J AIISH* 2: 34-39.
[63] Miller SA, Dykes DD, Polesky HF. (1988) A simple salting out procedure for extracting DNA from human nucleated cells. *Nucl Acids Res* 16: 1215-1224.
[64] Dudbridge F. (2003) Pedigree disequilibrium tests for multilocus haplotypes. *Genet Epidemiol* 25: 115-121.
[65] Spielman RS, McGinnis RE, Ewens WJ. (1993) Transmission test for linkage disequilibrium: the insulin gene region and insulin-dependent diabetes mellitus (IDDM). *Am J Hum Genet* 52: 506-516.
[66] Barrett JC, Fry B, Maller J, Daly MJ. (2005) Haploview: analysis and visualization of LD and haplotype maps. *Bioinformatics* 21: 263-265.
[67] Purcell S, Daly MJ, Sham PC. (2007) WHAP: haplotype-based association analysis. *Bioinformatics* 23: 255-256.
[68] Wong AHC, Buckle CE, Van Tol HHM. (2000) Polymorphisms in dopamine receptors: what do they tell us? *Eur J Pharmacol* 410: 183-203.
[69] Okuyama Y, Ishiguro H, Nankai M, et al. (2000) Identification of a polymorphism in the promoter region of DRD4 associated with the human novelty seeking personality trait. *Mol Psychiatry* 5: 64-69.
[70] Okuyama Y, Ishiguro H, Toru M, et al. (1999) A genetic polymorphism in the promoter region of DRD4 associated with expression and schizophrenia. *Biochem Biophys Res Commun* 258: 292-295.
[71] Mitsuyasu H, Hirata N, Sakai Y, et al. (2001) Association analysis of polymorphisms in the upstream region of the human dopamine D4 receptor gene (DRD4) with schizophrenia and personality traits. *J Hum Genet* 46: 26-31.
[72] Jönsson EG, Ivo R, Forslund K et al. (2001) No association between a promoter Dopamine D4 receptor gene variant and schizophrenia. *Am J Med Genet* 105B: 525-528.
[73] Lakatos K, Nemoda Z, Toth I, et al. (2002) Further evidence for the role of dopamine D4 receptor (DRD4) gene in attachment disorganization: interaction of the exon III 48-bp repeat and the –521 C/T promoter polymorphisms. *Mol Psychiatry* 7: 27-31.
[74] Gervai J, Nemoda Z, Lakatos K , et al. (2005) Transmission disequilibrium tests confirm the link between DRD4 gene polymorphism and infant attachment. *Am J Med Genet* 132B: 126-130.

[75] Kereszturi E, Király O, Csapó Z, et al. (2007) Analysis of the dopamine D4 receptor gene variants in attention deficit hyperactivity disorder. *Neuropsychopharmacol Hung* 9: 11-18.

[76] Paterson AD, Ying D-J, Petronis A, et al. (1996) A PstI restriction fragment length polymorphism in the 5'untranslated region of DRD4 is not associated with schizophrenia. *Psychiatric Genet* 6: 191-193.

[77] Todd RD, Neuman RJ, Lobos EA, et al. (2001) Lack of association of dopamine D4 receptor gene polymorphisms with ADHD subtypes in a population sample of twins. *Am J Med Genet* 105B: 432-438.

[78] Catalano M, Nobile M, Novelli E, et al. (1993) Distribution of a novel mutation in the first exon of the human dopamine D4 receptor gene in psychotic patients. *Biol Psychol* 34: 459-464.

[79] Barr CL, Wigg K, Bloom S, et al. (2000) Further evidence from haplotype analysis for linkage of the dopamine D4 receptor gene and attention-deficit hyperactivity disorder. *Am J Med Genet* 96B: 262-267.

[80] van Tol HH, Wu CM, Guan HC, et al. (1992) Multiple dopamine D4 receptor variants in the human population. *Nature* 358: 149-52.

[81] Bhaduri N, Das M, Sinha S, et al. (2006) Association of Dopamine D4 Receptor (DRD4) polymorphisms with Attention Deficit Hyperactivity Disorder in Indian population. *Am J Med Genet* 141B: 61 - 66.

[82] Chang FM, Kidd JR, Livak KJ, et al. (1996) The world wide distribution of allele frequencies at the human dopamine D4 receptor locus. *Human Genet* 98: 91-101.

[83] Ding Y-C, Chi H-C, Grady DL, et al. (2002) Evidence of positive selection acting at the human dopamine receptor D4 gene locus. *Proc Natl Acad Sci USA* 99: 309-314.

[84] Grady DL, Chi H-C, Ding Y-C, et al. (2003) High prevalence of rare dopamine receptor D4 alleles in children diagnosed with attention-deficit hyperactivity disorder. *Mol Psychiatry* 8: 536-545.

[85] Asghari V, Sanyal S, Buchwaldt S, et al. (1995) Modulation of intracellular cyclic AMP levels by different human dopamine D4 receptor variants. *J Neurochem* 65: 1157-1165.

[86] Faraone SV, Perlis RH, Doyle AE, et al. (2005) Advancing the neuroscience of ADHD: Molecular genetics of attention-deficit/hyperactivity disorder. *Biol Psychiatry* 57: 1313-1323.

[87] Swanson JM, Sunohara GA, Kennedy JL, et al. (1998) Association of the dopamine receptor D4 (DRD4) gene with a refined phenotype of attention deficit hyperactivity disorder (ADHD): a family-based approach. *Mol Psychiatry* 3: 38-41.

[88] Smalley SL, Bailey JN, Palmer CG, et al. (1998) Evidence that the dopamine D4 receptor is a susceptibility gene in attention deficit. *Mol Psychiatry* 3: 427-430.

[89] Mill J, Fischer N, Curran S, et al. (2003) Polymorphisms in the dopamine D4 receptor gene and attention deficit hyperactivity disorder. *Neuroreport* 14: 1463-1466.

[90] Strobel A, Lesch KP, Hohenberger K, et al. (2002) No association between dopamine D4 receptor gene exon III and –521 C/T polymorphism and novelty seeking. *Mol Psychiatry* 7: 537-538.

[91] Barr CL, Feng Y, Wigg KG, et al. (2001) 5'-untranslated region of the dopamine D4 receptor gene and attention-deficit hyperactivity disorder. *Am J Med Genet* 105: 84-90.

[92] Lowe N, Kirley A, Mullins C, et al. (2004) Multiple marker analysis at the promoter region of the DRD4 gene and ADHD: evidence of linkage and association with SNP –616. *Am J Med Genet* 131B: 33-37.

[93] Bellgrove MA, Hawi Z, Kirley A, et al. (2005) Association between dopamine transporter (DAT1) genotype, left-sided inattention, and an enhanced response to methylphenidate in attention-deficit hyperactivity disorder. *Neuropsychopharmacol* 30: 2290-2297.

[94] Giros B, el Mestikawy S, Godinot N, et al. (1992) Cloning, pharmacological characterization, and chromosome assignment of the human dopamine transporter. *Mol Pharmacol* 42: 383-390.

[95] Swanson JM, Flodman P, Kennedy J, et al. (2000) Dopamine genes and ADHD. *Neurosci and Behav Reviews* 24: 21-25.

[96] Mill J, Asherson P, Browes C, et al. (2002) Expression of the dopamine transporter gene is regulated by the 3' UTR VNTR: evidence from brain and lymphocytes using quantitative RT-PCR. *Am J Med Genet* 114B: 975-979.

[97] Das M, Mukhopadhyay K. (2007) DAT1 3'-UTR 9R allele: preferential transmission in Indian children with attention deficit hyperactivity disorder. *Am J Med Genet* 144B:826-829.

[98] Guindalini C, Howard M, Haddley K, et al. (2006) A dopamine transporter gene functional variant associated with cocaine abuse in a Brazilian sample. *Proc Natl Acad Sci USA* 103: 4552-4557.

[99] Brookes KJ, Mill J, Guindalini C, et al. (2006) A common haplotype of the dopamine transporter gene associated with attention-deficit/hyperactivity disorder and interacting with maternal use of alcohol during pregnancy. *Arch Gen Psychiatry* 63: 74-81.

[100] Bhaduri N, Sinha S, Chattopadhyay A, et al. (2005) Analysis of polymorphisms in the dopamine beta hydroxylase gene: association with attention deficit hyperactivity disorder in Indian children. *Ind Pediatrics* 42: 123-129.

[101] Smith KM, Daly M, Fischer M, et al. (2003) Association of the dopamine beta hydroxylase gene with attention deficit hyperactivity disorder: genetic analysis of the Milwaukee longitudinal study. *Am J Med Genet* 119: 77-85.

[102] Sabol SZ, Hu S, Hamer D. (1998) A functional polymorphism in the monoamine oxidase A gene promoter. *Human Genet* 103: 273-279.

[103] Deckert J, Catalano M, Syagailo YV, et al. (1999) Excess of high activity monoamine oxidase A gene promoter alleles in female patients with panic disorder. *Human Mol Genet* 8: 621-624.

[104] Manuck SB, Flory JD, Ferrel RE, et al. (2000) A regulatory polymorphism of monoamine oxidase-A gene may be associated with variability in aggression, impulsivity, and central nervous system serotonergic responsivity. *Psychiatr Res* 95: 9-23.

[105] Das M, Bhowmik AD, Sinha S, et al. (2006) MAOA promoter polymorphism and attention deficit hyperactivity disorder (ADHD) in Indian children. *Am J Med Genet* 141B: 637-642.

[106] Hotamisligil GS, Breakefield XO. (1991) Human monoamine oxidase A gene determines levels of enzyme activity. *Am J Hum Genet* 49: 383-392.

[107] Furlong RA, Luk H, Walsh C, Rubinsztein DC. (1999) Analysis of monoamine oxidase A (MAOA) gene in bipolar effective disorder by association studies, meta-analysis, and sequencing of the promoter. *Am J Med Genet* 88: 398-406.

[108] Lawson DC, Turic D, Langley K, et al. (2003) Association analysis of monoamine A and attention deficit hyperactivity disorder. *Am J Med Genet* 116: 84-89.

[109] Guan LL, Wang YF, Li J, et al. (2007) Association analysis of dopamine D4 receptor gene polymorphisms and attention deficit hyperactivity disorder with/without disruptive behavior disorder. *Beijing Da Xue Xue Bao* 39: 233-236.

[110] Kustanovich V, Merriman B, McGough J, et al. (2003) Biased paternal transmission of SNAP-25 risk alleles in attention-deficit hyperactivity disorder. *Mol Psychiatry* 8: 309-315.

[111] Feng Y, Crosbie J, Wigg K, et al. (2005) The SNAP25 gene as a susceptibility gene contributing to attention-deficit hyperactivity disorder. *Mol Psychiatry* 10: 998-1005.

[112] Hawi Z, Segurado R, Conroy J, et al. (2005) Preferential transmission of paternal alleles at risk genes in attention-deficit/hyperactivity disorder. *Am J Hum Genet* 77: 958-965.

[113] Roman T, Schmitz M, Polanczyk G, et al. (2001) Attention-deficit hyperactivity disorder: a study of association with both the dopamine transporter gene and the dopamine D4 receptor gene. *Am J Med Genet* 105B:471–478.

[114] Qian Q, Wang Y, Li J, et al. (2007) Evaluation of potential gene–gene interactions for attention deficit hyperactivity disorder in the Han Chinese population. *Am J Med Genet* 144B:200–206.

[115] Meyer UA. (2002) Introduction to pharmacogenomics: promises, opportunities, and limitations. In Licinio J, Wong M (eds): Pharmacogenomics. Weinherim, Germany: Wiley-VCH1-8.

[116] Faraone SV, Doyle AE. (2001) The nature and heritability of attention-deficit/hyperactivity disorder. *Child Adolesc Psychiatr Clin N Am* 10: 299-316.

[117] Stein MA, McGough JJ. (2008) The Pharmacogenomic Era: promise for personalizing attention deficit hyperactivity disorder therapy. *Child Adolesc Psychiatric Clin N Am* 17: 475–490.

[118] Das Banerjee T, Middleton F, Faraone SV. (2007) Environmental risk factors for attention-deficit hyperactivity disorder. *Acta Pœdiatrica* 96:1269–1274.

In: Attention Deficit Hyperactivity Disorder (ADHD)
Editors: Stuart M. Gordon and Aileen E. Mitchell
ISBN 978-1-60741-581-7

Chapter 5

Coercive Processes and Child Vagal Tone in Families of Preschoolers with Attention-Deficit/Hyperactivity Disorder

Emily Neuhaus, Theodore P. Beauchaine*, M. Jamila Reid and Carolyn Webster-Stratton
University of Washington, Seattle, WA, USA

Abstract

Longitudinal research indicates that early emerging attention-deficit/hyperactivity disorder (ADHD) can mark the beginning of a developmental pathway that ends in antisocial behavior. Parent-child interactions characterized by coercive cycles of escalation—the tendency to match or exceed a partner's level of aversiveness—may contribute to children's progression along this pathway. In this study, we explored coercive escalation among preschoolers both with and without ADHD. Parent-child interactions during a laboratory task were coded for escalation, and oppositional behavior was assessed via parent report and observational ratings. Respiratory sinus arrhythmia (RSA), a physiological marker of emotion dysregulation, was also collected. Escalation by the child was correlated with oppositional behavior, with a stronger relationship found for observational ratings than for parent reports. Escalation was not correlated with RSA. However, low RSA was associated with observed emotion dysregulation and opposition. Thus, escalation and RSA emerged as independent correlates of oppositional behavior in this high risk sample.

* Correspondence should be addressed to Theodore P. Beauchaine, University of Washington, Box 351525, Seattle, WA 98195-1525. E-mail may be sent to tbeaucha@u.washington.edu.

Attention-deficit/hyperactivity disorder (ADHD) in early childhood is among the most reliable predictors of more severe externalizing behaviors in later childhood and adolescence (Campbell, Shaw, and Gilliom, 2000). Among children with ADHD, up to 60% will meet criteria for oppositional defiant disorder (ODD) by age 7, and up to 50% will eventually qualify for a diagnosis of conduct disorder (CD; Barkley, 1990; Biederman, Faraone, and Lapey, 1992). By adulthood, as many as 25% of clinic-referred children with ADHD meet criteria for antisocial personality disorder (Biederman et al., 1992). Thus, for many children, early emerging ADHD marks the beginning of a problematic developmental trajectory—one characterized by increasing antisocial behavior, with potentially large costs to both individuals and society (Patterson, DeGarmo, and Knutson, 2000).

Once serious externalizing behaviors are established, they are exceedingly difficult to treat. In preschool and early childhood, about two thirds of children with conduct problems benefit from current intervention approaches (Webster-Stratton and Hammond, 1997). Yet interventions become increasingly less effective in later childhood and adolescence (Dishion and Patterson, 1992). Given this, specification of etiological factors involved in the progression of ADHD to more serious externalizing behaviors, and early identification of those at highest risk for adverse outcomes, are critical (Beauchaine, Neuhaus, Brenner, and Gatzke-Kopp, 2008).

Behavioral genetics studies indicate that hyperactivity/impulsivity, the core behavioral trait underlying ADHD (Barkley, 1997), is roughly 80% heritable (Levy, Hay, McStephen, Wood, and Waldman, 1997; Price, Simonoff, Waldman, Asherson, and Plomin, 2001; Krueger et al., 2002). However, environmental influences play a strong role in determining whether trait impulsivity leads to ADHD only, or whether it is shaped into more serious externalizing behaviors later in development (Beauchaine and Neuhaus, 2008; Krueger and Markon, 2006; Lynam et al., 2000; Patterson et al., 2000). Clearly, not all children with ADHD develop more serious externalizing disorders, but nearly all individuals who eventually display serious antisocial behavior begin with marked hyperactivity and progress through stages of increasingly serious conduct problems (Patterson, DeGarmo, and Knutson, 2000). Thus, further specification of environmental potentiators of inherited vulnerability may provide key insights into etiology and suggest possible points for intervention.

Considerable evidence identifies parenting as a key mechanism through which children's impulsive behaviors progress from ADHD to more severe externalizing problems. Families of children further along the antisocial trajectory exhibit a number of common characteristics, including coercive discipline strategies (Patterson et al., 2000). Mothers of impulsive preschoolers suggest fewer positive and preventive strategies and more negative and controlling strategies for managing their children's behavior (Cunningham and Boyle, 2002), and mothers of aggressive sons demonstrate a restricted range of competent responses to child noncompliance (Beauchaine, Strassberg, Kees, and Drabick, 2002).

According to the coercion theory advanced by Patterson and colleagues (e.g., Patterson, 1982), instances of aversive behavior in the families of externalizing children are frequently reinforced by the reactions of others within the household. In such exchanges, aversive behaviors by one dyad member (e.g., mother yells) are met with aversive behaviors from the other member (e.g., child yells and kicks). If the mother then ceases the original aversive behavior, the child's increased aversiveness is negatively reinforced.

Such patterns are repeated thousands of times in the families of many children with conduct problems, resulting in escalating levels of aversiveness from both members as each is reinforced for their use of negative tactics by the termination of their partner's aversiveness. This escalation may result eventually in physical aggression and thus contribute to the development of further behavioral problems culminating in emotional lability and psychopathology (Patterson, 1982; see also Beauchaine, Gatzke-Kopp, and Mead, 2007; Snyder et al., 1997, 2000).

Coercive behavior patterns characterize many families of children who are on an antisocial trajectory. Snyder, Edwards, McGraw, Kilgore and Holton (1994) found higher rates of escalation in dyads of mothers and their 5-year-old aggressive sons than in a group of nonaggressive dyads. Beauchaine and colleagues (2002) found similar group differences when comparing interaction patterns of mothers and their 4-6-year-old aggressive sons versus mothers and their nonaggressive sons, even after controlling for children's noncompliance.

Compared with typically-developing youth, children with ADHD represent a group at especially high risk for initiating this pattern. The hyperactivity, impulsivity, and motor activity associated with ADHD produce behaviors that many find aversive. Parents of children with ADHD experience increased parenting stress compared with controls (Fischer, 1990), suggesting that their children's ADHD behaviors prove especially challenging to manage. When children with ADHD exhibit higher rates of escalation-initiating behaviors, the stage may be set for the negative reinforcement and coercive family processes described by Patterson (1982). These children and their families therefore represent an important opportunity to examine putative mechanisms through which ADHD progresses to more serious externalizing behaviors—such as coercive family processes (see Patterson et al., 2000).

Given the importance of coercive family processes in a child's progression toward increasingly antisocial behavior, evidence of these interaction styles early in the developmental trajectory might suggest a possible point of intervention and prevention. Although some research has focused on younger children (e.g., Beauchaine et al., 2002; Snyder et al., 1994), most research relevant to this trajectory has focused on later childhood, adolescence, and adulthood (e.g., Snyder, Schrepferman and St. Peter, 1997; Patterson, DeGarmo and Knutson, 2000). The fact that coercive patterns of interaction have been demonstrated repeatedly in families in which the child has already progressed some distance along the antisocial trajectory of ADHD to ODD to CD suggests that levels of escalation in families of younger at-risk children may already be elevated compared with control families. In the current study, we examined patterns of escalation in parent-child dyads in which the children were of preschool age, with the hypothesis that dyads with children with ADHD would display more escalation than dyads with children without ADHD.

In addition, if escalation reflects a risk factor for the progression of antisocial behavior, then the degree of escalation should correlate with the degree to which behavior problems are already being displayed in other settings. Thus, escalation rates should be correlated with the amount of ODD-consistent behaviors displayed by the child. Given that ODD reflects the next step along the antisocial trajectory, emerging indicators of antisocial behavior should appear first on measures of ODD. Accordingly, we also explored the associations between the degree of escalation exhibited by parent-child dyads and the degree to which children displayed ODD-consistent behaviors, predicting that children from dyads higher in escalation would be higher in oppositional behavior.

In addition to reinforcing negative interactions, the coercive pattern of escalation described by Patterson (1982) might also serve to reinforce additional behaviors of children with ADHD. Coercive interactions are also characterized by significant emotional arousal on the part of both parents and children (Snyder et al., 1994, 1997). Over time, this pattern may reinforce emotional lability, interfering with the development of important emotion regulation capabilities of at-risk children (Beauchaine et al., 2007). Put another way, dyadic interactions of non-escalating families likely provide opportunities for emotion regulation rehearsal that the children of escalating families forego. As a result, children of families in which escalation is common may have difficulty developing consistent emotion regulation abilities, further amplifying emotional lability that is shaped directly in aversive interactions.

To date, research suggests that children with early ADHD experience problems with emotion regulation. According to parent reports, children with ADHD are more reactive emotionally than control children, particularly with regard to negative emotions (Jensen and Rosén, 2004). Observational data support these findings; even when instructed to hide signs of frustration during a challenging task, boys with ADHD display more negative emotion than control children (Walcott and Landau, 2004).

In contrast to these reports, other models speculate that temperamental negative affectivity is distinct from hyperactivity, reflecting separate vulnerability factors for the development of ADHD (Martel and Nigg, 2006). In addition, the extent to which emotion dysregulation characterizes all subtypes of ADHD is unclear, as children with the primarily inattentive subtype may not demonstrate the increased reactivity often found in children with the hyperactive/impulsive and combined subtypes (Maedgen and Carlson, 2000). Finally, questions persist over the extent to which deficits in emotion regulation are specific to ADHD versus later emerging aggression and oppositionality that often accompany the diagnosis (Melnick and Hinshaw, 2000; Walcott and Landau, 2004).

One objective means of inferring emotional lability or regulation is via respiratory sinus arrhythmia (RSA; see Beauchaine, 2001). RSA quantifies the magnitude of cyclic increases and decreases in heart rate over the respiratory cycle, and reflects cholinergic activity of the parasympathetic nervous system. Both baseline RSA and RSA reactivity (change from baseline under various stimulus conditions) have been used as markers of emotional lability. Across a number of studies, low baseline RSA has been observed among emotionally labile individuals, whereas high baseline RSA appears to mark emotional stability (Beauchaine et al., 2007; Crowell et al., 2006; Friedman and Thayer, 1998; Gottman and Katz, 2002; Yeragani et al., 1993). Evidence also indicates that excessive RSA reactivity (i.e., vagal withdrawal) during emotional challenge is associated with emotional lability (Crowell et al., 2005; Beauchaine, 2001; Gottman et al., 1995), though some degree of vagal withdrawal appears to be adaptive (Beauchaine, 2001). Accordingly, we assessed both baseline RSA and RSA reactivity during an emotional challenge.

Given that coercive processes are associated with reinforcement of emotional lability (Snyder et al, 1997), such processes may also be associated with compromises in children's RSA. Behavioral genetics studies indicate that RSA is about 50% heritable and 50% environmentally determined (Kupper et al., 2005; Sneider, Boomsma, van Doornen and

DeGeus, 1997). Negative reinforcement of emotional lability may be one mechanism through which environment shapes RSA (Beauchaine et al., 2007). If this is the case, high levels of escalation should be associated with low levels of baseline RSA and greater RSA reactivity. Following from this discussion, our goal in conducting this study was to explore links between (a) escalation within parent-child interactions, (b) oppositional child behaviors, and (c) RSA, a physiological marker of emotion dysregulation in children.

In examining these associations, the preschool age range was chosen for a number of reasons. First, preschool children are the least far along the antisocial trajectory, so escalation at this early age would support the supposition that coercive processes serve as a risk factor for, rather than a result of, later conduct problems or heightened aggression. Furthermore, the preschool period reflects a critical stage in the development of emotion regulation, which is socialized primarily by parents when children are very young (Maccoby, 1992). Accordingly, ineffective or problematic parenting during this time might be particularly influential in determining a child's future behavior. Finally, the preschool age range is a particularly stressful time for parents of hyperactive children (Mash and Johnston, 1983), so the potential for aversive interactions might be especially high.

In this study, we explored escalation processes in a group of preschool children with and without ADHD, and their parents. We hypothesized that dyads with an ADHD child would exhibit more instances of escalation during a semi-structured parent-child interaction than control dyads. In addition, we hypothesized that across dyads, escalation would correlate with ODD-consistent behaviors displayed by the child. Finally, we hypothesized that escalation would correlate negatively with RSA.

Method

All procedures in the current study were approved by the Human Subjects Division at the University of Washington.

Participants

Thirty seven children between the ages of 4 and 7 participated in the study (15 female, 22 male). At the time of testing, no children were taking stimulants (an entry criterion). The racial/ethnic composition of the sample included 29 participants who identified as Caucasian, 2 who identified as African American, 2 who identified as Asian American, 1 who identified as Latino, and 3 who did not identify with any racial/ethnic group. No difference in racial/ethnic composition was observed between the ADHD and control groups, described immediately below. All parents provided informed consent prior to participating.

Approximately half (n = 20) of the sample was recruited for high levels of hyperactivity/impulsivity as part of a larger study examining treatment outcomes and patterns of physiological responding of preschool children with ADHD. In order to avoid any confound with intervention effects, all participants completed their assessments prior to beginning treatment. Participants in the ADHD group were required to (a) score at or above the 98th percentile on the attention problems subscale of the Child Behavior Checklist (Achenbach, 1991) and (b) meet full *DSM-IV* (APA, 2000) criteria for the hyperactive/impulsive or combined subtype of ADHD, as assessed using the Child Symptom Inventory (CSI; Gadow and Sprafkin, 1997, see below). As shown in Table 1, the mean *T*-score on the attention problems scale of the CBCL for this group was 75.9 (SD=6.59), and their mean raw score on the CSI was 37.8 (SD = 5.87). Thus, all children in this group qualified for an ADHD diagnosis. The mean age of children in the ADHD group was 5.63 (SD = .95) years.

The remaining 17 children were community controls. Children in this group were required to score below the 60th percentile on the attention problems subscale of the CBCL. In addition, inclusion required that parents endorsed no more than two criteria for ADHD or ODD on the CSI. The mean CBCL *T*-score for the group was 53.18 (SD = 3.26), and their mean CSI score was 10.12 (SD = 3.76). The mean age of children in the control group was 4.79 (SD = .46) years. Because the difference in age between ADHD participants and controls was significant, $F(1, 35) = 11.2$, $p < .01$, $d = 1.10$, all group comparisons were run with age as a covariate[1]. Psychopathology scores are reported by group in Table 1.

Table 1. Psychopathology and Observed Respiratory Sinus Arrhythmia by Group

	ADHD (n = 20)	Control (n = 17)		
Variable	Mean (*SD*)	Mean (*SD*)	Effect size (*d*)	*F*-ratio
CBCL attention problems (*T*)	75.9 (6.6)	53.2 (3.3)	4.4	148.2***
CSI ADHD raw score	37.8 (5.9)	10.1 (3.8)	5.6	199.8***
CSI ODD raw score	12.1 (4.6)	4.9 (1.6)	2.1	29.9***
Observed ODD composite score	9.58 (4.0)	7.9 (2.4)	0.5	2.1
Observed emotion dysregulation	2.15 (1.4)	1.35 (1.0)	0.7	2.85
Baseline RSA [log(beats/min^2/Hz.)]	6.4 (1.3)	6.9 (1.3)	0.4	2.3
RSA reactivity – Free play	-.53 (1.04)	-.84 (.67)	0.4	.54
RSA reactivity – Block building	-.88 (.92)	-.88 (.71)	0.0	.14
RSA reactivity – Clean up	-.89 (-1.1)	-1.4 (1.3)	0.4	.26

Notes. CBCL = Child Behavior Checklist; CSI = Child Symptom Inventory; ADHD = attention-deficit/hyperactivity disorder; ODD = oppositional defiant disorder; RSA = respiratory sinus arrhythmia. All group comparisons were conducted controlling for age at time of assessment.
***$p < .001$.

1 Because children in the control group were younger than children in the ADHD group, age-related effects on behavior are likely to have worked against study hypotheses, as oppositional behavior declines with increasing age in normal samples. Nevertheless, we covaried age in all group comparisons.

Measures

Attention problems. As noted above, the attention problems subscale of the Child Behavior Checklist (Achenbach, 1991) was used to assess problems with hyperactivity and inattention. The CBCL is a well-established parent-report measure on which parents rate their child's behavior on 3-point scales ranging from 0 (*not true*) to 2 (*very true or often true*). The CBCL has been normed among children ages 18 months and older (Achenbach and Rescorla, 2001), and provides continuous symptom scores for each domain assessed. Internal consistency values for the CBCL are high, ranging from .66 to .92, with similar test-retest reliabilities (.63 to .97).

In addition, the Child Symptom Inventory (CSI; Gadow and Sprafkin, 1997) was used to assess ADHD behaviors for each *DSM-IV* (APA, 2000) criterion. Parents rated their child's symptoms on 4-point scales (0 = *never*, 1 = *sometimes*, 2 = *often*, 3 = *very often*). When using the CSI, ratings of 2 or higher are considered positive for each diagnostic criterion. Internal consistency for the ADHD scale is .87 (Sprafkin, Gadow, Salisbury, Schneider and Loney, 2002), and test-retest reliabilities exceed .65 for intervals up to four months. The correlation between the attention problems subscale of the CBCL and the CSI ADHD scale (combined subtype) was .65, indicating good convergent validity between the measures.

Oppositional behavior. Oppositional behavior was assessed in two ways. First, parents completed the ODD subscale of the CSI (Gadow and Sprafkin, 1997), which has an internal consistency of .86 (Sprafkin et al., 2002). This provided a measure of each child's oppositional and defiant behavior during the course of normal daily activities. Oppositional behavior was also assessed behaviorally during a structured parent-child interaction (described below). Using a scale of 1 (*never*) to 5 (*very often*), coders rated each child on a number of items created to capture behavior consistent with ODD, including (1) was negative or critical, (2) was hostile or threatening, (3) used sarcasm in an aversive way, and (4) used aversive techniques to get his or her way. For each behavior, separate ratings for each of three lab tasks (described below) were averaged, producing a single rating on each behavior for each child. In addition, two items were rated across the entire set of tasks, including the frequency with which each child (1) seemed irritable or angry, and (2) complied with parental commands (reverse scored). These 6 ratings were then summed to create a behavioral opposition score for each child.

Parasympathetic nervous system (PNS) activity. Individual differences in PNS activity were captured by measuring baseline RSA, as well as RSA reactivity during segments of the interaction task. Baseline RSA was recorded during a 2-min quiet time during which children sat alone in a sound-attenuated room. Throughout the baseline period and interaction task, the EKG signal was acquired through electrodes arranged in a modified Lead II configuration. Because the attached leads allowed participants a relatively unrestricted range of movement, electrodes were rarely disturbed over the course of data collection. Parasympathetic-linked cardiac activity was indexed by spectral-analyzing the R-wave time series with software developed by Richard Sloan and his colleagues at Columbia University. High frequency spectral densities (>0.15 Hz) were computed in 30 s epochs. As is standard with such data, RSA values were natural log-transformed prior to group comparisons. Cholinergic blockade studies have supported the validity of RSA as a marker of parasympathetic-linked cardiac activity (see Berntson et al., 1997).

Physiological reactivity was computed by comparing RSA collected throughout the interaction task with the values collected during the baseline period. For each segment of the interaction task, a reactivity value was computed to reflect change relative to baseline functioning. Positive RSA reactivity values indicate increases from baseline, and negative RSA reactivity values indicate decreases from baseline.

Task

Each parent-child dyad participated in a three-part interaction task lasting approximately 20 min. Throughout the interaction, parents wore a small "bug in the ear" device that allowed research assistants to communicate with them. In the first segment of the interaction, each dyad engaged in freeplay with a set of foam blocks in a small playroom. After 7 min elapsed, parents were cued to begin a structured block-building task with their children. This task required participants to build a series of complex structures from two-dimensional pictures. During the task children were required to do all of the physical work, with only verbal assistance from their parents, who were prohibited from touching the blocks. This task was designed to be challenging, and no dyads completed it within the time allotted. Following 7 min of block-building, parents were cued to begin the clean up segment of the interaction. As in the preceding segment, parents were not allowed to touch the blocks. The interaction ended when 7 min of clean up had elapsed, or when the parent and child had put all of the blocks away. All segments of the parent-child interaction were videotaped for later coding.

Coding

Microsocial coding. Parent-child interactions were coded using the Family and Peer Process code (FPP code; Stubbs, Crosby, Forgatch and Capaldi, 1998), developed and used by the Oregon Social Learning Center. FPP code is a microsocial system that categorizes all verbal and most nonverbal behaviors performed by each participant in a given interaction. Behaviors receive a 5-digit code that includes information about the initiator (speaker/actor), the content, the recipient, and the affective valence of the behavior. Content is coded into one of 24 categories (e.g., positive interpersonal, self-disclose, disagree to directive), and affective valence is coded into one of six categories (happy, caring, neutral, distressed, aversive, or sad). All of the interactions were coded onsite by a trained coder. Approximately one fourth of the interactions were also coded by the experienced FPP coding team at the Oregon Social Learning Center. Reliability statistics were good (content κ = .77; affect κ = .66).

Codes were reduced using a method adapted from Snyder and colleagues (1994). This method combines content and affect ratings, collapsing them along a single dimension of "aversiveness", allowing direct comparisons between behaviors. For each individual, escalation was calculated as the conditional probability that the individual offered an aversive response given an aversive behavior from his/her interaction partner. That is, escalation was operationalized as a person's likelihood of responding aversively to an aversive behavior.

Emotion dysregulation. In addition to the microsocial coding system described above, interactions were also assigned global ratings along a number of dimensions. These ratings spanned the entire interaction period, using a 5-point scale ranging from "never" to "very often". The item "How often did [the child] display emotion that appeared to be uncontrolled?" was extracted as an indicator of emotion dysregulation. Although RSA has been construed as a psychophysiological marker of emotion regulation (Beauchaine, 2001; Beauchaine et al., 2007), it was important to include a behavioral measure as well.

Results

Descriptive statistics for both parent-reports and observational measures of oppositional behavior are reported in Table 1. As discussed above, all group comparisons were conducted while controlling for age at time of assessment; however we report raw means for ease of interpretation. As shown, the two groups differed significantly on parent ratings of ADHD and oppositional behavior, all $Fs(1, 34) \geq 29.9$, all $ps \leq .001$, all $ds \geq 2.1$. However, the groups did not differ on the observational measure of oppositional behavior during the interaction task, $F(1, 34) = 2.08$, $p = .16$, $d = 0.5$, although the difference in group means was of medium effect size and in the expected direction. The two groups did not differ in ratings of observed emotion dysregulation, $F(1, 34) = 2.85$, $p = .10$, $d = 0.7$

Table 1 displays group means for baseline respiratory sinus arrhythmia. When controlling for age, children with ADHD did not differ from controls, $F(1, 34) = 2.27$, $p = .14$, $d = 0.4$. This finding is consistent with our previous work comparing RSA between children with ADHD/ODD and controls in this age range (e.g., Crowell et al., 2006). Table 1 also displays group means for RSA reactivity across the segments of the interaction task. When controlling for age, children with ADHD did not differ in RSA reactivity from children in the control group during any of the three interaction segments, all $Fs(1,34) < 0.6$, all $ps > .46$.

Levels of aversive behavior during the parent-child interaction task are shown for both groups of participants in Table 2. Because the task consisted of three segments (freeplay, block building, and clean up), we assessed behavior for each dyad within each segment individually, and across the interaction as a whole. We also characterized behavior for each member of the dyad (parent and child) individually. Thus, each dyad received eight values reflecting aversive behavior (4 ratings × 2 members). Proportions of aversive behavior to total behavior by each participant in each segment of the task are reported in Table 2. As shown, the only group difference that emerged was during clean up, when children in the ADHD group exhibited a larger proportion of aversive behavior than children in the control group, $F(1, 34) = 12.84$, $p < .001$, $d = 0.91$. Thus, consistent with previous research, behavioral differences in oppositional behavior emerged when task demands were highest.

Our first hypothesis was that dyads in which the child had ADHD would display more escalation than dyads in which the child did not have ADHD. As described earlier, escalation was defined as any aversive behavior by one dyad member given aversive behavior by the other dyad member. The conditional probabilities for escalation are reported in Table 3. As shown, the groups differed on a number of values. During the task as a whole, children with ADHD exhibited more instances of responding to a parent's aversive behavior with their own aversive behavior, $F(1, 34) = 15.9$, $p < .001$, $d = 1.1$. As expected, this effect was driven largely by behavior during block building, $F(1, 34) = 8.5$, $p = .006$, $d = 0.8$, and clean up, $F(1, 34) = 17.6$, $p < .001$, $d = 1.1$. In contrast with the child data, escalation by parents did not differ across groups during any of the tasks, all *F*s < 0.9, all *p*s > .34. Thus, the first hypothesis was partially supported; although rates of parent escalation did not differ according to the presence of ADHD, escalation by the child was more frequent in dyads in which the child had ADHD.

Table 2. Proportions of Aversive Behavior by Group and Condition

	ADHD ($n = 20$)	Control ($n = 17$)		
Task	Mean (*SD*)	Mean (*SD*)	Effect size (*d*)	*F*-ratio
Free play				
Parent	.09 (.05)	.08 (.06)	0.2	0.5
Child	.14 (.15)	.12 (.17)	0.1	0.7
Block building				
Parent	.08 (.05)	.06 (.03)	0.5	0.1
Child	.19 (.10)	.18 (.10)	0.1	0.2
Cleanup				
Parent	.10 (.07)	.11 (.07)	0.1	0.2
Child	.28 (.20)	.14 (.09)	0.9	12.9***
Overall				
Parent	.09 (.04)	.07 (.03)	0.6	0.5
Child	.20 (.13)	.16 (.12)	0.3	2.8

Notes. All group comparisons were conducted controlling for age at time of assessment.
***$p < .001$.

Table 3. Conditional Probabilities of Aversive Responding to Aversiveness (Escalation)

	ADHD ($n = 20$)	Control ($n = 17$)		
Task	Mean (*SD*)	Mean (*SD*)	Effect size (*d*)	*F*-ratio
Free play				
Parent	.03 (.54)	.09 (.24)	0.1	0.5
Child	.05 (.12)	.03 (.09)	0.2	1.6
Block building				
Parent	.09 (.09)	.05 (.08)	0.5	0.2
Child	.12 (.17)	.02 (.05)	0.8	8.5**
Cleanup				
Parent	.04 (.06)	.03 (.12)	0.1	0.5

Child	.17 (.22)	.00 (.00)	1.1	17.6***
Overall				
Parent	.07 (.05)	.05 (.07)	0.3	0.9
Child	.11 (.11)	.02 (.05)	1.1	15.9***

Notes. All group comparisons were conducted controlling for age at time of assessment.
*p < .05. **p < .01 ***. p < .001.

Our second hypothesis was that across dyads, escalation during the parent-child interaction would correlate positively with oppositional behavior by the child. This hypothesis was first tested with regard to parent-reported oppositional behavior. Correlations between escalation and parents' reports of children's oppositional behavior are reported in Table 4. As indicated, the only significant correlation was for the clean up segment of the interaction task, $r = .33$, $p = .048$. During clean up, children who were rated as more oppositional displayed more escalation. In addition, the correlation between child escalation during block building and parent-reported oppositional behavior approached significance, $r = .27$, $p = .10$. Escalation by the parent was not associated with reported oppositional behavior in any segment of the interaction task.

Next, the hypothesized relation between escalation and opposition was tested with regard to oppositional behavior observed during the parent-child interaction. Across the interaction task, child oppositional behavior was correlated with child escalation, $r = .50$, $p = .002$. This pattern was driven by the correlations observed during free play, $r = .54$, $p = .001$, and clean up, $r = .35$, $p = .03$. As with parent-reported oppositional behavior, there were no significant associations between observed opposition and escalation by the parent in any parts of the task (see Table 4). Thus, our second hypothesis, that escalation would be correlated positively with oppositional behavior, was supported for child behavior but not for parent behavior. Links between child escalation and oppositional behavior were stronger for observed oppositional behavior than for parent-reported oppositional behavior.

Our third hypothesis was that escalation during the parent-child interaction would be correlated negatively with the child's baseline RSA. Associations between escalation and RSA were examined across the entire interaction, and during each individual task. Contrary to predictions, there were no significant correlations between baseline RSA and escalation, or between RSA reactivity and escalation in any of the segments of the parent-child interaction task (see Table 4). This pattern applied to both child and parent escalation. Thus, our third hypothesis was not supported in this sample of parent-child dyads.

Although uncorrelated with escalation, children's RSA was associated with several behavioral variables of interest, as shown in Table 4. First, baseline RSA was correlated negatively with observed oppositional behavior, $r = -.38$, $p = .02$. This finding is consistent with research on older children further along the antisocial pathway (Beauchaine et al., 2001, 2007; Mead et al., 2004; Mezzacappa et al., 1997). Additionally, observed oppositional behavior was correlated with changes in RSA during the clean up segment of the interaction task, $r = .38$, $p = .02$). Thus, children who displayed more oppositional behavior exhibited smaller reductions in RSA during clean up.

RSA was also associated with observational ratings of emotion dysregulation during the interaction. Baseline RSA was correlated negatively with observed emotion dysregulation ($r = -.35$, $p = .03$). Thus, children with lower baseline RSA exhibited more uncontrolled emotion during the task. In addition, RSA reactivity during clean up was associated with observed emotion dysregulation (r = .35, p = .04). These findings are also consistent with previous research (Beauchaine et al., 2001, 2007; Crowell et al., 2006; Gottman and Katz, 2002). Thus, even though RSA was not associated with escalation, it was associated with behavioral dysregulation, replicating results from several previous studies.

Discussion

A number of related hypotheses were explored in this study, with varying degrees of support found for each. First, we predicted that during a structured parent-child interaction, families with a child with ADHD would display more instances of escalation than families with a child without ADHD. This hypothesis was partially supported. Although parents' levels of escalation did not differ across the groups, children with ADHD were more likely than children without ADHD to engage in escalation.

The lack of group differences within parent behavior is surprising in light of the existing research on family interactions among children with attention and conduct problems. Compared to parents of typically-developing children, Tripp, Schaughency, Langlands, and Mouat (2007) found that parents of children with ADHD received lower global ratings of warmth, engagement, and communication during a problem solving task with their children. Similarly, Johnston and colleagues (2002) found a relationship between maternal responsiveness and fewer child behavior problems. However, their analyses indicated that this link was specific to child conduct problems, offering one possible explanation for the lack of parenting differences in our ADHD sample. Furthermore, these studies did not explore escalation directly.

The inconsistency between our findings and other reports in the literature may also be an artifact of our recruitment methods. Families of children with ADHD who participated in our study were recruited from a larger intervention effort targeting children with attentional difficulties and emerging conduct problems. Thus, they may not fully represent the population of parents of children with ADHD. Instead, they may represent a subset of parents who are especially motivated to enhance their parenting skills, due perhaps to the severity of their children's symptoms, or to their own responsiveness to the conflicts within their families. Such parent characteristics might account for the similarity across groups in rates of escalation.

Our second hypothesis predicted that the level of escalation observed during the parent-child interaction would be correlated positively with the child's level of oppositional behavior. This hypothesis was supported for children, but not for parents. Children who displayed more escalation also exhibited more oppositional behavior, particularly with regard to oppositional behavior assessed through observational means. In contrast to our hypothesis, and to findings reported with older children (Snyder et al., 1997; Patterson et al., 2000), no significant relations emerged between parental escalation and any other variables.

Table 4. Correlations between Escalation, Oppositional Behavior, Emotion Dysregulation, and Child RSA

	Escalation—Overall		Escalation—Free play		Escalation—Block building		Escalation—Clean up		Observed oppositional behavior	Observed emotion dysregulation
	Parent	Child	Parent	Child	Parent	Child	Parent	Child		
Parent-reported opposition	-.04	.14	-.19	-.18	-.06	.27	.06	.33*	.08	.19
Observed oppositional behavior	.14	.50**	-.07	.54**	-.01	.10	.19	.35*	—	.94***
RSA—Baseline	-.09	-.25	-.06	-.18	-.01	-.20	.22	-.13	-.38*	-.35*
RSA reactivity—Free play	-.12	.18	-.21	.19	-.03	.14	.09	-.08	.29	.29
RSA reactivity—Block building	.03	.03	-.17	.08	-.01	.16	.17	-.18	.26	.22
RSA reactivity—Clean up	-.15	-.08	-.13	.05	-.27	.10	-.01	.01	.38*	.35*

*$p < .05$. *** $p < .001$.

The discrepancy between our findings and the established literature on the role of parent-child interactions in the development of conduct problems is intriguing, and may be due to a number of factors. As discussed previously, it may be that the parents in this sample did not represent the parents typically included in similar research. Alternatively, the lack of association between parent and child behavior may be related to the developmental stage during which the data were collected. In the model originally proposed by Patterson (1992), Snyder and colleagues (1997), and others, escalation by both the parent and child shapes the behavior of the other via negative reinforcement. Each time an escalation in aversiveness terminates an unpleasant interaction, the cycle is strengthened. Accordingly, it was expected that escalation by parents would be associated with oppositional behavior by their children. However, this hypothesis assumes that the cycle of negative reinforcement has been enacted with sufficient frequency to become well established within a family, which likely requires many instances over many interactions. In fact, Sagvolden, Aase, Johansen, and Russell (2005) argue that the reinforcement gradient for children with ADHD differs from that of typically-developing children, such that they require more learning trials than their peers without ADHD to acquire learned behaviors. Perhaps families in our study are only beginning to shape one another through the cycle described by Patterson et al. and Snyder et al., and links between parental escalation and child opposition will become apparent in time. Although speculative, this possibility would reconcile differences between our findings and those in the published literature with older children.

Perhaps the most likely explanation for the inconsistencies between our current findings and the existing literature relates to the diagnostic status of the participating children. Much of the existing literature on mechanisms contributing to early conduct problems has been conducted with groups of children meeting criteria for both ADHD and a disruptive behavior disorder such as ODD (e.g., Schrepferman and Snyder, 2002). In the current study, typically-developing children were compared with children who met criteria for either the primarily hyperactive or combined subtypes of ADHD and demonstrated significant attention problems. Although it is likely that a number of these children would have also met criteria for ODD (given the comorbidity rates discussed previously), inclusion in the current study did not require such a diagnosis. This approach was pursued in order to allow emerging conduct problems to serve as a continuous outcome variable, increasing statistical power over group-comparison designs with categorical outcomes. However, the discrepancy between our current findings and those reported traditionally may be the result of the discrepancy between the diagnostic criteria chosen.

Our third hypothesis was that children's physiological dysregulation, as indexed by baseline RSA, would be associated with escalation by the parent. Had the proposed relation been found, it would have supported the notion that escalation reinforces dysregulation not only at the behavioral (Patterson, 1982) and emotional (Snyder et al., 1994) levels, but at the physiological level as well. However, the proposed correlation did not emerge, and the hypothesis was not supported by our data.

Although our results did not support the hypothesized link between escalation and RSA, RSA was associated with several other variables of interest. Children who displayed more oppositional behavior had lower baseline RSA. This relation is consistent with existing literature in which children and adolescents further along the antisocial trajectory differ from typically-developing peers on measures of autonomic functioning. In both middle-school-aged and adolescent males with conduct disorder, baseline RSA is significantly lower than that of controls (Beauchaine et al., 2001, 2007; Mead et al., 2004; Mezzacappa et al., 1997). Although we did not find RSA differences between groups of preschool children with and without ADHD, the negative correlation between RSA and observed oppositional behaviors is consistent with previous findings in studies of older children.

In addition, children who displayed higher levels of dysregulated emotion during the interaction task had lower baseline RSA. This finding adds to the substantial body of literature supporting RSA as a psychophysiological marker of emotion regulation (e.g., Beauchaine, 2001; Porges, Doussard-Roosevelt, and Maiti, 1994). Previous research has revealed attenuated RSA among individuals who engage in self-injury (Crowell et al., 2005), those who are anxious (Lyonfields et al., 1995), and those with aggression and CD (Beauchaine et al., 2001, 2007; Mezzacappa et al., 1997). Furthermore, given the widespread difficulties inherent in defining emotion regulation at the cognitive and experiential levels (Cole, Martin and Dennis, 2004), neurobiological markers such as RSA are especially valuable. Our findings support the feasibility of collecting RSA with a sample of young children who may not have the developmental capacity or introspection required to provide self-report data on their emotional experiences and capabilities.

Links between RSA reactivity and behavioral measures were somewhat less clear in our data. Change in RSA was correlated positively with both dysregulated emotion and observed oppositional behavior. Greater decreases in RSA were associated with less observed dysregulation, both emotionally and behaviorally. Initially, this finding is somewhat puzzling, as it indicates that children who displayed less dysregulation experienced the greatest degree of change in RSA. However, it is consistent with existing theories which suggest that optimal behavioral and emotional functioning is associated with moderate changes in RSA during demanding tasks (Beauchaine, 2001; Calkins, Graziano and Keane, 2007). That is, changes in RSA that are either very large or very small are thought to reflect emotion regulation capabilities that are insufficient to adapt appropriately to changing environmental conditions. In contrast, moderate changes in RSA are thought to reflect a system that is appropriately responsive to the environment (Porges, Doussard-Roosevelt, and Maiti, 1994). Of course, what constitutes "very large," "very small," or "moderate" amounts of change is dependent upon the task in question, the age of participants, and other factors, but it may be that the larger decreases in RSA experienced by the children who displayed the least behavioral and emotional dysregulation represent such a "moderate" change; the absence of such a decrease was associated with greater emotional and behavioral dysregulation, perhaps indicating a suboptimal parasympathetic response.

As a whole, findings from this study highlight several important issues at both conceptual and practical levels. With regard to children's physiological functioning, RSA is emerging as an important indicator of risk for psychopathology. Recent findings indicate that low baseline RSA represents a biologically-based vulnerability to the negative effects of maladaptive environmental influences. For instance, within a sample of children and adolescents, high RSA offered partial protection against the development of psychopathology in the context of parental psychopathology (Shannon et al., 2007). Among participants with fathers high in antisocial features, children with high RSA were less likely to develop conduct problems than those with low RSA. Similar findings indicate that high RSA predicts fewer behavior problems and better emotion regulation abilities in children exposed to marital conflict (Katz and Gottman, 1997). Thus, high baseline RSA appears to protect children from maladaptive outcomes under a variety of stressful environmental conditions, whereas low baseline RSA indicates vulnerability to negative environmental conditions.

These findings have direct implications for prevention and intervention of conduct problems in young children. For example, RSA may prove to moderate children's responses to intervention, as it has in some contexts (e.g., Beauchaine, Gartner, and Hagen, 2000). Assuming that RSA is indeed a physiological marker of emotion regulation, treatment programs that target emotion regulation skills may have differential effects on children according to their baseline functioning. Although this possibility has not yet been tested empirically, existing research highlights the moderating effect of other biological markers on treatment response (Beauchaine et al., 2008). Within the autonomic nervous system, skin conductance activity during gambling tasks predicts response to preventive substance use interventions for adolescents (Fishbein, Hyde, Coe, and Paschall, 2004). Similarly, heart rate variability moderates treatment outcome for adolescent males with depression and conduct problems (Beauchaine et al., 2000). As a potential marker of vulnerability, attenuated RSA may indicate children whose biological functioning renders them particularly susceptible to the coercive effects of conflictual family interactions. Accordingly, interventions that target coercive family interactions may prove especially beneficial for those families in which children's oppositional behavior is driven by a combination of parenting and physiological factors.

Furthermore, associations such as those found here between child escalation and opposition may indicate that intervention efforts targeting family interaction patterns are well-placed. Many current interventions, such as the Incredible Years series (Webster-Stratton, 2005) and McMahon and Forehand's (2003) Helping the Noncompliant Child treatment, emphasize improvement in parent-child interactions as a primary treatment goal for families in which children have established conduct problems. However, our results indicate that such efforts might also be beneficial for children who are only begin to develop significant conduct problems. In our sample, children with ADHD displayed more instances of escalation throughout the course of the interaction task relative to the control group. This heightened level of aversive responding suggests the need for strategies addressing parent-child interactions within treatment programs aimed at ADHD, and not only those interventions that target conduct problems explicitly.

Conclusions

Taken together, these findings suggest that children's RSA and escalation during parent-child interactions provide independent prediction of oppositional behavior in preschool children. Although the role of coercive parenting has been appreciated for some time (e.g., Patterson, 1982), far less is known regarding the role of autonomic vulnerabilities in the progression to antisocial behavior. Given the longitudinal nature of these relationships, it is likely that the relative contributions of different factors change over time. That is, individual factors may play greater or lesser roles at various points across development. Indeed, current conceptualizations of the etiology and progression of ADHD and conduct problems posit a transactional model in which behavioral and environmental factors interact over the course of years. These findings highlight the potential role of biological factors within such a model. If this supposition is supported by further research, RSA may become an important index of vulnerability to externalizing psychopathology.

Acknowledgment

Work on this article was supported by Grants MH63699 and MH067192 from the National Institute of Mental Health. We express thanks to Jane Chipman for her helpful contributions.

References

Achenbach, T. M. (1991). *Manual for the Child Behavior Checklist/4-18 and 1991 profile.* Burlington, VT: University of Vermont Department of Psychiatry.

Achenbach, T. M., and Rescorla, L. A. (2001). *Manual for ASEBA School-Age Forms and Profiles.* Burlington, VT: University of Vermont, Research Center for Children, Youth, and Families.

American Psychiatric Association (2000). *Diagnostic and statistical manual of mental disorders* (4th ed. Text revision). Washington, DC: Author.

Arnold, D. S., O'Leary, S. G., Wolff, L. S., and Acker, M. M. (1993). The Parenting Scale: A measure of dysfunctional parenting in discipline situations. *Psychological Assessment, 5,* 137-144.

Barkley, R. A. (1996). Attention-deficit/hyperactivity disorder. In E. J. Mash and R. A. Barkley (Eds.). *Child psychopathology* (pp. 63-112). New York, NY: Guilford Press.

Barkley, R.A. (1997). Behavioral inhibition, sustained attention, and executive functions: Constructing a unifying theory of ADHD. *Psychological Bulletin, 121*, 65-94.

Beauchaine, T. P. (2001). Vagal tone, development, and Gray's motivational theory: Toward an integrated model of autonomic nervous system functioning in psychopathology. *Development and Psychopathology, 13,* 183-214.

Beauchaine, T. P., Gartner, J., and Hagen, B. (2000). Comorbid depression and heart rate variability as predictors of aggressive and hyperactive symptom responsiveness during inpatient treatment of conduct-disordered, ADHD boys. *Aggressive Behavior, 26,* 425-441.

Beauchaine, T. P., Gatzke-Kopp, L., and Mead, H. (2007). Polyvagal Theory and developmental psychopathology: Emotion dysregulation and conduct problems from preschool to adolescence. *Biological Psychology, 74*, 174-184.

Beauchaine, T. P., Katkin, E. S., Strassberg, Z., and Snarr, J. (2001). Disinhibitory psychopathology in male adolescents: Discriminating conduct disorder from attention-deficit/hyperactivity disorder through concurrent assessment of multiple autonomic states. *Journal of Abnormal Psychology, 110,* 610-624.

Beauchaine, T. P., and Neuhaus, E. (2008). Behavioral disinhibition and vulnerability to psychopathology. In T. P. Beauchaine and S. P. Hinshaw (Eds.), *Child psychopathology* (pp. 129-156). Hoboken, NJ: Wiley.

Beauchaine, T. P., Neuhaus, E., Brenner, S. L., and Gatzke-Kopp, L. (2008). Ten good reasons to consider biological variables in prevention and intervention research. *Development and Psychopathology, 20,* 745-774.

Beauchaine, T. P., Strassberg, Z. , Kees, M. R., and Drabick, D. A. G. (2002). Cognitive response repertoires to child noncompliance by mothers of aggressive boys. *Journal of Abnormal Child Psychology, 30,* 89-101.

Berntson, G. G., Bigger, T., Eckberg, D. L., Grossman, P., Kaufman, P. G., Malik, M., et al. (1997). Heart rate variability: Origins, methods, and interpretive caveats. *Psychophysiology, 34*, 623–648.

Biederman, J., Faraone, S. V. and Lapey, K. (1992). Comorbidity of diagnosis in attention-deficit hyperactivity disorder. In G. Weiss (Ed.), *Child and adolescent psychiatric clinics of North America: Attention-deficit hyperactivity disorder* (pp. 335-360). Philadelphia: Saunders.

Brown, S. A., Myers, M. G., Lippke, L., Tapert, S. F., and Stewart, D. G. (1998). Psychometric evaluation of the Customary Drinking and Drug Use Record (CDDR): A measure of adolescent alcohol and drug involvement. *Journal of Studies on Alcohol, 59,* 427-438.

Calkins, S. D., Graziano, P. A., and Keane, S. P. (2007). Cardiac vagal regulation differentiates among children at risk for behavior problems. *Biological Psychology, 74*, 144-153.

Campbell, S. B., Shaw, D. S., and Gilliom, M. (2000). Early externalizing behavior problems: Toddlers and preschoolers at risk for later maladjustment. *Development and Psychopathology, 12*, 467-488.

Cole, P.M., Martin, S.E. and Dennis, T.A. (2004). Emotion regulation as a scientific construct: Methodological challenges and directions for child development research. *Child Development, 75*, 317-333.

Crowell, S., Beauchaine, T. P., Gatzke-Kopp, L., Sylvers, P., Mead, H., and Chipman-Chacon, J. (2006). Autonomic correlates of attention-deficit/hyperactivity disorder and oppositional defiant disorder in preschool children. *Journal of Abnormal Psychology, 115*, 174-178.

Crowell, S., Beauchaine, T. P., McCauley, E., Smith, C. J., Stevens, A. L., and Sylvers, P. (2005). Psychological, autonomic, and serotonergic correlates of parasuicide among adolescent girls. *Development and Psychopathology, 17,* 1105-1127.

Cunningham, C.E. and Boyle, M.H. (2002). Preschoolers at risk for attention-deficit hyperactivity disorder and oppositional defiant disorder: Family, parenting, and behavioral correlates. *Journal of Abnormal Child Psychology, 30*, 555-569.

Danforth, J. S., Barkley, R. A., and Stokes, T. F. (1991). Observations of parent-child interactions with hyperactive children: Research and clinical implications. *Clinical Psychology Review,* 11, 703-727.

Dishion, T. J., and Patterson, G. R. (1992). Age effects in parent training outcome. *Behavior Therapy, 23*, 719–729.

Fischer, M. (1990). Parenting stress and the child with attention deficit hyperactivity disorder. *Journal of Clinical Child Psychology, 19,* 337-346.

Friedman, B. H. and Thayer, J. F. (1998). Anxiety and autonomic flexibility: a cardiovascular approach. *Biological Psychology, 49*, 303-323.

Gadow, K. D. and Sprafkin, J. (1997). *Child Symptom Inventory-4 norms manual.* Stony Brook, New York: Checkmate Plus.

Gottman, J. M., Jacobson, N. S., Rushe, R. H., Shortt, J. W., Babcock, J., La Taillade, J. J., and Waltz, J. (1995). The relationship between heart rate reactivity, emotionally aggressive behavior, and general violence in batterers. *Journal of Family Psychology, 9*, 227–248.

Gottman, J. M. and Katz, L. F. (2002). Children's emotional reactions to stressful parent-child interactions: The link between emotion regulation and vagal tone. *Marriage and the Family Review, 34*, 265–283.

Jensen, S.A. and Rosén, L.A. (2004). Emotional reactivity in children with Attention-Deficit/Hyperactivity Disorder. *Journal of Attention Disorders, 8*, 53-61.

Johnston, C., Murray, C., Hinshaw, S. P., Pelham, W., and Hoza, B. (2002). Responsiveness in interactions of mothers and sons with ADHD: Relations to maternal and child characteristics. *Journal of Abnormal Child Psychology, 30*, 77-88.

Katz, L. F. and Gottman, J. M. (1997). Buffering children from marital conflict and dissolution. *Journal of Clinical Child Psychology, 26*, 157-171.

Kilgore, K., Snyder, J. and Lentz, C. (2000). The contribution of parental discipline, parental monitoring, and school risk to early-onset conduct problems in African American boys and girls. *Developmental Psychology, 36*, 835-845.

Krueger, R.F., Hicks, B.M., Patrick, C.J., Carlson, S.R., Iacono, W.G. and McGue, M. (2002). Etiologic connections among substance dependence, antisocial behavior, and personality: Modeling the externalizing spectrum. *Journal of Abnormal Psychology, 111,* 411-424.

Krueger, R. F., and Markon, K. E. (2006). Reinterpreting comorbidity: A model-based approach to understanding and classifying psychopathology. *Annual Review of Clinical Psychology, 2, 111-133.*

Kupper, N., Willemsen, G., Posthuma, D., De Boer, D., Boomsma, D. I., and De Geus, E. J. C. (2005). A genetic analysis of ambulatory cardiorespiratory coupling. *Psychophysiology, 42*, 202–212.

Levy, F., Hay, D. A., McStephen, M., Wood, C. and Waldman, I. (1997). Attention-deficit hyperactivity disorder: A category or a continuum? Genetic analysis of a large-scale twin study. *Journal of the American Academy of Child and Adolescent Psychiatry, 36*, 737-744.

Lynam, D., Caspi, A., Moffitt, T. E., Wikström, P-O. H., Loeber, R. and Novak, S. (2000). The interaction between impulsivity and neighborhood context on offending: The effects of impulsivity are stronger in poorer neighborhoods. *Journal of Abnormal Psychology, 109*, 563-574.

Maccoby, E. E. (1992). The role of parents in the socialization of children: An historical overview. *Developmental Psychology, 28,* 1006-1017.

Maedgen, J. W. and Carlson, C. L. (2000). Social functioning and emotional regulation in the attention deficit hyperactivity disorder subtypes. *Journal of Clinical Child Psychology, 29*, 30-42.

Martel, M. M. and Nigg, J. T. (2006). Child ADHD and personality/temperament traits of reactive and effortful control, resiliency, and emotionality. *Journal of Child Psychology and Psychiatry, 47*, 1175-1183.

Mash, E. J. and Barkley, R. A. (Eds.). (1996). *Child psychopathology.* New York, NY: Guilford Press.

Mash, E. J. and Johnston, C. (1983). Parental perceptions of child behavior problems, parenting self-esteem, and mothers' reported stress in younger and older hyperactive and normal children. *Journal of Consulting and Clinical Psychology, 51,* 86-99.

McMahon, R.J. and Forehand, R. L. (2003). *Helping the noncompliant child: Family-based treatment for oppositional behavior.* New York, NY: Guilford Press.

Mead, H., Beauchaine, T. P., Brenner, S. L., Crowell, S., Gatzke-Kopp, L., and Marsh, P. (2004). Autonomic response patterns to reward and negative mood induction among children with conduct disorder, depression, and both psychiatric conditions. Poster presented at the annual meeting of the Society for Psychophysiological Research, Santa Fe, NM.

Melnick, S. M. and Hinshaw, S. P. (2000). Emotion regulation and parenting in AD/HD and comparison boys: Linkages with social behaviors and peer preference. *Journal of Abnormal Child Psychology, 28*, 73-86.

Mezzacappa, E., Tremblay, R. E., Kindlon, D., Saul, J. P., Arseneault, L., Seguin, J., et al., (1997). Anxiety, antisocial behavior, and heart rate regulation in adolescent males. *Journal of Children Psychology and Psychiatry, 38*, 457-469.

Patterson, G. R. (1982). *Coercive family process.* Eugene, OR: Castalia.

Patterson, G. R., DeGarmo, D. S., and Knutson, N. (2000). Hyperactive and antisocial behaviors: Comorbid or two points in the same process? *Development and Psychopathology, 12,* 91-106.

Porges, S.W., Doussard-Roosevelt, J.A. and Maiti, A.K. (1994). Vagal tone and the physiological regulation of emotion. *Monographs of the Society for Research in Child Development, 59* (2-3, Serial No. 240).

Price, T. S., Simonoff, E., Waldman, I., Asherson, P. and Plomin, R. (2001). Hyperactivity in pre-school children is highly heritable. *Journal of the American Academy of Child and Adolescent Psychiatry, 40*, 1342-1364.

Sagvolden, T., Johansen, E. B., Aase, H. and Russell, V. A. (2005). A dynamic developmental theory of attention-deficit/hyperactivity disorder (ADHD) predominantly hyperactive/impulsive and combined subtypes. *Behavioral and Brain Sciences, 28*, 397-468.

Sarason, I. G., Johnson, J. H., and Siegel, J. M. (1978). Assessing the impact of life changes: Development of the Life Experiences Survey. *Journal of Consulting and Clinical Psychology, 46,* 932-946.

Schrepferman, L. and Snyder, J. (2002). Coercion: The link between treatment mechanisms in behavioral parent training and risk reduction in child antisocial behavior. *Behavior Therapy, 33*, 339-359.

Sneider, H., Boomsma, D.I., van Doornen, L.J.P., DeGeus, E.J.C., 1997. Heritability of respiratory sinus arrhythmia: Dependency on task and respiration rate. *Psychophysiology 34*, 317–328.

Snyder, J., Edwards, P., McGraw, K., Kilgore, K., and Holton, A. (1994). Escalation and reinforcement in mother-child conflict: Social processes associated with the development of physical aggression. *Development and Psychopathology, 6,* 305-321.

Snyder, J., Schrepferman, L., and St. Peter, Carolyn. (1997) Origins of antisocial behavior: Negative reinforcement and affect dysregulation of behavior as socialization mechanisms in family interaction. *Behavior Modification, 21*, 187-215.

Spanier, G. B. (1989). Measuring dyadic adjustment: New scales for assessing the quality of marriage and similar dyads. *Journal of Marriage and the Family, 38*, 15-28.

Sprafkin, J., Gadow, K. D., Salisbury, H., Schneider, J. and Loney, J. (2002). Further evidence of reliability and validity of the Child Symptom Inventory-4: Parent Checklist in clinically referred boys. *Journal of Clinical Child and Adolescent Psychology, 21*, 513-524.

Stubbs, J., Crosby, L., Forgatch, M., and Capaldi, D. M. (1998). *Family and peer process code: Training manual: A synthesis of three OSLC behavior codes.* Available from the Oregon Social Learning Center, 160 E. 4th Ave., Eugene, OR 97401.

Tripp, G., Schaughency, E.A., Langlands, R. and Mouat, K. (2007). Family interactions in children with and without ADHD. *Journal of Child and Family Studies, 16*, 385-400.

Walcott, C. M. and Landau, S. (2004). The relation between disinhibition and emotion regulation in boys with attention deficit hyperactivity disorder. *Journal of Clinical Child and Adolescent Psychology, 33*, 772-782.

Webster-Stratton, C. (2005). The Incredible Years: A Training Series for the Prevention and Treatment of Conduct Problems in Young Children. In E.D. Hibbs and P.S. Jensen (Eds.). *Psychosocial Treatments for Child and Adolescent Disorder: Empirically Based Strategies for Clinical Practice*, 2nd ed, (pp. 507-556). Washington, D.C.: American Psychological Association.

Webster-Stratton, C., and Hammond, M. (1997). Treating children with early-onset conduct problems: A comparison of child and parent training interventions. *Journal of Consulting and Clinical Psychology, 65*, 93–109.

Webster-Stratton, C., Reid, M. J., and Hammond, M. (2001). Preventing conduct problems, promoting social competence: A parent and teacher training partnership in Head Start. *Journal of Clinical Child Psychology, 30,* 283-302.

Yeragani, V. K., Pohl, R., Berger, R., Balon, R., Ramesh, C., Glitz, D., Srinivasan, K., and Weinberg, P. (1993). Decreased heart rate variability in panic disorder patients: a study of power-spectral analysis of heart rate. *Psychiatry Research, 46*, 89-103.

In: Attention Deficit Hyperactivity Disorder (ADHD)
Editors: Stuart M. Gordon and Aileen E. Mitchell
ISBN 978-1-60741-581-7

Chapter 6

A Review of the Dopamine System in the Animal Models of Attention-Deficit Hyperactivity Disorder

LiQi*[1] *and Yew DT*[2]

1. The Department of Psychiatry, Faculty of Medicine, The University of Hong Kong, 21 Sassoon Road, Pokfulam, Hong Kong.
2. School of Biomedical Sciences, Faculty of Medicine, The Chinese University of Hong Kong, Shatin, N.T., Hong Kong.

Abstract

Attention-deficit hyperactivity disorder (ADHD) is characterized by age-inappropriate inattention, impulsiveness, and hyperactivity. Experimental models, in addition to mimicking syndromal features, should resemble the clinical condition in pathophysiology, and predict potential new treatments. In this review, we summarized the different animal models of ADHD which are established from genetic and environmental alterations, and compared their similarities and differences to clinical ADHD. However, none is fully comparable to clinical ADHD. The pathophysiology involved varies, in this review we focused on the dopaminergic system in ADHD. Because, the most compelling evidence that dopaminergic mechanisms were involved in ADHD was pharmacological challenge in both animals and humans. However, the question was that whether any other central factors which regulated the process of dopaminergic neurotransmission involved in the origins of ADHD. We speculated that "synaptogenesis hypotheses" might be involved in ADHD. Above all, any improved models as well as further testing of their ability to predict treatment responses are required.

1.1. Introduction

Attention-deficit hyperactivity disorder (ADHD) is characterized by age-inappropriate inattention, impulsiveness, and hyperactivity (Wilens et al., 2002). Approximately 5-10 % of school-aged children worldwide have ADHD, with the incidence being 3 times higher in boys than girls (Barkley and Biederman, 1997; Brown et al., 2001; Hinshaw, 1992; Scahill and Schwab-Stone, 2000). Unfortunately, the disease continues into adulthood in 30-70 % of patients (Silver, 2000). It has been proposed that ADHD may lead to memory deficits, delinquency, substance abuse, and problematic personality disorders, in addition to being one of the highest risk factors for other mental illnesses (Taylor, 1998). Accumulating data indicate that genetics may influence its incidence. For example, studies focusing on twins show that the heritability of ADHD is 0.80, indicating a strong genetic predisposition (Faraone and Biederman, 1998). Genes studies of ADHD show that ADHD might be due to the interaction of several different genes involved in the function of several different neurotransmitters such as dopamine D4 receptor (DRD4), dopamine transporter (DAT), dopamine D5 receptor (DRD5) and serotonin transporter and so on (Bobb et al., 2005a). Besides, many magnetic resonance imaging (MRI) morphometric studies have identified reductions in total brain volume and in the various regions of the brain (such as the prefrontal lobe, caudate nucleus, corpus callosum and cerebellum) that involved in the regulation of attention and impulsivity (Voeller, 2004). Functional neuroimaging studies such as positron emission tomography (PET) revealed that lower activity in the right frontal cortex and right temporal cortex (Ernst et al., 1994). Also the other relevant neuroimaging studies showed that the dopaminergic system is dysfunction in ADHD children (Forssberg et al., 2006). In clinical trials, psychostimulants (e.g., methylphenidate, d-amphetamine and pemoline) are the most common treatments for ADHD (Solanto, 1998). Even though, the precise etiology and pathological mechanisms underlying ADHD are poorly understood.

1.2. Animal Models of Attention-Deficit Hyperactivity Disorder

Animal models could help to simplify and promote the understanding of disorders. Studies using animal models of ADHD have provided some inherent advantages over human studies and could establish causal effects resulting from documented exposure or treatment. In addition, they permit invasive manipulations in order to investigate underlying neurochemical or neuropathological alterations and allow assessment of potential new pharmacological therapeutics or behavioral interventions (Fisch, 2007; Rorick-Kehn et al., 2007).

1.2.1. Criteria for Animal Models of ADHD

Sarter et al (Sarter et al., 1992) developed the general validation criteria for animal models in neuropsychology. Recently, an optimal animal model of ADHD was suggested by

Sagvolden et al (Sagvolden, 2000b), which included (1) Face validity: the model should have similar fundamental behavioral characteristics of ADHD. Hyperactivity should not be observed in a novel environment, but should develop over time and impulsiveness should develop gradually over time, Attention deficit should be demonstrated when stimuli are widely spaced in time. (2) Construct validity: the model should conform to a theoretical rationale for ADHD. It is hard to conclude on the construct validity of ADHD, because the theoretical rationale for ADHD has little agreement. Even though, similar alterations in genetics, neurophysiology and neurobiology of ADHD children should be found in the animal models. (3) Predictive validity: the ability to predict previously unknown aspects of behavior, genetics, and neurobiology of the disorder from the model. This review considers conditions in laboratory animals that have been used as models of ADHD in the context of these criteria. Construct validity is especially important in view of advances in understanding the genetic and pathophysiology of ADHD (see Figure1).

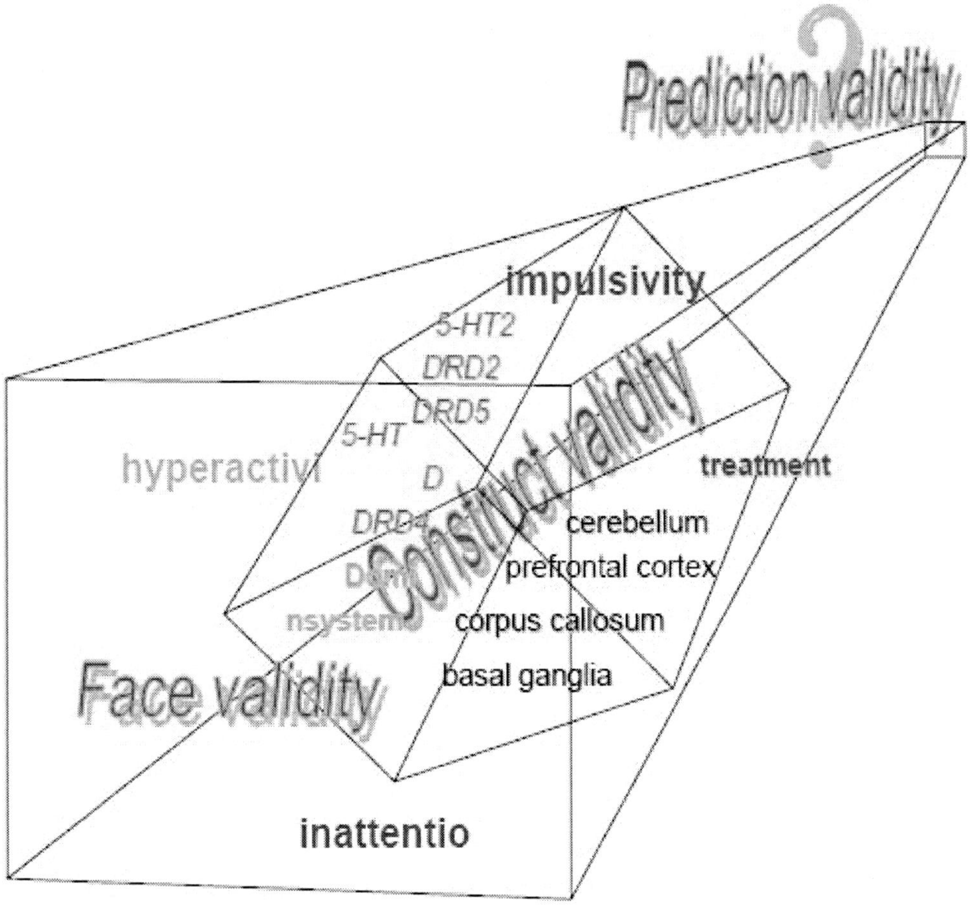

Figure 1. On the surface of this 3D cartoon, it represents face validity, one criteria for ADHD, including hyperactivity, inattention and /or impulsivity. Inside this 3D cartoon, it represents construct validity which is an essential criteria for ADHD including genes correlated with ADHD, dopamine hypotheses in ADHD, brain areas involved in ADHD and treatment in ADHD. The outside of this 3D cartoon represents prediction validity, which means any unknown parts of ADHD studied from animal models.

1.2.2. Major Rodent models of ADHD

1.2.2.1. Genetic Models

Spontaneously Hypertensive Rats

The spontaneously hypertensive rats are the most frequently used model of ADHD (Sagvolden, 2000c). It is a genetic model bred from progenitor Wistar Kyoto rats (WKY)(OKAMOTO and AOKI, 1963). Selecting for hypertension of SHR in early 1960s, the model has also been reported for unexpectedly high spontaneous motor activity (Moser et al., 1988). Over several decades, Sagvolden and colleagues studied the SHR extensively and established it as one of the most widely used animal models of ADHD.

The ADHD patients have three major characteristics – hyperactivity, impulsive and attention deficit. SHR showed several features characteristics of ADHD, including motor hyperactivity that was not present in novel, non-threatening situations but developed over time (Sagvolden, 2000a). SHR exhibited sensitive to immediate reinforcement and delayed reinforcement than WKY (Hand et al., 2006; Sagvolden et al., 1992). SHR showed sustained attention deficit because SHR resumed responding after a short time in the extinction component of the fixed interval (FI) / extinction (Ext) schedule, a behavioral paradigm for testing activity level, discrimination behavior and impulsiveness (Sagvolden, 2000d; Sagvolden et al., 2005b). SHR also showed sex differences similar to the ADHD children (Berger and Sagvolden, 1998). In summary, behavioral studies supported the face validity of the SHR as a model of ADHD.

The "dopamine hypothesis" was one of the most widely accepted hypothesis of ADHD, which was based on the amelioration of symptoms by medicines acting at the dopamine synapses. Three dopaminergic genes, DRD2, DRD4 and DAT1, in the SHR and WKY were sequenced, and only DAT1 gene was found to show several variations in the SHR (Mill et al., 2005). The dopamine release in prefrontal cortex and caudate-putamen slices was also significantly lower in SHR than in corresponding slices of WKY (Russell et al., 1995). Dopamine 1 receptor (DRD1) and dopamine 5 receptor (DRD5) in the caudate-putamen (CPU), the nucleus aaccumbens (NAc) and the olfactory tubercle (OT) exhibited lower affinity in SHR (Carey et al., 1998b). In addition, treatment with methylphenidate (MP) normalized the DRD1 and DRD5 receptors by increasing the affinity to the normal level (Carey et al., 1998a). Systematic dosage injection of DRD1 agonist showed that motor behavior changes and alteration of the frontal-striatal circuity of SHR were involved in these changes (Diaz and Castellanos, 2006). Alpha (2)-adrenoreceptor which mediated inhibition of norepinephrine (NE) was deficient in prefrontal cortex of SHR (Russell et al., 2000). In addition, calcium metabolism and N-methyl-D-aspartate (NMDA) receptor function were disturbed in the cortex of SHR (Lehohla et al., 2001; Lehohla et al., 2004). These findings were consistent with the hypothesis that the behavioral disturbances in ADHD were the results of an imbalance between NE and DA systems in the prefrontal cortex.

Further, histamine H(3) receptor antagonists which have been proposed as potential useful therapeutic agents for the treatment of ADHD could improve SHR performance(Fox et al., 2002).

Wistar-kyoto Hyperactive Rats (WKHA)

Development of WKHA started in the late 1970s from progenitor, SHR and WKY rats. WKHA expressed hyperactivity in a novel environment, as did SHR, but their blood pressure was normal, thus they were potentially be a more promising model of ADHD. WKHA, compared with Wistar rats, exhibited specific abnormalities in attention processing as well as in learning stimulus-reward tests (Chess et al., 2005). Molecular genetic studies of WKHA showed that DRD4 and dopamine-β-hydroxylase (DBH) associated with exploratory activity in WKHA (Moisan et al., 2003). Besides, there was an evidence support that 5-HT_{1B} receptors play a key role in the increased locomotion activity in WKHA (Chaouloff et al., 1999). However, WKHA were less aggressive, habituated more readily to a novel environment, and were less exploratory in a familiar environment than the SHR (Hendley and Ohlsson, 1991). In the view of possible dopaminergic defects, Drolet et al. concluded that WKHA might not be a suitable model of ADHD (Drolet et al., 2002).

Naples High Excitability Rats

The Naples high- (NHE) and low-excitability (NLE) were two rat lines, selectively bred for high and low activity levels in a Lat-maze and a hexagonal tunnel maze with asymmetric radial arms, respectively (Gonzalez-Lima and Sadile, 2000b). Both NHE and NLE demonstrated lower metabolism in the cortex and the amygdala, which led to a potential learning impairment (Gonzalez-Lima and Sadile, 2000a). Only NHE demonstrated a significant sensitivity to acute inhibition in the production of nitric oxide (NO) which appeared to play a role in attention processes (Aspide et al., 1998). This meant that NHE rats had the problem of attention as well. On the other hand, NHE rats exhibited an increased number of dopamine neurons in the VTA but not in the substantial nigra, with an increased number of axonal varicosities in the prefrontal cortex as well as the down regulation of DRD1 in the prefrontal cortex (Viggiano et al., 2002b; Viggiano et al., 2003; Viggiano and Sadile, 2000). It appeared that NHE rats had a hypertrophic mesocorticolimbic system and a normal mesostriatal system. The NHE rats might also be a possible model for attention deficit disorder (ADD) because they were inattentive with learning and memory deficit, but they did not exhibit hyperactive or impulsive behavior typical of ADHD (Viggiano et al., 2002a).

Dopamine Transporter Knockout Mouse (DAT-KO)

Dopamine transporter (DAT) knockout mice were hyperactivity, had inhibition deficit and learning and memory deficits. Psychostimulants such as amphetamine could attenuate the hyperlocomotion of the mutants DAT-KO, but stimulated activity in the wild type (WT) controls. These paradoxical effects of psychostimulants in $DAT^{-/-}$ mice had been explained by an action on the 5-HT system (Gainetdinov et al., 1999; Rocha et al., 1998). Further, only the limbic areas mediated responses to psychostimulants in the mutants (Trinh et al., 2003), and there was no dopamine involvement.

Coloboma Mutant Mouse

Coloboma mutant mice displayed a variety of behavioral, neurophysiological and developmental deficits. They showed hyperactivity which was mediated by a deficiency in synaptic release of dopamine input to the striatum (Raber et al., 1997). This hyperlocomotion could be reversed by low dose of amphetamine (Steffensen et al., 1999b). In addition, the deficit in SNAP-25 expression seen in these mutants may also be link to deficiency of learning and hippocampal physiology (Steffensen et al., 1999a). Because the 25 kDa synaptosomal-associated protein (SNAP - 25) is essential for neurotransmitter storage and release (Kataoka et al., 2006); (Sorensen et al., 2006). However, the Coloboma mouse was predominantly hyperactive, lacked impulsiveness and sustained attention deficit.

1.2.2.2. Neurotoxin-Exposed Animal Models

Six-Hydroxydopamine-Lesioned Rat

Juvenile animals lesioned with neurotoxin 6-hydroxydopamine (6-OHDA) had destruction of the DA projections to forebrain, and the severe depletion of DA very early in development increased motor activity and learning deficits in juvenile animals (Kostrzewa et al., 1994). Hyperactivity started to wear off at puberty, although impulsion and inattention persisted throughout adulthood. Psychostimulants including amphetamine and methylphenidate could reverse hyperactivity resulting from neonatal 6-OHDA lesions (Davids et al., 2002a; Davids et al., 2002c). DRD4 was a part of the motor and emotional changes in the 6-OHDA lesioned model of ADHD (Avale et al., 2004). Besides the dopamine studies of 6-OHDA, the NE or 5-HT release might mediate certain behavioral changes using psychostimulants (Davids et al., 2002b).

Nucleus Accumbens Core (ACB) Lesions Rats

Behavioral changes associated with ADHD and ADD might be produced by the selective brain lesions as well as by neurotoxin induced dysfunction of neurotransmitters. Cardinal reports indicated that Acb was involved in the pathogenesis of impulsive choice, which suggested that Acb dysfunction may contribute to ADHD (Cardinal et al., 2001). Recent evidence suggested that Acb-lesioned rats were hyperactive, but were unimpaired in spatial attention (Cardinal et al., 2004). Amphetamine enhanced the hyper-locomotion induced by Acb lesions, but shell lesions of nucleus accumbens could attenuate amphetamine-induced activity (Parkinson et al., 1999).

Hippocampal Irradiation

Focal x-irradiation of the hippocampus in an infant rat exhibited hippocampal agenesis, also showed hyperactivity and working memory deficit (az-Granados et al., 1994; Highfield et al., 1998a). Amphetamine could alleviate the short-term memory deficit induced by x-irradiation of the hippocampus (Highfield et al., 1998b).

Environmental Toxins

Exposure to environmental toxins including lead and polychlorinated biphenyls (PCBs) had been implicated in some cases of human ADHD (Safe, 1994; Taylor et al., 1998). Mice were exposed to lead could cause hyperactivity and psychostimulants suppressed their abnormal activity (Silbergeld and Goldberg, 1974). Developmental exposure to lead or PCBs resulted in a behavioral impairment in monkeys. These abnormal behavior included impaired ability to organize behavior temporally and had an inability to learn from consequences of previous actions (Rice, 2000).

A summary of animal models reviewed here as ADHD models, with similarities and differences when compared with clinical disorders, is shown in Table 1.

Table 1. Comparison of animal models of ADHD

Models	Similarities to ADHD	Differences to ADHD	Comments
Spontaneously Hypertensive Rats	Hyperactivity, impulsive, attention deficit, imbalance between NE and DA systems in the prefrontal cortex with some responses to psychostimulants. Sex differences in SHR.	Developmental hypertension with ADHD.	Most studied animal model; Need to choose an appropriate control.
Wistar-kyoto Hyperactive Rats	Hyperactivity, inattention. Dopaminergic genes associated with their abnormal behavior.	Less aggression, no response to amphetamine, no dopaminergic deficit.	Not an appropriate model of ADHD.
Naples High Excitability Rats	Inattentive, learning and memory deficit.	No hyperactivity and impulsive behavior. Normal mesostriatal system.	A possible model of the attention deficit disorder (ADD).
DAT-KO Mice	Hyperactive, inattention and exhibit learning, memory deficit. Psychostimulants could attenuate the hyperlocomotion.	Only the limbic system was involved in its abnormal behavior and treatment, but not dopamine system.	No evidence of dopamine functional changes.
Coloboma Mutant Mice	Hyperactivity, dopamine release defect. Amphetamine alleviated the hyperactivity.	No attention problem or impulsion. No responses to methylphenidate.	No specific neural deficits. The cognitive behavior was not well evaluated.
Six-Hydroxydo-pamine-Lesiond Rats	Increased motor activity and learning deficits. Have responses to the psychostimulants.	Hyperactivity ware off early at puberty.	Need more assessment of attention and impulsivity.
Nucleus accumbens core (Acb) lesions rats	Hyperactivity with impulsion. Dysfunction of neurotransmitters has been shown.	Amphetamine could not attenuate their hyperactivity.	Attention problem need to be assessed.
Hippocampal Irradiation	Hyperactivity and working memory deficit. Amphetamine alleviated the short-term memory deficit.	Radiation not implicated in ADHD.	Cognitive behaviors should be assessed.

Table 1. (Continued)

Models	Similarities to ADHD	Differences to ADHD	Comments
Environmental toxins	Hyperactivity and working memory deficit, response to the psychostimulants.	Relationships between toxins and ADHD was not proven.	Attention problem and impulsion needed further studies.

1.3. Dopamine System and Attention-Deficit Hyperactivity Disorder

Dopamine is believed to play an important role in the pathophysiology of ADHD. Bobb et al.(Bobb et al., 2005b) reviews 113 articles about ADHD studies spanning 14 years, including 3 genome-wide linkage studies, and association studies of 94 polymorphisms of 33 different candidate genes. They summarized the genes related to ADHD as follows: The dopamine system: dopamine transporter (DAT1), dopa decarboxylase (DDC), dopamine receptor D1 (DRD1), dopamine receptor D2 (DRD2), dopamine receptor D3 (DRD3), dopamine receptor D4 (DRD4), dopamine receptor D5 (DRD5), tyrosine hydroxylase (TH); the serotonin system: serotonin transporter (5-HTT), serotonin 1B receptor (5-HT1B), serotonin 2A receptor (5-HT2A), serotonin 2C receptor (5-HT2C); the noradrenalin system: alpha 1C adrenergic receptor (ADRA1C), alpha 2A adrenergic receptor (ADRA2A), alpha 2C adrenergic receptor (ADRA2C), catechol – o-methyltransferase(COMT), dopamine beta-hydroxylase (DBH), monoamine oxidase A (MAOA), monoamine oxidase B (MAOB), norepinephrine transporter (NET1). Other candidate genes also included: the α-4, 7 subunit of nicotinic acetylcholine receptors (CHRNA4 and CHRNA7); N-methl-D-aspartate (NMDA) receptor; synaptosomal - associated protein 25 (SNAP25).

Above all, candidate gene studies of ADHD produced substantial evidence implicating several genes have been involved in the etiology of the disorder. Indeed, there are at least seven genes which show significant evidence of association with ADHD, which are DRD4, DRD5, DAT, DBH, 5-HTT, 5-HT1B and SNAP25 (Lowe et al., 2004). The dopamine D4 receptor gene has been one of the most studied genes in ADHD, with a recent quantitative trait study showing that a 7-repeat allele may be linked to locomotor activity and other associated behaviors give rise to a new phenotype of ADHD (Swanson et al., 1998). Obviously, genes involved in regulating dopamine system play a key role in the etiology of ADHD. Here we attempt to summarize anatomical and functional studies of dopamine systems in ADHD.

1.3.1. The Anatomical Dopamine Pathways

There are four dopamine pathways which include the nigrostriatal dopamine pathway, mesolimbic dopamine pathway, mesocortical and tuberoinfundibular dopamine pathways.

Nigrostriatal dopamine pathway begins in the substantia nigra and projects axons to the striatum, the caudate and the putamen. This system is concerned with the initiation and maintenance of motor behavior (Straughan and James, 1979). The striatum and the substantial nigra are both key players in a group of structures called the basal ganglia. The basal ganglia, as well as the cerebellum, are the center of motor coordination, movement and initiation of movement. It is this pathway that is thought to be greatly altered in patients with Parkinson's disease. Increasingly, researchers are realizing that the basal ganglia may play a role in cognitive functioning, although the precise nature of this role remains unclear (Chudasama and Robbins, 2006b). Neuroscientists have posed many and varied speculations as to the cognitive role of the basal ganglia, while most suggested an inhibitory function that served to augment executive control of the frontal lobes. The prefrontal lobes send projections to the basal ganglia, which in turn, direct projections back to the prefrontal lobes via thalamic nuclei, forming a neural circuitry (Afifi, 2003; Chudasama and Robbins, 2006c).

The mesolimbic dopamine pathway projects from midbrain ventral tegmental area (VTA) to the nucleus accumbens, amygdala, hippocampus which belong to the limbic system of brain and are involved in many behaviors, such as drug abuse, pleasurable sensation, impulsivity and so on (Funada et al., 2006; Totterdell, 2006).

The mesocortical dopamine pathway has cell bodies located in the ventral tegmental area as well, but this pathway terminates in the prefrontal cortex. These neurons have an excitatory effect on the frontal cortex and affect such functions as formation of working memories, long-term memories, planning or strategy and preparations for problem solving (Chudasama and Robbins, 2006a).

The tuberoinfundibular dopamine pathway projects from the hypothalamus to anterior pituitary gland. It inhibits the release of prolactin (Emiliano and Fudge, 2004).

1.3.2. Dopamine Receptors

The first evidence for the existence of dopamine receptors in the central nervous system (CNS) comes from biochemical studies showing that dopamine is able to stimulate adenylyl cyclase (Kebabian and Calne, 1979). The dopamine D1 receptor gene is located at chromosome 5q35.1, and is composed of two exons separated by a small intron in the 5' untranslated region (Grandy et al., 1990).Dopamine D2-like receptor (D2R) gene is located on chromosome 11q22-23, and is included in two forms of the receptors $D2_L$ (Long) and $D2_S$ (Short) (Grandy et al., 1989). Dopamine D3-like receptor (D3R) sites on chromosome 3q13.3 (Griffon et al., 1996). Dopamine D4 receptor (D4R) sites on chromosome 11p15.5, and contains a number of polymorphic regions (Petronis et al., 1993). Dopamine D5 receptor (D5R) is located on chromosome 4p15.1-p15.3, and contains two pseudogenes $D5\psi1$ and $D5\psi2$ that do not direct the synthesis of a functional receptor (Sherrington et al., 1993). For decades, dopamine receptors are intensively studied in the field of pharmacology, biochemistry, physiology and anatomy.

Dopamine (DA) modulates the initiation of locomotor activity and the integration of goal-oriented behaviors, through the stimulation of five distinct G-protein-coupled receptors. However, once activated, they lead to different downstream molecular events, and can be classified as two groups. The dopamine D1-like (D1R and D5R) receptors, which are coupled to G_s, activate adenyl cyclase leading to the production of cyclic adenosine monophosphate (cAMP). On the other side, D2-like (D2R, D3R and D4R) receptors, which are coupled to G_i will inhibit adenyl cyclase (see Figure 2 and Table 2). cAMP is a second messenger, which in turn activates cAMP-dependent protein kinase (PKA), and phosphorylates several substrates, including L-type calcium channels, transcription factors such as cAMP response element binding protein (CREB), as well as other intracellular signaling components. CREB is involveed in a large variety of processes in both developing and mature nervous system, such as proliferation of neuronal precursors and outgrowth of neuronal processes (Kandel, 2001).

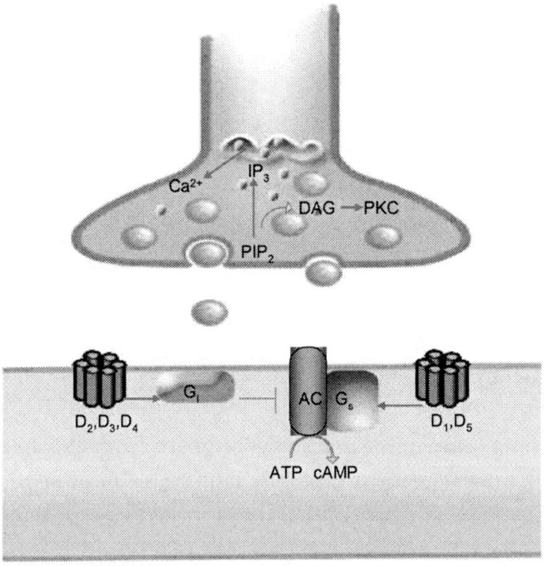

Figure 2. At the pre-synaptic area, the phosphatidyl-4,5-bisphosphate (PIP2), a membrane phospholipids, is hydrolyzed to the intracellular second messengers 1,4,5-inositoltrisphosphate (IP3) and diacylglycerol (DAG). IP3 leads to mobilization of intracellular calcium through binding IP3 receptor on the smooth ER (endoplasmic reticulum), and DAG is the physiological activator of protein kinase C (PKC). An increase of calcium (shown by the little red dots) within the cell is a common trigger for the release of a neurotransmitter. At the post-synaptic area, neurotransmitters such as dopamine could activate a G- protein- coupled receptor. D1 and D5 receptors could activate G_s which leads to the production of cAMP. D2, D3 and D4 receptors could inhibit the production of cAMP through activating the G_i protein.

1.3.3. Distribution of Dopamine Receptors in the Brain

The D1R is the most widespread DA receptor and is expressed at higher levels than any other DA receptors. In situ hybridization is often used to study the distribution of dapamine receptors mRNAs in brain. D1R is mainly expressed in the corpus callosum (CPu), nucleus accumbens (Acb), olfactory tract (OT), cortex (Cx) and amygdala (Jackson and Westlind-Danielsson, 1994). D1R mRNA is also found in the hypothalamus and thalamus. On the other hand, in the entopeducular nucleus and the substantia nigra pars reticulate where the D1R protein is highly expressed, no mRNA has been detected (Gerfen et al., 1990; Le et al., 1991). This suggests that in these areas D1R is mainly present in projections. D5R, however, is expressed in the lateral mammillary nucleus, cerebellum, cerebral cortex, lateral thalamus, striatum and to a lesser extent, the substantial nigra, medial thalamus, and hippocampus. (Choi et al., 1995; Huntley et al., 1992b; Huntley et al., 1992a; Zelenin et al., 2002). D2R mRNA is expressed mainly in the corpus callosum, olfactory tract, ventral tegmental area (VTA) of the midbrain, hypothalamus, the substantial nigra pars compacta, and nucleus accumbens (Acb) (Bouthenet et al., 1991b; Weiner et al., 1991). D2R mRNA is also present in the septal region, amygdala, and in the granule cells of the hippocampal formation (Bouthenet et al., 1991a). Distribution of D3 mRNA indicated that these receptors are mainly expressed in subcortical limbic regions including islands of Calleja, nucleus accumbens and olfactory tubercle, with low levels of expression in the basal ganglia (Bouthenet et al., 1991c). D4 dopamine receptors are abundant in the globus pallidus and in GABAergic internreurons inside the prefrontal cortex, amygdala, hippocampus, hypothalamus, and mesencephalon (Mrzljak et al., 1996; O'Malley et al., 1992; Van Tol et al., 1991). Significant levels of D4R are also found in the retina (Cohen et al., 1992). Several laboratories have described the mRNA distributions of the dopamine receptors in the CNS, while no total agreement have been reached. Differences may be methodological or in some cases reflect technical differences.

A summary of particularities of the different dopamine receptor subtypes is shown in Table 2.

Table 2. Particularities of the different dopamine receptor subtypes

	D1-LIKE		D2-LIKE		
	D1	D5	D2	D3	D4
Chromosomal Localization Special Characteristic	5q 35.1	4p 15.1-16.1 Human pseudogenes D5ψ1 and D5ψ2	11q 22-23 Alternative splicing $D2_S/D2_L$	3q 13.3	11p 15.5 Polimorphism in human
G-protein cAMP	Gs +	Gs +	Gi —	Gi —	Gi —
Distribution in CNS	corpus callosum (CPu), nucleus accumbens (Acb), olfactory tract (OT), cortex and amygdale, thalamus hypothalamus, entopeducular, nucleus and the substantia nigra pars reticulate.	lateral mammillary nucleus, cerebellum, cerebral cortex, lateral thalamus, striatum and substantial nigra, medial thalamus, and hippocampus.	corpus callosum (CPu), olfactory tract(OT), ventral tegmental area (VTA) of the midbrain and nucleus accumbens (Acb), the septal region, amygdale, and hippocampal formation.	islands of Calleja, nucleus accumbe ns, basal ganglia and olfactory tubercle.	globus pallidus and prefrontal cortex, amygdale, hippocampus, hypothalamus, and mesencephalon, retina.

1.3.4. Dopamine Systems and ADHD

Many theories have postulated the involvement of brain dopamine pathways in the attention and executive functions which are altered in ADHD. Indeed, it had been hypothesized that the hyperactivity (and possibly impulsivity) might be the result of the hypodopaminergic state in the prefrontal cortex. Furthermore, the cognitive impairments associated with ADHD might also result from a hypodopaminergic state in the prefrontal cortex (Solanto, 2002). Functional alterations of the different dopamine pathways induce the different ADHD symptoms. A hypofunctioning mesolimbic dopamine pathway produced increased behavioral variability and disinhibition. A hypofunctioning mesocortical dopamine pathway caused attention deficit and poor behavioral planning. A hypofunctioning nigrostriatal dopamine pathway gave rise to impaired modulation of motor function and deficient non-declarative learning and memory. These impairments would cause apparent developmental delay (Sagvolden et al., 2005a).

The dopamine D4 receptor (D4R) is predominantly expressed in the frontal cortex (FC), a brain region that receives dense input from the basal ganglia and midbrain dopamine neurons and is associated with executive function. The frontal lobe theory of ADHD had suggested that children with ADHD had a delayed maturation and thus immaturity of the frontal lobe, which resulted in inefficient inhibition of both irrelevant stimuli and behavioral impulses as well as difficulties with selective attention. D4R was involved in the regulation of cortical excitability, possibly through inhibitory influences on glutamatergic (Rubinstein et al., 2001) and GABAergic activity (Wang et al., 2002; Wedzony et al., 2000). Stimulation of the D4 receptors inhibited adenyl cyclase activity and activated release of arachidonic acid in brain neurons (Meador-Woodruff et al., 1994). Additional support for possible involvement of D4R in ADHD was provided by recent findings that transgenic mice lacking D4R showed increased sensitivity to psychostimulants and increased metabolic turnover of striatal dopamine compared to wild type mice(Rubinstein et al., 1997). However the significance of the D3, D4 and D5 subtypes receptors in the central nervous system (CNS) was unclear, largely due to the fact that no specific agonists or antagonists for these subtypes were available.

Currently, the primary form of treatment for ADHD was the prescription of stimulant medication, such as methylphenidate or amphetamine. These drugs stimulated release and inhibited uptake of catecholamines and thus enhance the activity of this neurotransmitter system, reducing the symptomatology in ADHD. Methlphenidate could block more than 50% of the dopamine transporters in the striatum (Volkow et al, 2000). Mice lacking the dopamine transporter gene, for example, induced a spontaneous hyperlocomotion (Biala, 2004). This hyperactivity was novelty-driven, long lasting, and persisted after repeated exposure to the same environment (Spielewoy et al., 2000b; Spielewoy et al., 2000a).

1.4. Synaptogenesis Hypotheses in ADHD

Over the past 10 years, the vast majority of psychiatric studies have focused almost exclusively on the “dopamine hypotheses” and dopamine genes. This is also the case in

ADHD studies. The most compelling evidence that dopaminergic mechanisms were involved in ADHD was pharmacological challenge in both animals and humans. However, the question was that whether any other central factors which regulated the process of dopaminergic neurotransmission involved in the origins of ADHD. We speculated that "synaptogenesis hypotheses" might be involved in ADHD (Fossella et al., 2003).

As we know, calcium entry into nerve terminals via voltage gated calcium channels was an essential step in neurotransmission (Atwood and Karunanithi, 2002). The arrival of a nerve impulse at a nerve terminal led to an opening of voltage-gated $Ca2^+$ channels and a rapid influx of $Ca2^+$. The increase in calcium concentration at the active zone triggered the fusion of docked synaptic vesicles and led to the neurotransmitter release. A large number of proteins had been identified at nerve terminals to be involved in the cycling of synaptic vesicles. Studies had revealed that the SNARE core complex, consisting of synaptobrevin VAMP, a synaptic vesicle-associated protein, syntaxin and SNAP-25, played essential roles in synaptic vesicle exocytosis (Mochida, 2000). The SNARE complex interacted with calcium channels which provided calcium for triggering exocytosis in the central nervous system (CNS) (Rettig et al., 1996). Disruption of this interactions altered the $Ca2^+$-dependence of neurotransmitter release at the neuromuscular junctions (Rettig et al., 1997). Therefore, SNARE complex appeared to participate in the calcium-dependent regulation of exocytosis. Besides, SNAP-25 not only played a key role in presynaptic regulation of synaptogenesis (Fossella et al., 2003), but was also involved in the regulation of neuronal excitability via controlling calcium responsiveness to depolarization (Verderio et al., 2004). SNAP-25 was therefore a multifunctional protein that participated in exocytotic function both at the mechanistic and at the regulatory level.

The "synaptogenesis hypotheses" in ADHD might be the dysfunction of SNARE complex which reduced the affinity between SNARE complex and calcium channel in the presynaptic area, thereby damaged the synaptic vesicle docking and fusion processes and finally reduced the neurotransmitters release. Therefore, we speculated that the "synaptogenesis hypotheses" might involve these biochemical changes in ADHD. However, further studies should be done to demonstrate this in detail to find bench marker to improve ADHD treatment.

1.5. Summary

In this review, we summarized the different animal models of ADHD which are established from genetic and environmental alterations, and compared their similarities and differences to clinical ADHD. Despite the many advances in developing and analyzing animal models of ADHD, an ideal laboratory model for it has yet to be established. The pathophysiology involved varies, in this review we focused on the dopaminergic system in ADHD. Because, the most compelling evidence that dopaminergic mechanisms were involved in ADHD was pharmacological challenge in both animals and humans. However, the question was that whether any other central factors which regulated the process of dopaminergic neurotransmission involved in the origins of ADHD. We speculated that "synaptogenesis hypotheses" might be involved in ADHD. The "synaptogenesis hypotheses" in ADHD might be the dysfunction of SNARE complex which reduced the affinity between SNARE complex and calcium channel in the presynaptic area, thereby damaged the synaptic vesicle docking and fusion processes and finally reduced the neurotransmitters release. Above all, any improved models as well as further testing of their ability to predict treatment responses are required.

References

Afifi, A.K., 2003. The basal ganglia: a neural network with more than motor function. Semin.Pediatr.*Neurol.* 10, 3-10.

Aspide, R., Gironi Carnevale, U.A., Sergeant, J.A., Sadile, A.G., 1998. Non-selective attention and nitric oxide in putative animal models of Attention-Deficit Hyperactivity Disorder. *Behav.Brain Res.* 95, 123-133.

Atwood, H.L., Karunanithi, S., 2002. Diversification of synaptic strength: presynaptic elements. *Nat.Rev.Neurosci.* 3, 497-516.

Avale, M.E., Falzone, T.L., Gelman, D.M., Low, M.J., Grandy, D.K., Rubinstein, M., 2004. The dopamine D4 receptor is essential for hyperactivity and impaired behavioral inhibition in a mouse model of attention deficit/hyperactivity disorder. *Mol.Psychiatry* 9, 718-726.

az-Granados, J.L., Greene, P.L., Amsel, A., 1994. Selective activity enhancement and persistence in weanling rats after hippocampal X-irradiation in infancy: possible relevance for ADHD. *Behav.Neural Biol.* 61, 251-259.

Barkley, R.A., Biederman, J., 1997. Toward a broader definition of the age-of-onset criterion for attention-deficit hyperactivity disorder. *J.Am.Acad.Child Adolesc.Psychiatry* 36, 1204-1210.

Berger, D.F., Sagvolden, T., 1998. Sex differences in operant discrimination behaviour in an animal model of attention-deficit hyperactivity disorder. *Behav.Brain Res.* 94, 73-82.

Biala, G., 2004. [Behavioral and pharmacological characteristics of mice lacking the dopamine transporter]. Postepy Hig.Med.Dosw.(Online.) 58, 560-564.

Bobb, A.J., Castellanos, F.X., Addington, A.M., Rapoport, J.L., 2005a. Molecular genetic studies of ADHD: 1991 to 2004. Am.J.Med.Genet.B Neuropsychiatr.*Genet.* 132, 109-125.

Bobb, A.J., Castellanos, F.X., Addington, A.M., Rapoport, J.L., 2005b. Molecular genetic studies of ADHD: 1991 to 2004. *Am.J.Med.Genet.B Neuropsychiatr.Genet.* 132, 109-125.

Bouthenet, M.L., Souil, E., Martres, M.P., Sokoloff, P., Giros, B., Schwartz, J.C., 1991a. Localization of dopamine D3 receptor mRNA in the rat brain using in situ hybridization histochemistry: comparison with dopamine D2 receptor mRNA. *Brain Res.* 564, 203-219.

Bouthenet, M.L., Souil, E., Martres, M.P., Sokoloff, P., Giros, B., Schwartz, J.C., 1991c. Localization of dopamine D3 receptor mRNA in the rat brain using in situ hybridization histochemistry: comparison with dopamine D2 receptor mRNA. *Brain Res.* 564, 203-219.

Bouthenet, M.L., Souil, E., Martres, M.P., Sokoloff, P., Giros, B., Schwartz, J.C., 1991b. Localization of dopamine D3 receptor mRNA in the rat brain using in situ hybridization histochemistry: comparison with dopamine D2 receptor mRNA. *Brain Res.* 564, 203-219.

Brown, R.T., Freeman, W.S., Perrin, J.M., Stein, M.T., Amler, R.W., Feldman, H.M., Pierce, K., Wolraich, M.L., 2001. Prevalence and assessment of attention-deficit/hyperactivity disorder in primary care settings. *Pediatrics* 107, E43.

Cardinal, R.N., Pennicott, D.R., Sugathapala, C.L., Robbins, T.W., Everitt, B.J., 2001. Impulsive choice induced in rats by lesions of the nucleus accumbens core. *Science* 292, 2499-2501.

Cardinal, R.N., Winstanley, C.A., Robbins, T.W., Everitt, B.J., 2004. Limbic corticostriatal systems and delayed reinforcement. *Ann.N.Y.Acad.Sci.* 1021, 33-50.

Carey, M.P., Diewald, L.M., Esposito, F.J., Pellicano, M.P., Gironi Carnevale, U.A., Sergeant, J.A., Papa, M., Sadile, A.G., 1998a. Differential distribution, affinity and plasticity of dopamine D-1 and D-2 receptors in the target sites of the mesolimbic system in an animal model of ADHD. *Behav.Brain Res.* 94, 173-185.

Carey, M.P., Diewald, L.M., Esposito, F.J., Pellicano, M.P., Gironi Carnevale, U.A., Sergeant, J.A., Papa, M., Sadile, A.G., 1998b. Differential distribution, affinity and plasticity of dopamine D-1 and D-2 receptors in the target sites of the mesolimbic system in an animal model of ADHD. *Behav.Brain Res.* 94, 173-185.

Chaouloff, F., Courvoisier, H., Moisan, M.P., Mormede, P., 1999. GR 127935 reduces basal locomotor activity and prevents RU 24969-, but not D-amphetamine-induced hyperlocomotion, in the Wistar-Kyoto hyperactive (WKHA) rat. Psychopharmacology (Berl) 141, 326-331.

Chess, A.C., Keene, C.S., Wyzik, E.C., Bucci, D.J., 2005. Stimulus processing and associative learning in Wistar and WKHA rats. *Behav.Neurosci.* 119, 772-780.

Choi, W.S., Machida, C.A., Ronnekleiv, O.K., 1995. Distribution of dopamine D1, D2, and D5 receptor mRNAs in the monkey brain: ribonuclease protection assay analysis. *Brain Res.Mol.Brain Res.* 31, 86-94.

Chudasama, Y., Robbins, T.W., 2006b. Functions of frontostriatal systems in cognition: comparative neuropsychopharmacological studies in rats, monkeys and humans. *Biol.Psychol.* 73, 19-38.

Chudasama, Y., Robbins, T.W., 2006a. Functions of frontostriatal systems in cognition: comparative neuropsychopharmacological studies in rats, monkeys and humans. *Biol.Psychol.* 73, 19-38.

Chudasama, Y., Robbins, T.W., 2006c. Functions of frontostriatal systems in cognition: comparative neuropsychopharmacological studies in rats, monkeys and humans. *Biol.Psychol.* 73, 19-38.

Cohen, A.I., Todd, R.D., Harmon, S., O'Malley, K.L., 1992. Photoreceptors of mouse retinas possess D4 receptors coupled to adenylate cyclase. *Proc.Natl.Acad.Sci.U.S.A* 89, 12093-12097.

Davids, E., Zhang, K., Kula, N.S., Tarazi, F.I., Baldessarini, R.J., 2002b. Effects of norepinephrine and serotonin transporter inhibitors on hyperactivity induced by neonatal 6-hydroxydopamine lesioning in rats. *J.Pharmacol.Exp.Ther.* 301, 1097-1102.

Davids, E., Zhang, K., Kula, N.S., Tarazi, F.I., Baldessarini, R.J., 2002a. Effects of norepinephrine and serotonin transporter inhibitors on hyperactivity induced by neonatal 6-hydroxydopamine lesioning in rats. *J.Pharmacol.Exp.Ther.* 301, 1097-1102.

Davids, E., Zhang, K., Tarazi, F.I., Baldessarini, R.J., 2002c. Stereoselective effects of methylphenidate on motor hyperactivity in juvenile rats induced by neonatal 6-hydroxydopamine lesioning. *Psychopharmacology (Berl)* 160, 92-98.

Diaz, H.R., Castellanos, F.X., 2006. Differential effects of a selective dopamine D1-like receptor agonist on motor activity and c-fos expression in the frontal-striatal circuitry of SHR and Wistar-Kyoto rats. *Behav.Brain Funct.* 2, 18.

Drolet, G., Proulx, K., Pearson, D., Rochford, J., Deschepper, C.F., 2002. Comparisons of behavioral and neurochemical characteristics between WKY, WKHA, and Wistar rat strains. *Neuropsychopharmacology* 27, 400-409.

Emiliano, A.B., Fudge, J.L., 2004. From galactorrhea to osteopenia: rethinking serotonin-prolactin interactions. *Neuropsychopharmacology* 29, 833-846.

Ernst, M., Liebenauer, L.L., King, A.C., Fitzgerald, G.A., Cohen, R.M., Zametkin, A.J., 1994. Reduced brain metabolism in hyperactive girls. *J.Am.Acad.Child Adolesc.Psychiatry* 33, 858-868.

Faraone, S.V., Biederman, J., 1998. Neurobiology of attention-deficit hyperactivity disorder. *Biol.Psychiatry* 44, 951-958.

Fisch, G.S., 2007. Animal models and human neuropsychiatric disorders. *Behav.Genet.* 37, 1-10.

Forssberg, H., Fernell, E., Waters, S., Waters, N., Tedroff, J., 2006. Altered pattern of brain dopamine synthesis in male adolescents with attention deficit hyperactivity disorder. *Behav.Brain Funct.* 2, 40.

Fossella, J.A., Sommer, T., Fan, J., Pfaff, D., Posner, M.I., 2003. Synaptogenesis and heritable aspects of executive attention. *Ment.Retard.Dev.Disabil.Res.Rev.* 9, 178-183.

Fox, G.B., Pan, J.B., Esbenshade, T.A., Bennani, Y.L., Black, L.A., Faghih, R., Hancock, A.A., Decker, M.W., 2002. Effects of histamine H(3) receptor ligands GT-2331 and ciproxifan in a repeated acquisition avoidance response in the spontaneously hypertensive rat pup. *Behav.Brain Res.* 131, 151-161.

Funada, M., Sato, M., Aoo, N., Wada, K., 2006. [Role of the monoamine system in the brain on the development of psychological dependence on toluene]. Nihon Arukoru Yakubutsu Igakkai Zasshi 41, 31-38.

Gainetdinov, R.R., Wetsel, W.C., Jones, S.R., Levin, E.D., Jaber, M., Caron, M.G., 1999. Role of serotonin in the paradoxical calming effect of psychostimulants on hyperactivity. *Science* 283, 397-401.

Gerfen, C.R., Engber, T.M., Mahan, L.C., Susel, Z., Chase, T.N., Monsma, F.J., Jr., Sibley, D.R., 1990. D1 and D2 dopamine receptor-regulated gene expression of striatonigral and striatopallidal neurons. *Science* 250, 1429-1432.

Gonzalez-Lima, F., Sadile, A.G., 2000b. Network operations revealed by brain metabolic mapping in a genetic model of hyperactivity and attention deficit: the naples high- and low-excitability rats. *Neurosci.Biobehav.Rev.* 24, 157-160.

Gonzalez-Lima, F., Sadile, A.G., 2000a. Network operations revealed by brain metabolic mapping in a genetic model of hyperactivity and attention deficit: the naples high- and low-excitability rats. *Neurosci.Biobehav.Rev.* 24, 157-160.

Grandy, D.K., Marchionni, M.A., Makam, H., Stofko, R.E., Alfano, M., Frothingham, L., Fischer, J.B., Burke-Howie, K.J., Bunzow, J.R., Server, A.C., ., 1989. Cloning of the cDNA and gene for a human D2 dopamine receptor. *Proc.Natl.Acad.Sci.U.S.A* 86, 9762-9766.

Grandy, D.K., Zhou, Q.Y., Allen, L., Litt, R., Magenis, R.E., Civelli, O., Litt, M., 1990. A human D1 dopamine receptor gene is located on chromosome 5 at q35.1 and identifies an EcoRI RFLP. *Am.J.Hum.Genet.* 47, 828-834.

Griffon, N., Crocq, M.A., Pilon, C., Martres, M.P., Mayerova, A., Uyanik, G., Burgert, E., Duval, F., Macher, J.P., Javoy-Agid, F., Tamminga, C.A., Schwartz, J.C., Sokoloff, P., 1996. Dopamine D3 receptor gene: organization, transcript variants, and polymorphism associated with schizophrenia. *Am.J.Med.Genet.* 67, 63-70.

Hand, D.J., Fox, A.T., Reilly, M.P., 2006. Response acquisition with delayed reinforcement in a rodent model of attention-deficit/hyperactivity disorder (ADHD). *Behav.Brain Res.* 175, 337-342.

Hendley, E.D., Ohlsson, W.G., 1991. Two new inbred rat strains derived from SHR: WKHA, hyperactive, and WKHT, hypertensive, rats. *Am.J.Physiol* 261, H583-H589.

Highfield, D.A., Hu, D., Amsel, A., 1998a. Alleviation of x-irradiation-based deficit in memory-based learning by D-amphetamine: suggestions for attention deficit-hyperactivity disorder. *Proc.Natl.Acad.Sci.U.S.A* 95, 5785-5788.

Highfield, D.A., Hu, D., Amsel, A., 1998b. Alleviation of x-irradiation-based deficit in memory-based learning by D-amphetamine: suggestions for attention deficit-hyperactivity disorder. *Proc.Natl.Acad.Sci.U.S.A* 95, 5785-5788.

Hinshaw, S.P., 1992. Academic underachievement, attention deficits, and aggression: comorbidity and implications for intervention. *J.Consult Clin.Psychol.* 60, 893-903.

Huntley, G.W., Morrison, J.H., Prikhozhan, A., Sealfon, S.C., 1992b. Localization of multiple dopamine receptor subtype mRNAs in human and monkey motor cortex and striatum. *Brain Res.Mol.Brain Res.* 15, 181-188.

Huntley, G.W., Morrison, J.H., Prikhozhan, A., Sealfon, S.C., 1992a. Localization of multiple dopamine receptor subtype mRNAs in human and monkey motor cortex and striatum. *Brain Res.Mol.Brain Res.* 15, 181-188.

Jackson, D.M., Westlind-Danielsson, A., 1994. Dopamine receptors: molecular biology, biochemistry and behavioural aspects. Pharmacol.Ther. 64, 291-370.

Kandel, E.R., 2001. The molecular biology of memory storage: a dialogue between genes and synapses. *Science* 294, 1030-1038.

Kataoka, M., Kuwahara, R., Matsuo, R., Sekiguchi, M., Inokuchi, K., Takahashi, M., 2006. Development- and activity-dependent regulation of SNAP-25 phosphorylation in rat brain. *Neurosci.Lett.* 407, 258-262.

Kebabian, J.W., Calne, D.B., 1979. Multiple receptors for dopamine. Nature 277, 93-96.

Kostrzewa, R.M., Brus, R., Kalbfleisch, J.H., Perry, K.W., Fuller, R.W., 1994. Proposed animal model of attention deficit hyperactivity disorder. Brain Res.Bull. 34, 161-167.

Le, M.C., Normand, E., Bloch, B., 1991. Phenotypical characterization of the rat striatal neurons expressing the D1 dopamine receptor gene. *Proc.Natl.Acad.Sci.U.S.A* 88, 4205-4209.

Lehohla, M., Kellaway, L., Russell, V.A., 2004. NMDA receptor function in the prefrontal cortex of a rat model for attention-deficit hyperactivity disorder. *Metab Brain Dis.* 19, 35-42.

Lehohla, M., Russell, V., Kellaway, L., 2001. NMDA-stimulated Ca2+ uptake into barrel cortex slices of spontaneously hypertensive rats. *Metab Brain Dis.* 16, 133-141.

Lowe, N., Kirley, A., Hawi, Z., Sham, P., Wickham, H., Kratochvil, C.J., Smith, S.D., Lee, S.Y., Levy, F., Kent, L., Middle, F., Rohde, L.A., Roman, T., Tahir, E., Yazgan, Y., Asherson, P., Mill, J., Thapar, A., Payton, A., Todd, R.D., Stephens, T., Ebstein, R.P., Manor, I., Barr, C.L., Wigg, K.G., Sinke, R.J., Buitelaar, J.K., Smalley, S.L., Nelson, S.F., Biederman, J., Faraone, S.V., Gill, M., 2004. Joint analysis of the DRD5 marker concludes association with attention-deficit/hyperactivity disorder confined to the predominantly inattentive and combined subtypes. *Am.J.Hum.Genet.* 74, 348-356.

Meador-Woodruff, J.H., Grandy, D.K., Van Tol, H.H., Damask, S.P., Little, K.Y., Civelli, O., Watson, S.J., Jr., 1994. Dopamine receptor gene expression in the human medial temporal lobe. *Neuropsychopharmacology* 10, 239-248.

Mill, J., Sagvolden, T., Asherson, P., 2005. Sequence analysis of Drd2, Drd4, and Dat1 in SHR and WKY rat strains. *Behav.Brain Funct.* 1, 24.

Mochida, S., 2000. Protein-protein interactions in neurotransmitter release. *Neurosci.Res.* 36, 175-182.

Moisan, M.P., Llamas, B., Cook, M.N., Mormede, P., 2003. Further dissection of a genomic locus associated with behavioral activity in the Wistar-Kyoto hyperactive rat, an animal model of hyperkinesis. *Mol.Psychiatry* 8, 348-352.

Moser, M.B., Moser, E.I., Wultz, B., Sagvolden, T., 1988. Component analyses differentiate between exploratory behaviour of spontaneously hypertensive rats and Wistar Kyoto rats in a two-compartment free-exploration open field. *Scand.J.Psychol.* 29, 200-206.

Mrzljak, L., Bergson, C., Pappy, M., Huff, R., Levenson, R., Goldman-Rakic, P.S., 1996. Localization of dopamine D4 receptors in GABAergic neurons of the primate brain. *Nature* 381, 245-248.

O'Malley, K.L., Harmon, S., Tang, L., Todd, R.D., 1992. The rat dopamine D4 receptor: sequence, gene structure, and demonstration of expression in the cardiovascular system. *New Biol.* 4, 137-146.

OKAMOTO, K., AOKI, K., 1963. Development of a strain of spontaneously hypertensive rats. *Jpn.Circ.J.* 27, 282-293.

Parkinson, J.A., Olmstead, M.C., Burns, L.H., Robbins, T.W., Everitt, B.J., 1999. Dissociation in effects of lesions of the nucleus accumbens core and shell on appetitive pavlovian approach behavior and the potentiation of conditioned reinforcement and locomotor activity by D-amphetamine. *J.Neurosci.* 19, 2401-2411.

Petronis, A., Van Tol, H.H., Lichter, J.B., Livak, K.J., Kennedy, J.L., 1993. The D4 dopamine receptor gene maps on 11p proximal to HRAS. *Genomics* 18, 161-163.

Raber, J., Mehta, P.P., Kreifeldt, M., Parsons, L.H., Weiss, F., Bloom, F.E., Wilson, M.C., 1997. Coloboma hyperactive mutant mice exhibit regional and transmitter-specific deficits in neurotransmission. *J.Neurochem.* 68, 176-186.

Rettig, J., Heinemann, C., Ashery, U., Sheng, Z.H., Yokoyama, C.T., Catterall, W.A., Neher, E., 1997. Alteration of Ca2+ dependence of neurotransmitter release by disruption of Ca2+ channel/syntaxin interaction. *J.Neurosci.* 17, 6647-6656.

Rettig, J., Sheng, Z.H., Kim, D.K., Hodson, C.D., Snutch, T.P., Catterall, W.A., 1996. Isoform-specific interaction of the alpha1A subunits of brain Ca2+ channels with the presynaptic proteins syntaxin and SNAP-25. *Proc.Natl.Acad.Sci.U.S.A* 93, 7363-7368.

Rice, D.C., 2000. Parallels between attention deficit hyperactivity disorder and behavioral deficits produced by neurotoxic exposure in monkeys. *Environ.Health Perspect.* 108 Suppl 3, 405-408.

Rocha, B.A., Fumagalli, F., Gainetdinov, R.R., Jones, S.R., Ator, R., Giros, B., Miller, G.W., Caron, M.G., 1998. Cocaine self-administration in dopamine-transporter knockout mice. *Nat.Neurosci.* 1, 132-137.

Rorick-Kehn, L.M., Johnson, B.G., Burkey, J.L., Wright, R.A., Calligaro, D.O., Marek, G.J., Nisenbaum, E.S., Catlow, J.T., Kingston, A.E., Giera, D.D., Herin, M.F., Monn, J.A., McKinzie, D.L., Schoepp, D.D., 2007. Pharmacological and Pharmacokinetic Properties of a Structurally Novel, Potent, and Selective Metabotropic Glutamate 2/3 Receptor Agonist: In Vitro Characterization of Agonist (-)-(1R,4S,5S,6S)-4-Amino-2-sulfonylbicyclo[3.1.0]-hexane-4,6-dicarboxylic Acid (LY404039). *J.Pharmacol.Exp.Ther.* 321, 308-317.

Rubinstein, M., Cepeda, C., Hurst, R.S., Flores-Hernandez, J., Ariano, M.A., Falzone, T.L., Kozell, L.B., Meshul, C.K., Bunzow, J.R., Low, M.J., Levine, M.S., Grandy, D.K., 2001. Dopamine D4 receptor-deficient mice display cortical hyperexcitability. *J.Neurosci.* 21, 3756-3763.

Rubinstein, M., Phillips, T.J., Bunzow, J.R., Falzone, T.L., Dziewczapolski, G., Zhang, G., Fang, Y., Larson, J.L., McDougall, J.A., Chester, J.A., Saez, C., Pugsley, T.A., Gershanik, O., Low, M.J., Grandy, D.K., 1997. Mice lacking dopamine D4 receptors are supersensitive to ethanol, cocaine, and methamphetamine. *Cell* 90, 991-1001.

Russell, V., Allie, S., Wiggins, T., 2000. Increased noradrenergic activity in prefrontal cortex slices of an animal model for attention-deficit hyperactivity disorder--the spontaneously hypertensive rat. *Behav.Brain Res.* 117, 69-74.

Russell, V., de Villiers, A., Sagvolden, T., Lamm, M., Taljaard, J., 1995. Altered dopaminergic function in the prefrontal cortex, nucleus accumbens and caudate-putamen of an animal model of attention-deficit hyperactivity disorder--the spontaneously hypertensive rat. *Brain Res.* 676, 343-351.

Safe, S.H., 1994. Polychlorinated biphenyls (PCBs): environmental impact, biochemical and toxic responses, and implications for risk assessment. *Crit Rev.Toxicol.* 24, 87-149.

Sagvolden, T., 2000d. Behavioral validation of the spontaneously hypertensive rat (SHR) as an animal model of attention-deficit/hyperactivity disorder (AD/HD). *Neurosci.Biobehav.Rev.* 24, 31-39.

Sagvolden, T., 2000c. Behavioral validation of the spontaneously hypertensive rat (SHR) as an animal model of attention-deficit/hyperactivity disorder (AD/HD). *Neurosci.Biobehav.Rev.* 24, 31-39.

Sagvolden, T., 2000b. Behavioral validation of the spontaneously hypertensive rat (SHR) as an animal model of attention-deficit/hyperactivity disorder (AD/HD). *Neurosci.Biobehav.Rev.* 24, 31-39.

Sagvolden, T., 2000a. Behavioral validation of the spontaneously hypertensive rat (SHR) as an animal model of attention-deficit/hyperactivity disorder (AD/HD). *Neurosci.Biobehav.Rev.* 24, 31-39.

Sagvolden, T., Johansen, E.B., Aase, H., Russell, V.A., 2005a. A dynamic developmental theory of attention-deficit/hyperactivity disorder (ADHD) predominantly hyperactive/impulsive and combined subtypes. *Behav.Brain Sci.* 28, 397-419.

Sagvolden, T., Metzger, M.A., Schiorbeck, H.K., Rugland, A.L., Spinnangr, I., Sagvolden, G., 1992. The spontaneously hypertensive rat (SHR) as an animal model of childhood hyperactivity (ADHD): changed reactivity to reinforcers and to psychomotor stimulants. *Behav.Neural Biol.* 58, 103-112.

Sagvolden, T., Russell, V.A., Aase, H., Johansen, E.B., Farshbaf, M., 2005b. Rodent models of attention-deficit/hyperactivity disorder. *Biol.Psychiatry* 57, 1239-1247.

Sarter, M., Hagan, J., Dudchenko, P., 1992. Behavioral screening for cognition enhancers: from indiscriminate to valid testing: Part I. *Psychopharmacology* (Berl) 107, 144-159.

Scahill, L., Schwab-Stone, M., 2000. Epidemiology of ADHD in school-age children. *Child Adolesc.Psychiatr.Clin.N.Am.* 9, 541-55, vii.

Sherrington, R., Mankoo, B., Attwood, J., Kalsi, G., Curtis, D., Buetow, K., Povey, S., Gurling, H., 1993. Cloning of the human dopamine D5 receptor gene and identification of a highly polymorphic microsatellite for the DRD5 locus that shows tight linkage to the chromosome 4p reference marker RAF1P1. *Genomics* 18, 423-425.

Silbergeld, E.K., Goldberg, A.M., 1974. Hyperactivity: a lead-induced behavior disorder. Environ.Health Perspect. 7, 227-232.

Silver, L.B., 2000. Attention-deficit/hyperactivity disorder in adult life. Child *Adolesc.Psychiatr.Clin.N.Am.* 9, 511-523.

Solanto, M.V., 1998. Neuropsychopharmacological mechanisms of stimulant drug action in attention-deficit hyperactivity disorder: a review and integration. *Behav.Brain Res.* 94, 127-152.

Solanto, M.V., 2002. Dopamine dysfunction in AD/HD: integrating clinical and basic neuroscience research. *Behav.Brain Res.* 130, 65-71.

Sorensen, J.B., Wiederhold, K., Muller, E.M., Milosevic, I., Nagy, G., de Groot, B.L., Grubmuller, H., Fasshauer, D., 2006. Sequential N- to C-terminal SNARE complex assembly drives priming and fusion of secretory vesicles. *EMBO J.* 25, 955-966.

Spielewoy, C., Gonon, F., Roubert, C., Fauchey, V., Jaber, M., Caron, M.G., Roques, B.P., Hamon, M., Betancur, C., Maldonado, R., Giros, B., 2000a. Increased rewarding properties of morphine in dopamine-transporter knockout mice. *Eur.J.Neurosci.* 12, 1827-1837.

Spielewoy, C., Roubert, C., Hamon, M., Nosten-Bertrand, M., Betancur, C., Giros, B., 2000b. Behavioural disturbances associated with hyperdopaminergia in dopamine-transporter knockout mice. *Behav.Pharmacol.* 11, 279-290.

Steffensen, S.C., Henriksen, S.J., Wilson, M.C., 1999b. Transgenic rescue of SNAP-25 restores dopamine-modulated synaptic transmission in the coloboma mutant. *Brain Res.* 847, 186-195.

Steffensen, S.C., Henriksen, S.J., Wilson, M.C., 1999a. Transgenic rescue of SNAP-25 restores dopamine-modulated synaptic transmission in the coloboma mutant. *Brain Res.* 847, 186-195.

Straughan, D.W., James, T.A., 1979. Inhibitory mechanisms in the substantia nigra and the dopamine pathway. *Int.J.Neurol.* 13, 81-93.

Swanson, J.M., Sunohara, G.A., Kennedy, J.L., Regino, R., Fineberg, E., Wigal, T., Lerner, M., Williams, L., LaHoste, G.J., Wigal, S., 1998. Association of the dopamine receptor D4 (DRD4) gene with a refined phenotype of attention deficit hyperactivity disorder (ADHD): a family-based approach. *Mol.Psychiatry* 3, 38-41.

Taylor, E., 1998. Clinical foundations of hyperactivity research. Behav.Brain Res. 94, 11-24.

Taylor, E., Sergeant, J., Doepfner, M., Gunning, B., Overmeyer, S., Mobius, H.J., Eisert, H.G., 1998. Clinical guidelines for hyperkinetic disorder. European Society for Child and Adolescent Psychiatry. *Eur.Child Adolesc.Psychiatry* 7, 184-200.

Totterdell, S., 2006. The anatomy of co-morbid neuropsychiatric disorders based on cortico-limbic synaptic interactions. *Neurotox.Res.* 10, 65-85.

Trinh, J.V., Nehrenberg, D.L., Jacobsen, J.P., Caron, M.G., Wetsel, W.C., 2003. Differential psychostimulant-induced activation of neural circuits in dopamine transporter knockout and wild type mice. *Neuroscience* 118, 297-310.

Van Tol, H.H., Bunzow, J.R., Guan, H.C., Sunahara, R.K., Seeman, P., Niznik, H.B., Civelli, O., 1991. Cloning of the gene for a human dopamine D4 receptor with high affinity for the antipsychotic clozapine. *Nature* 350, 610-614.

Verderio, C., Pozzi, D., Pravettoni, E., Inverardi, F., Schenk, U., Coco, S., Proux-Gillardeaux, V., Galli, T., Rossetto, O., Frassoni, C., Matteoli, M., 2004. SNAP-25 modulation of calcium dynamics underlies differences in GABAergic and glutamatergic responsiveness to depolarization. *Neuron* 41, 599-610.

Viggiano, D., Grammatikopoulos, G., Sadile, A.G., 2002b. A morphometric evidence for a hyperfunctioning mesolimbic system in an animal model of ADHD. *Behav.Brain Res.* 130, 181-189.

Viggiano, D., Grammatikopoulos, G., Sadile, A.G., 2002a. A morphometric evidence for a hyperfunctioning mesolimbic system in an animal model of ADHD. *Behav.Brain Res.* 130, 181-189.

Viggiano, D., Sadile, A.G., 2000. Hypertrophic A10 dopamine neurones in a rat model of attention-deficit hyperactivity disorder (ADHD). *Neuroreport* 11, 3677-3680.

Viggiano, D., Vallone, D., Ruocco, L.A., Sadile, A.G., 2003. Behavioural, pharmacological, morpho-functional molecular studies reveal a hyperfunctioning mesocortical dopamine system in an animal model of attention deficit and hyperactivity disorder. *Neurosci.Biobehav.Rev.* 27, 683-689.

Voeller, K.K., 2004. Attention-deficit hyperactivity disorder (ADHD). *J.Child Neurol.* 19, 798-814.

Wang, X., Zhong, P., Yan, Z., 2002. Dopamine D4 receptors modulate GABAergic signaling in pyramidal neurons of prefrontal cortex. *J.Neurosci.* 22, 9185-9193.

Wedzony, K., Chocyk, A., Mackowiak, M., Fijal, K., Czyrak, A., 2000. Cortical localization of dopamine D4 receptors in the rat brain--immunocytochemical study. *J.Physiol Pharmacol.* 51, 205-221.

Weiner, D.M., Levey, A.I., Sunahara, R.K., Niznik, H.B., O'Dowd, B.F., Seeman, P., Brann, M.R., 1991. D1 and D2 dopamine receptor mRNA in rat brain. *Proc.Natl.Acad.Sci.U.S.A* 88, 1859-1863.

Wilens, T.E., Biederman, J., Spencer, T.J., 2002. Attention deficit/hyperactivity disorder across the lifespan. *Annu.Rev.Med.* 53, 113-131.

Zelenin, S., Aperia, A., Diaz, H.R., 2002. Calcyon in the rat brain: cloning of cDNA and expression of mRNA. *J.Comp Neurol.* 446, 37-45.

In: Attention Deficit Hyperactivity Disorder (ADHD)
Editors: Stuart M. Gordon and Aileen E. Mitchell
ISBN 978-1-60741-581-7

Chapter 7

Homeopathic Treatment of Children with Attention Deficit Hyperactivity Disorder: Results of a Long-Term Study over 5 Years, Including a Randomized, Double-Blind Placebo Controlled Crossover Trial [1,2,3,4]

Heiner Frei[1], *Klaus von Ammon*[2], *André Thurneysen*[2], *Regula Everts*[3], *Franz Kaufmann*[3], *Daniel Walther*[3], *Maja Steinlin*[3], *Shu-Fang Hsu-Schmitz*[4] *and Marco Collenberg*[4]

[1]University of Berne, Switzerland,
[2]Institute for Complementary and Alternative Medicine, KIKOM, University of Berne, Switzerland
[3]Division of Pediatric Neurology, University Childrens Hospital Berne Switzerland
[4]Institute of Mathematical Statistics (IMSV), University of Berne, Switzerland

Abstract

Introduction: An increasing number of parents turn to homeopathy for treatment of their children with attention defict hyperactivity disorder (ADHD). The Swiss ADHD-study aimed at obtaining scientific evidence for the effectiveness of homeopathy in hyperactive children by a randomized placebo controlled double blind trial, followed by five years of open label observation.

Methods: A total of 83 children, aged 6-16 years, with ADHD diagnosed using the Diagnostic and Statistical Mannual of Mental Disorders-IV (DSM-IV), were recruited. Their mean Conners Global Index (CGI)-rating was 19 points. Prior to the randomised double blind placebo controlled crossover study, they were treated with individually prescribed homeopathic medications (screening phase). 70 patients achieved an improvement of 50% or more in the CGI, which was confirmed by neuropsychological testing. 62 patients participated in the crossover trial. They were split into two groups and received either verum for 6 weeks followed by placebo for 6 weeks (group A), or vice versa (group B). CGI-evaluations were performed at the beginning of the trial and after each crossover period. The Conners Parent and Teacher Raing Scales were evaluated at diagnosis and again after the crossover trial, and CGI ratings were obtained at 18 and 60 months after treatment start.

Results: At the end of the open label *screening phase* cognitive performance such as visual global perception, impulsivity and divided attention, had improved significantly ($p<0.0001$). The comparison of suboptimal and optimal homeopathic prescriptions revealed a highly significant difference in the mean CGI-improvement per month ($p<0.0001$), showing that (optimal) remedies, which perfectly cover the patients symptoms, cause a much stronger improvement than (suboptimal) remedies with an insufficient coverage of the symptoms. During the *crossover trial* CGI parent-ratings were significantly lower under verum than under placebo ($p=0.0479$). Five years after treatment start mean CGI- ratings by parents reached 7 points (64% improvement, $p<0.0001$) in 28 patients who had continued homeopathy, and 9 points (53% improvement, $p=0.0001$) in 25 patients who had stopped any treatment. Seven participants had changed to Methylphenidate (MPD) after the crossover trial. Their final mean CGI-parent rating under MPD was 11 points.

Conclusion: The trial reveals specific effects of homeopathic treatment in ADHD, particularly in the areas of behavioural and cognitive functions. In longtime follow up 74% of all patients benefited from homeopathy without needing any other treatment.

Keywords: *Attention deficit hyperactivity disorder, homeopathy, randomized controlled trial, long-term effects.*

Introduction

The attention-deficit disorder is a combination of impaired attention (visual, tactile, auditory and proprioceptive) and hyperactivity/impulsivity or passivity (ADHD/ADD). Diagnostic criteria for the disorder are six or more symptoms of either inattention, hyperactivity/impulsivity, or both [5]. ADHD is one of the most common disorders of childhood, occurring in 3-5% of children, with male to female ratios ranging from 3:1 to 9:1 [6]. Common medical treatments are stimulants such as Methylphenidate (MPD), which fall under the legislation for narcotics. Parents who do not want such medication for their child, seek increasingly homeopathic alternatives [7,8]. Homeopathy relies on highly diluted substances, chosen according to the characteristic individual symptoms of the patient, to cause a positive therapeutic effect. The aim of the homeopathic physician is to find the specific remedy that corresponds most closely to the individual symptoms of the patient [9] Since this process depends on precise observations by patients or parents, the initial phase of treatment is often characterised by the use of different medications until an optimal response is reached. The effectiveness of homeopathy, in which the active substance is no longer traceable due to its high dilution, is contested. Two large meta analyses have concluded that the clinical effects of homeopathic treatments should not be interpreted merely as a placebo effect [10,11]. A third study [12], although widely criticised for its methodology [13,14,15,16], postulates that the clinical effects of homeopathy equal that of placebo. This shows that the issue remains controversial. The suggestion that better trials in specific clinical diseases are necessary to establish scientific evidence for the effectiveness of homeopathy led to the Swiss ADHD study, encompassing an initial open-label treatment phase (screening phase), a double-blind crossover trial and an open label long-term follow-up over five years

The *objectives* of this study were to find answers to the following questions:

A) Screening phase:

1 How many patients respond to homeopathic treatment?

2 How long do responding patients need until they reach a sufficient treatment effect (i.e. an improvement of Conners Global Index (CGI)-ratings[2]* of 50% or more [17]?

3 Do neuropsychological parameters change in successfully treated patients?

4 How do CGI-ratings in responding patients change before and after the identification of the *individually optimal* homeopathic treatment? (I.e. is there a difference in CGI-improvement between suboptimal and optimal homeopathic prescriptions, or do all medications cause similar CGI-changes, suggesting a nonspecific treatment effect)?

B) Crossover trial

5 Is the effect of homeopathy significantly distinct and distinguishable from placebo in the treatment of ADHD?

C) Long-term follow up

6 How high is the percentage of patients successfully treated with homeopathy alone in a five-year follow up.

7 What CGI-values do the study participants reach with continued homeopathic treatment, what are the CGI-values after treatment stop, and what are they in patients who changed to stimulants?

Methods

Design

The need for individually prescribed homeopathic medication complicates the planning of a double blind clinical trial, as blinding is only possible *after* the correct individual medication for each patient has been found. Since this process is particularly difficult in ADHD patients, a straightforward randomised controlled trial was deemed impossible. In our previous study [18] we made the observation that in *early* phase of ADHD treatment with Q-potencies*, the improvement attained declines within four weeks after stopping the medication and reappears if treatment is restarted. The deterioration seen when early treatment is interrupted could therefore be used to test the difference between placebo and

2 The Conners Global Index is a 10 item rating scale encompassing the most important ADHD symptoms (see below). It is used in conventional medicine to monitor stimulant treatment.

* Liquid homeopathic medications produced by dilution steps of 1:50'000, administered daily [9].

verum in a crossover trial and led to the present study design. In the first phase of this study, children received individually prescribed homeopathic treatment (*screening phase*). Children who achieved a pre-defined level of improvement then participated in a randomised, double blind, placebo controlled crossover trial, to study deterioration under placebo.

The *double blind part* of the study consisted of two parallel groups of children who received verum (V) for six weeks followed by placebo (P) for six weeks (group A: VP), or placebo for six weeks followed by verum for six weeks (group B: PV). Both groups received another six weeks of open label treatment (group A: VPV, group B: PVV) and an additional follow-up under treatment up to 18 months after treatment start. The length of each crossover period was determined using the data from the previous study of the authors [16] and a preliminary study in four children which revealed that the carry-over effect was longer than four weeks after stopping treatment. Since a carry-over effect may be an obstacle for a crossover trial, relatively long crossover periods of six weeks were chosen. From previous experience this duration was thus considered long enough to minimize this problem. No wash-out time was therefore incorporated between the two crossover periods.

For *long-time follow-up* the parents had to evaluate the treatment course 6 and 14 weeks after the crossover trial, and at 18 and 60 months after treatment start. 18 months after treatment start they were free to choose either to go on with homeopathy, to stop any treatment at all or to change to MPD.

Eligibility

Eligibility criteria for screening phase: Age between 6 and 16 years, both genders, confirmed ADHD according to criteria of DSM-IV [5] and known neuropsychological correlates (greater difficulty on learning, memory, non-automated language tasks, and traditional frontal executive measures) [19,20], necessity for treatment, absence of any chronic physical, neurological or psychiatric disorders. Necessity for treatment was assumed if parents or teachers imperatively demanded an intervention in order to improve the integration and performance of the patient in family or school. A primary selection of possible candidates was made using the Conners Parent Rating Scale (CPRS), the Conners Teacher Rating Scale (CTRS) [17] and the Kinsbourne Attention Questionnaire [21]. Patients complying with the ADHD criteria in these questionnaires underwent neuropsychological and neurological testing at the Division of Paediatric Neurology of the University Children's Hospital Berne to confirm the ADHD diagnosis. Subjects taking methylphenidate were obliged to stop medication before neuropsychological testing. Candidates not conforming to rigorous ADHD criteria in the questionnaires were excluded. Patients were recruited between January 2002 and September 2003 by referral of informed paediatricians and by information of regional ADHD parent organisations. All parents previously knew about their participation in a study involving homeopathy.

Assessment for confirmation of diagnosis: A 2- to 4-hour neuropsychological examination was performed on patients by a paediatric psychologist and a paediatric neurologist between January 2002 and September 2003. The tests were always arranged in the same order. The organisation of the session and the time of day for testing were identical for all subjects in order to avoid effects of uncontrolled factors on performance. The investigation included the following tests: Checklist DSM-IV criteria [5], K-ABC [22] or WISC-III [23], TAP [24], motor function test of Largo [25] and general physical and neurological examination. Children conforming to all diagnostic ADHD criteria, including a parent-rated CGI [17] of at least 14 points without any treatment, were referred to the homeopathic paediatrician for individual treatment.

Eligibility criteria for crossover trial: Patients must reach an amelioration of 50% of the initial CGI value or at least 9 points during the screening phase. Written informed consent was obtained from the parents of each child.

Treatment and Assessments

Screening phase: Patients entered homeopathic treatment within one month after confirmation of diagnosis. Every eligible child was seen only once at the beginning of the screening phase by the homeopathic physician to minimize any further psychological support influencing ADHD symptoms. They received individually prescribed homeopathic treatment daily according to the guidelines of Hahnemann and Boenninghausen [9,26]. To cope with the special difficulties of homeopathic treatment of ADHD patients the applied procedure was slightly modified, as described in an earlier publication [3]. Any other ADHD treatment was prohibited throughout the whole study-period and had to stop immediately or subsequently. Compliance to this rule was checked by periodical inquiry during treatment controls and neuropsychological assessments. Treatment progress was clinically assessed with parents only, at intervals of four weeks by the homeopathic paediatrician including regular reporting of the CGI. No other counselling took place in these sessions. Adjustment of the medication was made as necessary. The duration of the screening phase was determined on an individual bases and not a priori limited by the study design.

Crossover trial: Participants eligible for the crossover trial were referred to the University Children's Hospital between September 2002 and February 2004 . Prior to their assignment at random to treatment groups A or B, they underwent neuropsychological testing again to document changes in performance between diagnosis and crossover trial, i.e. possible effects of homeopathic treatment in the screening phase. Patients, their parents, the investigators and the consulting physician were blind to the assigned treatments and the consulting physician had no contact with patients and parents during the crossover trial. Children with acute diseases, serious accidents and severe social changes in their life during the crossover trial were not assessed for all endpoints and were considered as dropouts; they were, however, included in the primary endpoint analysis according to the intention-to-treat principle.

Open label treatment follow-up: At the end of the second crossover period, all patients continued on open label verum-treatment for an unlimited period of time.

Endpoints

The primary endpoint for the crossover trial was the parents' rating of CGI, a 10-item rating scale containing the most important ADHD symptoms (i.e. temper outbursts / excitable, impulsive / overactive / cries often / inattentive / fidgeting / disturbs other children / easily frustrated / fails to finish things / moods change quickly. Rating: 0=never, 1=occasionally, 2=often, 3=very often) [15]. Baseline value for the *screening phase* was the CGI assessed before treatment start, and for the *crossover trial* the CGI assessed before entering the crossover trial. The CGI was evaluated again after each crossover period and six weeks after the crossover trial. For an additional long-time follow-up the CGI was assessed again 18 and 60 months after treatment start. Secondary endpoints were the CPRS and CTRS, completed by parents and teachers at diagnosis and 14 weeks after the crossover trial. Subtests of K-ABC[22] and TAP[24] performed at diagnosis and prior to entering the crossover trial served as additional neuropsychological endpoints.

Ethics

The study was conducted in accordance with the International Conference on Harmonisation, Guidelines for Good Clinical Practice [27], the Declaration of Helsinki with all its amendments [28], and in compliance with relevant regulations for informed consent and protection of subject rights in Switzerland. The study protocol was approved by the ethics committee of the Canton of Berne and Swissmedic. The sponsors had no influence on the design, implementation and publication of the study.

Statistics

Sample size: The sample size was calculated for the CGI, the primary endpoint in the crossover trial. A mean reduction of 11.25 points (SD 4.00) in CGI had been observed in a previous homeopathic study [18]. Four weeks after interruption of treatment, the CGI increased by only 5 points (unpublished observation), indicating a possible carry-over effect of verum. If this effect were strong, measurements obtained during the second period should be ignored [29]. A statistical test of carry-over effect is however not recommended [30]. To take into account the potential carry-over effect and drop-outs, the sample size was therefore estimated using the conservative approach of a t-test for two parallel groups in the first period. A reduction of 5 points from pre-treatment value due to verum was considered clinically relevant and a zero point reduction was assumed under placebo. Taking into account the possibly greater heterogeneity in this trial due to a different recruitment practice when compared with the previous study, the SD was inflated to 5 for verum and the same value was assumed for placebo. To achieve a 5% significance level and a 95% statistical power, 27 patients were required in each treatment group Hence, a total of approximate 50-60 patients was planned. No interim analyses were considered.

Randomisation

Patient stratification by age and CGI before treatment start was used in the crossover trial: Stratum 1: Age 6-11, baseline CGI 14-21

- Stratum 2: Age 6-11, baseline CGI 22-30
- Stratum 3: Age 12-16, baseline CGI 14-21
- Stratum 4: Age 12-16, baseline CGI 22-30

For each stratum, a randomisation list for 50 patients was computer generated with a block size of 4 by the Institute of Mathematical Statistics of the University of Berne. The random treatment assignments were sealed in consecutively numbered envelopes and given to the manufacturer Spagyros, who produced the homeopathic medications [9] and their placebos. Spagyros was informed in writing by the conculting physician when a child was eligible for the double blind crossover study. The appropriate medication for that child was then prepared according to the randomisation scheme. The medication was sent by mail to the participating family at the beginning of each crossover period. Placebos (20% alcohol, diluted 1:1000 when administered to the patients) were indistinguishable from verum in packaging, labelling, colour and taste. There was no contact between Spagyros, the investigators, the participants and the physician during the crossover trial, except when a child dropped out due to unexpected problems.

Statistical Methods

The data collected during the *screening phase*, including data from patients who were not enrolled in the subsequent crossover phase, were used in the analysis for answering the questions raised concerning the screening phase. The time to reach randomisation eligibility was estimated (median and 95% confidence intervals) for all patients using the Kaplan Meier method. Data from non-responding patients were censored at the time of study drop-out. For responders, the within-patient difference in CGI change rate (points/month) between the suboptimal and the optimal treatment phases was analysed by the signed rank test. For patients who immediately entered the optimal treatment phase, their CGI change rate was set to zero for the suboptimal treatment phase. For non-responders, the CGI change rate in the suboptimal treatment phase was analysed also by the signed rank test. All tests were two-sided.

For the evaluation of the *crossover trial* the assessments of each outcome variable recorded at the end of both crossover periods within a patient were not independent. To analyse such correlated data, a linear mixed model, including a random patient effect, a fixed treatment effect and a fixed period effect was applied using SAS® version 8 [31,32]. With this approach, patients who dropped out after the first crossover period could also be included in the analysis, by assuming missing at random. For other types of analyses, patients with missing values were excluded. For selected variables of behaviour and cognitive performance, the within-patient differences between diagnosis and the beginning of the crossover trial were analysed using the Wilcoxon signed rank test. The changes in CGI from diagnosis to later time points were analysed by paired t-test. All significance tests were two-sided. The statistician was blinded to the sequence of the two study groups.

Results

Recruitment, Participant Flow and Baseline Data

A total of 140 children were evaluated and 83 fulfilled the rigorous ADHD criteria to enter the screening process. Seventy children (84%) reached the eligibility for the crossover study *(Figure 1).* Eight children dropped out due to insufficient response to homeopathy (three no response at all, 5 partial responders with a median improvement of 7 points, range 6-8), and five patients dropped out due to compliance problems (median improvement 6 points, range 3-8). Eight patients, who had reached the eligibility did not enter the crossover trial (5 patient refusal, 3 reached eligibility after deadline for entering the crossover trial), i.e. 62 patients finally participated in the double blind trial. Summaries of their baseline data are presented in *Table 1 and 2*. Patient characteristics were similar between treatment groups (i.e. no statistically significant differences were found in baseline data between treatment groups with the exception of number recall [K-ABC], p=0.0284). The median CGI before treatment was 19 (range 15-25) in both treatment groups. As usual in groups of ADHD subjects, cognitive functions of the patients as a group did not deviate much from the normal population means (exception: short term memory, *Table 2*).

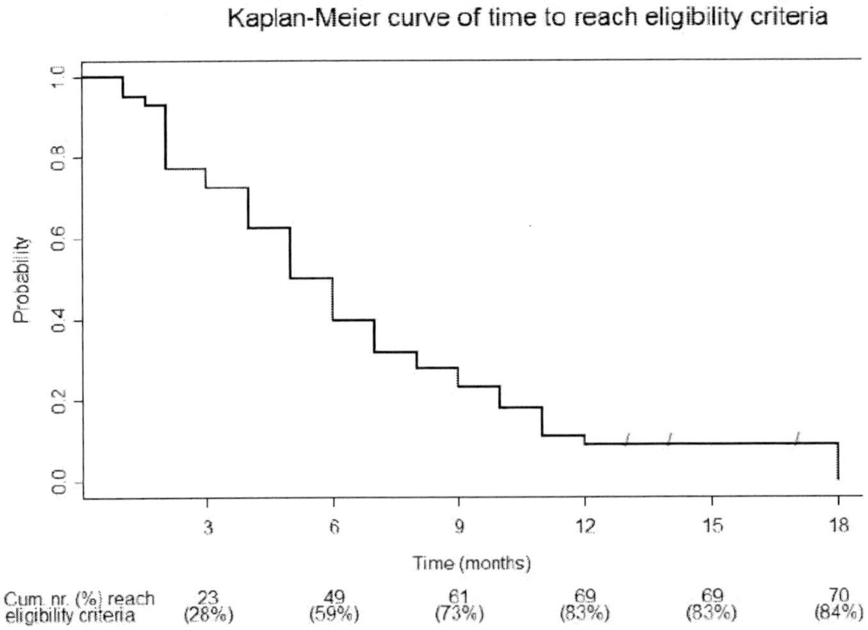

Figure 1 shows the time patients need to reach eligibility for the crossover trial (50% or 9 point improvement in their CGI rating). After 12 months of treatment 83 % of all patients are eligible.

Table 1. Baseline Data, Diagnostic Criteria and CGI Data

	Group A N = 31	Group B N = 31
Baseline data		
Gender (girls / boys)	4 / 27	3 / 28
Median age (range)	10 (7-15)	10 (7-15)
Social situation (intact family / single parent)	23 (74%) / 8 (26%)	20 (65%) / 11 (35%)
Prior stimulant treatment	7 (23%)	4 (13%)
Clinical characteristics at diagnosis		
DSM-IV criteria		
Inattention (n=56)	27 (87%)	29 (94%)
Hyperactivity / impulsivity (n=36)	19 (61%)	17 (55%)
Inattention and hyperactivity/impulsivity (n=31)	15 (48%)	16 (52%)
CGI data		
Median before treatment, cut-off <14 (range)	19 (15-25)	19 (15-25)
Median at end of screening phase (range)	8 (5-14)	8 (4-15)
Ratio of changes with respect to before-treatment value	58%	58%

No statistically significant differences have been found in baseline data between treatment arms.

Table 2. Baseline Data from Neuropsychological Tests

		Group A N = 31	Group B N = 31
	Normal Values	*Baseline Values*	*Mean ± SD*
Intelligence			
General intelligence (K-ABC)	100 ± 15	96.1 ± 11.8	95.2 ± 7.7
Sequential Processing Scale (K-ABC)	100 ± 15	88.4 ± 13.0	85.5 ± 10.0
Simultaneous Processing Scale (K-ABC)	100 ± 15	101.4 ± 13.1	101.8 ± 10.4
Memory			
Sequential short term memory (K-BC,HM)	10 ± 3	8.5 ± 3.2	8.7 ± 2.5
Auditory abstract STM (K-ABC, NR)	10 ± 3	7.6 ± 2.0	6.3 ± 1.8
Auditory semantic STM (K-ABC, WO)	10 ± 3	8.3 ± 2.9	8.1 ± 2.5
Spatial short term memory (K-ABC, BC)	10 ± 3	10.2 ± 2.5	9.7 ± 2.9
Perception			
Visual global (K-ABC, GC)	10 ± 3	10.0 ± 2.6	10.5 ± 2.1
Visual constructive (K-ABC, TR)	10 ± 3	10.4 ± 2.2	9.9 ± 2.5
Executive Functions			
Inferential thinking (K-ABC, MA)	10 ± 3	10.2 ± 2.5	10.5 ± 2.2

Table 2 (Continued)

Performance sequences (K-ABC, PS)	10 ± 3	10.1 ± 2.4	10.4 ± 2.5
Attention			
Divided attention (TAP, DA, m)	50 ± 10	48.4 ± 11.7	45.2 ± 12.4
Impulsivity (TAP, GN, m)	50 ± 10	41.8 ± 7.7	41.9 ± 11.6

STM:	short term memory	m:	mistakes	BC:	block counting
GC:	gestalt closure	PS:	photo series	HM:	hand movements
TR:	triangles	DA	divided attention	NR:	number recall
MA:	matrix analogies	GN:	Go/NoGo	WO:	word order

No statistically significant differences have been found in neuropsychological baseline data between treatment arms [exception attributable to coincidental: number recall (K-ABC) p 0.0284].

Screening Phase

The 62 children participating in the crossover trial attained the eligibility criteria after a mean treatment duration of 5.1 months (SD 3.20, range 1-18 months) with a median CGI of 8 (range 4-15). The following homeopathic medications were used in potencies between Q 3 and Q 42 with success (number of patients): Calcarea-carb. (15), Sulphur (8), Chamomilla (5), Lycopodium (5), Silica (5), Hepar-sulph. (4), Nux-vom. (4), China (3), Ignatia (3), Mercurius (3), Capsicum (1), Causticum (1), Hyoscyamus (1), Phosphorus (1), Phosphoric-ac. (1), Sepia (1), Staphysagria (1) [33]. The neuropsychological tests assessed at diagnosis and at entry to the crossover trial allow comparison of performance throughout the screening phase. Highly significant improvement in visual detection of details, impulsivity and divided attention were observed (*Table 3*).

During the *optimal treatment period* which led to eligibility for the randomised controlled phase, responding patients had a median rate of change in CGI of -4.50 points per month (range -14 to -1) compared with a rate of change of -0.53 points per month (range -7 to 2.5) during the preceding *suboptimal treatment period* ($p < 0.0001$). Once the optimal medication was identified, eligibility for the randomised controlled phase was reached quickly (median 1 month, range 1-3). Non responding patients, for whom an optimal medication was not identified, had a median improvement of only -0.57 CGI points per months (range -4 to 0.5), a rate of change similar to that observed in the responding patients during the suboptimal treatment period [2].

Crossover Trial

Four of the 62 randomised patients dropped out during the crossover trial, three during crossover period one and one during crossover period two (3 verum, 1 placebo).

Table 3. Results of Screening Phase: Total of observed differences in Cognitive Performance between Diagnosis and Crossover Period One (Wilcoxon signed rank test)

Outcome Variable	Median of Differences	Difference in %*	p-value**	Effect
Visual global perception (GC[A], K-ABC)	-3	10.1	0.0001	Improvement
Impulsivity (Go/NoGo, SD[B], TAP)	-13	17.0	0.1044	Improvement
Impulsivity (Go/NoGo, median[C], TAP)	17.5	16.2	0.0001	Improvement
Impulsivity (Go/NoGo, mistakes, TAP)	-43	104.2	0.0001	Improvement
Divided attention (SD[B], TAP)	-30.5	24.1	0.0001	Improvement
Divided attention (median[C], TAP)	-32	44.3	0.0001	Improvement
Divided attention (missings, TAP)	-29	24.6	0.0001	Improvement
Divided attention (mistakes, TAP)	-30.5	27.1	0.0001	Improvement

* Ratio of changes with respect to the before treatment values.

** If $p < 0.05$: difference in performance between diagnosis and crossover period one is significantly different from zero.

A gestalt closure

B standard deviation of reaction time

C median of reaction time

Reasons for drop out were increasing tics, behavioural problems and a reactive depression. Following the intention-to-treat principle, all 62 patients were included in the analysis.

Prior to the crossover trial, both treatment groups had similar CGI (8, range 3-16 in group A vs. 9, range 4-20 in group B). Within-patient comparison of treatment effect shows that the CGI, the primary endpoint, increased under placebo with a mean of 1.67 points (95% CI -3.316, -0.016) compared with verum, indicating a statistically significant improvement in ADHD symptoms with verum (p=0.0479) At the end of six weeks of open label treatment after the crossover trial, the ADHD symptoms of both treatment groups had returned to around their values at beginning of the crossover trial (8, range 2-16 in group A vs. 8, range 2-21 in group B).

Open Label Treatment Follow-Up

Comparison of CPRS scores between start of treatment and 14 weeks after crossover trial still revealed highly significant improvements in all subscales, in both mothers' and fathers' ratings. Teachers ratings (CTRS) showed a significant improvement of behaviour, and a trend to improvement of the CGI. Impulsivity/hyperactivity and passivity were improved, but didn't reach significance in teachers observations *(Table 4).* The median CGI of the 62 children dropped significantly from 19 (range 15-25) at treatment start to 8 (range 2-16), 6 weeks after the crossover trial (*Figure 2*). At follow-up 14 weeks after the crossover trial, however, a rise to 10 points (range 1-18) was observed *(Figure 2).* This rise may be attributable to lack of treatment compliance as both children and parents were less likely to follow the strict conditions of the crossover periods during continued open label treatment. At a further assessment (median duration of treatment 18 months, range 10-30 months: early entry into the trial led to longer follow-up times), 53 children reached a median CGI of 7 points (range 2-15) (*Figure 2*), corresponding to an overall improvement of 63% ($p < 0.0001$).

Long time observation: 60 of the 62 participants of the crossover-trial were available for a 5-year follow up. Long term *CGI* ratings by parents reached 7 points (63% improvement, $p<0.0001$) in 28 patients who continued homeopathic treatment, and 9 points (53% improvement, $p=0.0001$) in 25 patients who had stopped any treatment. Seven participants had changed to Methylphenidate (MPD) after the crossover trial. Their final CGI-parent rating under MPD was 11 points *(Figure 3)* [33].

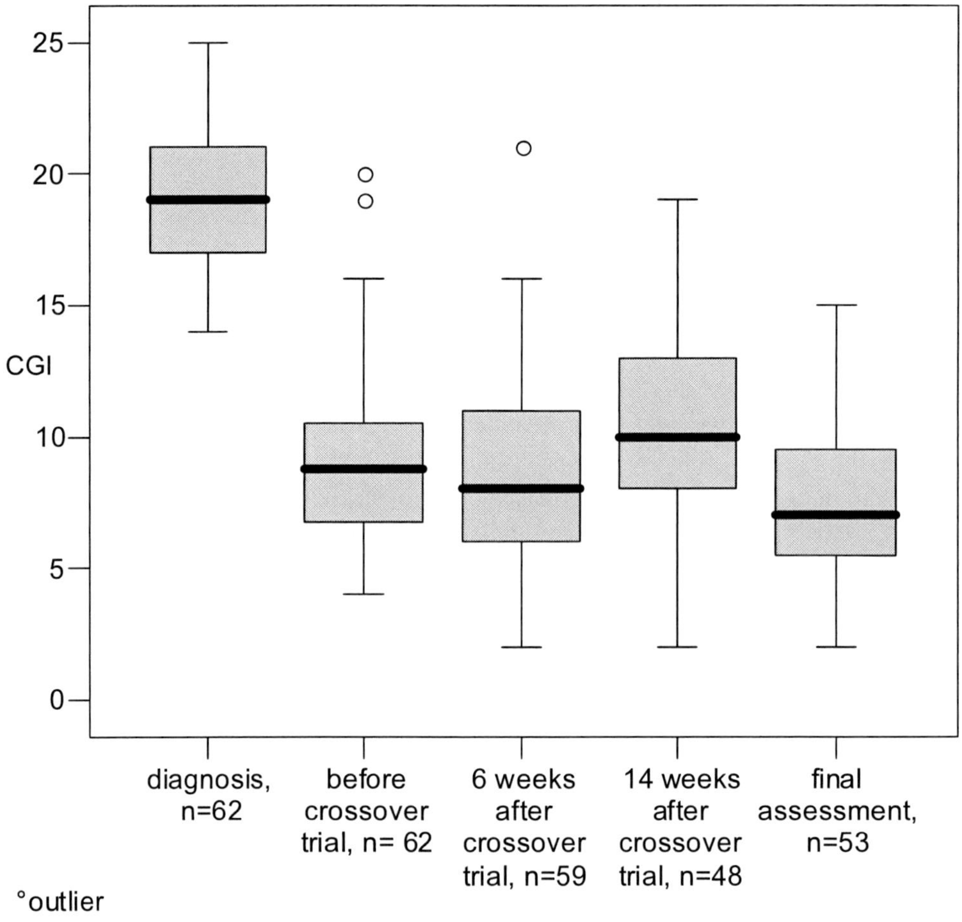

Figure 2. Course of CGI between diagnosis and follow-up (median, quartile, range)Alterations of CGI throughout screening-phase, crossover trial and long-time follow-up. Transient rise after crossover trial due to possible compliance problems. The latest follow-up during open label treatment showed a maximum amelioration of 12 points (63%).

Table 4. Long-term Treatment Effects: Differences in Conners' Parents Rating Scales between Diagnosis and Follow-up 14 Weeks after Crossover Trial (Wilcoxon signed rank test)

Parents' Rating	Median of Differences	Difference in %	p-value	Effect
Behaviour	3.5	42.5	0.0001	Improvement
Learning / Attention	3	36.5	0.0001	Improvement
Psychosomatics	1	46.7	0.0004	Improvement
Impulsivity / Hyperactivity	3	41.5	0.0001	Improvement
Shyness / Anxiety	1	39.5	0.0001	Improvement
Conners' Global Index	7	43.3	0.0001	Improvement
Behaviour	3	36.4	0.0347	Improvement
Impulsivity / Hyperactivity	2	28.0	0.1932	Improvement
Passivity	2	27.8	0.1184	Improvement
Conners' Global Index	3	30.8	0.0561	Improvement

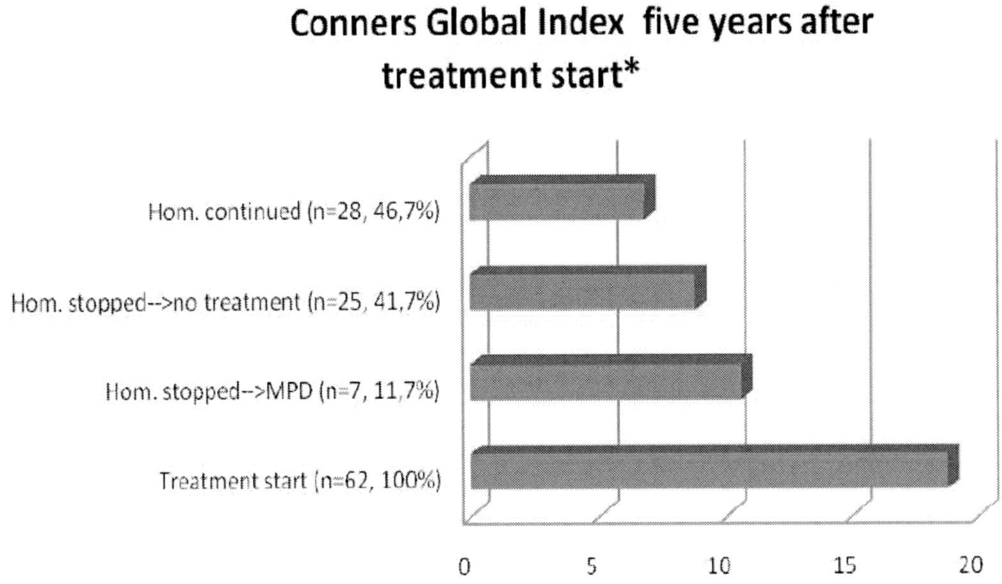

Figure 3.* Participants of crossover-trial, 60 of 62 patients traceable. Improvement of CGI with continued homeopathic treatment (63% of initial CGI-value). Persitent imprrovemnet of CGI after treatment stop (53% of initial CGI-value).

Conclusion

The necessity of individual prescriptions in homeopathy is a severe obstacle for any double blind trial. The present study design, including a screening phase prior to the crossover trial, and analysing deterioration instead of improvement during crossover trial, enabled us to use individually prescribed medication in a double blind trial. Since it is known, that homeopathic medications may produce strong carryover effects, and that these effects may compromise the results of a crossover trial, placebo-phases had to be of a duration, which was at the limits of tolerance for a number of participating families. Another limitation of the study design was the necessity to exclude patients from the crossover trial who showed an inadequate response to homeopathic treatment during the screening phase. This means that the intention to treat principle could not be followed through all the way. The implications of this obstacle are discussed below. Patients participating in the study have been selected by a rigorous diagnostic evaluation, ruling out any other diagnosis but ADHD. In addition, strict inquiries at periodical controls were performed to prevent the application of any other treatment but homeopathy. The long duration of observation of an average of 60 months was chosen to make sure that observed changes are not just of transitory nature.

The time needed to reach the eligibility criteria for the crossover trial (mean 5,1 months) shows, that the study design with an initial open label screening phase was essential, if one wants to compare a real effect of homeopathy with placebo. If one would choose a randomisation and blinding at treatment start, the evaluation of homeopathic treatment in children with ADHD should take place after 12 months of treatment, when 83 % of the study participants have reached the eligibility criteria (as in our screening phase). The problem of such a study design is, that an ethic commission would hardly allow placebo-treatment for twelve months.

Due to the fact that homeopathic physicians make extended explorations of patient histories and inquiries about the family and social environment of their patients, sceptics often assume, that the effects of homeopathic treatment are merely psychological, caused by the time the physician devotes to the patient. On the other hand homeopathy claims, that only homeopathic remedies which perfectly cover the specific patient symptoms have an effect on the disease of the patients. If this is correct, suboptimal homeopathic prescriptions, i.e. medications which do not optimally cover the patient symptoms, should have little effect on the disease (i.e. near placebo-effect), while optimally chosen medications will cause a considerable improvement. – The highly significant difference in CGI-change/month between suboptimal prescriptions and the final optimal one ($p< 0.0001$) supports the hypothesis that a correctly chosen homeopathic medication has a specific effect, while suboptimal prescriptions act similar to placebos.

Comparison of some of the cognitive tests at diagnosis and at the beginning of the crossover trial after the initial open label homeopathic therapy reveal highly significant treatment effects. Since every other treatment was stopped during the screening phase, this improvement is only explicable by the homeopathic intervention. The question arises whether the 8 patients who dropped out of the screening phase due to insufficient treatment response cause a selection bias influencing the results considerably. Five of these dropouts still had a partial amelioration under treatment. Their influence on the high significance of the results of the screening phase and the long time follow up would therefore have been minimal. Thus, it is unlikely, that they would have caused very different results. Improvements in cognitive deficits following stimulant treatment of ADHD patients, especially spatial working memory, attention-set shifting and visual search performance have been reported in the literature [34]. The effects of homeopathy observed in this study are similar. To gain a better insight into the quantitative aspects of cognitive improvements following treatment, a comparison of matched patients receiving stimulants, homeopathy or placebo would be worthwhile.

Effects of homeopathy in children with ADHD have been demonstrated in the present randomised double blind crossover trial. The within-patient difference in CGI between treatment with verum or placebo was statistically significant ($p=0.0479$) and supports the positive effect of homeopathy. However, CGI increased under placebo by only 17 percent (1.67 CGI points), less than that expected from the results of an earlier study [18]. This may be due to more precisely prescribed individual homeopathic medication in this trial, with a consequently stronger carry-over effect (persistence of two thirds of the improvements reached under homeopathy throughout the placebo phase). Following an additional six weeks of open label treatment, both groups had CGI values similar to those at the beginning of the crossover trial, an indirect confirmation of the appropriateness of the study design. The validity of the CGI has been proven over time across many studies and therefore its application in this study is well supported [35].

The CGI and the CPRS-scores (parent ratings) have decreased between 37% and 63% 14 weeks after the crossover trial, most probably related to treatment induced adjustment of behaviour. The CTRS improvement ratings by teachers at this time were smaller (between 28% and 37%) than those of the parents, reflecting the higher cognitive stress for patients in school situations. However, as a whole, the overall-intensity of ADHD symptoms is lower during treatment and results in an improvement in the children's social, emotional and scholastic behaviour. The question whether these long-term improvements are a treatment effect or merely due to a spontaneous change in development of the children cannot by definitely answered by our trial data. However, the authors have observed that stopping treatment after prolonged medication leads to a *slow* partial decline of previous improvements over a time-period of several months in most children. Such a course cannot just be explained by spontaneous evolution and is highly suggestive of a treatment effect.

The five-year follow-up in the participants of the crossover trial showed that 88% of the patients still did well in school and family, either with continued homeopathic treatment, or without any treatment at all. Considering the improvement in 84% of the patients in the screening phase, and the long-term improvement in 88% of the participants of the crossover trial, one may conclude that 74% of the initially recruited patients were benefited by homeopathy.

The results of this trial thus point to the effectiveness of homeopathy in treatment of ADHD. Factors limiting the widespread use of this method in the treatment of ADHD are the time needed for amelioration of symptoms, excluding this treatment from use in emergency situations, and the necessity of accurate observation and recording of symptoms by the parents.

References

[1] Frei H, Everts R, Ammon K v, Kaufmann F, Walther D, Hsu-Schmitz SF, Collenberg M, Fuhrer K, Hassink R, Steinlin M, Thurneysen A. Homeopathic treatment of children with attention deficit disorder: a randomised, double blind, placebo controlled trial. *Eur J Pediatr* (2005) 164:758-767.

[2] Frei H, Everts R, Ammon K v, Kaufmann F, Walther D, Hsu-Schmitz SF, Collenberg M, Steinlin M, Lim C, Thurneysen A. Randomised controlled trials of homeopathy in hyperactive children: treatment procedure leads to an unconventional study design. *Homeopathy* (2007) 96, 35-41.

[3] Frei H, von Ammon K, Thurneysen A. Treatment of hyperactive children: Increased efficiency through modifications of homeopathic diagnostic procedure. *Homeopathy* 2006, 95, 163-170.

[4] Von Ammon K, Sauter U, Thurneysen A, Everts R, Hsu Schmitz S, Steinlin M, Frei H. Long-term effects and costs of homeopathic treatment in children with attention deficit hyperactivity disorder (publication in preparation).

[5] American Psychiatric Association. Diagnostic and statistical manual of mental disorders, DSM-IV. 4th edition. Washington DC: American Psychiatric Association, 1994.

[6] Lahey BB, Applegate B, McBurnett K, Biederman J, Greenhill L, Hynd GW, Barkley RA, Newcorn J, Jensen P, Richters J. DSM-IV field trials for attention deficit hyperactivity disorder in children and adolescents. *Am J Psychiatry* 1994; 151: 1673-85.

[7] Brue AW, Oakland TD. Alternative treatments for attention deficit/hyperactivity disorder: does evidence support their use? *Altern Ther Health Med* 2002; 8: 68-70, 72-4. Review.

[8] Gross-Tsur V, Lahad A, Shalev R. Use of complementary medicine in children with attention deficit hyperactivity disorder and epilepsy. *Ped Neurol* 2003; 29: 53-55.

[9] Hahnemann CFS. Organon der Heilkunst, 6th edition. Heidelberg: Haug, 1989.

[10] Kleijnen J, Knipschild P. Clinical trials of homeopathy. *Brit Med J* 1991; 302: 316-323.

[11] Linde K, Clausius N, Ramirez G, Melchart D, Eitel F, Hedges LV, Jonas WB. Are the clinical effects of homeopathy placebo effects? A meta-analysis of controlled trials. *Lancet* 1997; 350: 834-843.

[12] Shang A, Huwiler-Müntener K, Nartey L, Jüni P, Dörig S, Sterne JA, Pewsner D, Egger M. Are the clinical effects of homeopathy placebo effects? Comparative study of placebo-controlled trials of homeopathy and allopathy. *Lancet* 2005, 366 (9487): 726-732.

[13] Fisher P, Berman B, Davidson J, Reilly D, Thompson T. Are the clinical effects of homeopathy placebo effects? *Lancet* 2005, 366 (9503):2082-2083.

[14] Kiene H, Kienle GS, von Schön-Angerer T. Failure to exclude false negative bias: a fundamental flaw in the trial of Shang et al. *J Altern Complement Med.* 2005 Oct;11(5):783

[15] Lüdtke R, Rutten AL. The conclusions on the effectiveness of homeopathy highly depend on the set of analyzed trials. *J Clin Epidemiol.* 2008. Doi:10.1016/j.jclinepi.2008.06.015
[16] Rutten AL, Stolper CF. The 2005 meta-analysis of homeopathy: the importance of post publication data. *Homeopathy* 2008; 97:169-177.
[17] Conners CK. Conners rating scales (revised), technical manual. Toronto: MHS; 1997.
[18] Frei H, Thurneysen A. Treatment for hyperactive children: homeopathy and methylphenidate compared in a family setting. *Brit Hom J* 2001; 90: 183-188.
[19] Carte ET, Nigg JT, Hinshaw SP. Neuropsychological functioning, motor speed, and language processing in boys with and without ADHD. *J Abnorm Child Psychol* 1996; 24: 481-98.
[20] Seidman LJ, Biederman J, Monuteaux MC, Weber W, Faraone SV. Neuropsychological functioning in nonreferred siblings of children with attention deficit/hyperactivity disorder. *J Abnorm Psychol* 2000: 109: 252-65.
[21] Kinsbourne M. School problems. *Paediatrics* 1973; 52: 679-710.
[22] Kaufman AS, Kaufman NL. Kaufman Assessment Battery for Children (K-ABC). Circle Pines: AGS Publishing, 1983.
[23] Tewes U, Schallberger U, Rossmann K. Hamburg Wechsler Intelligenztest für Kinder III (HAWIK-III). Göttingen: Hogrefe, 1999.
[24] Zimmermann P, Fimm B. Testbatterie zur Aufmerksamkeitsprüfung TAP, Handbuch. Freiburg: Psychologische Testsysteme PsyTest, 1992.
[25] Largo R. Zürcher neuromotorische Untersuchung. Zürich: Abteilung für Wachstum und Entwicklung Universitäts-Kinderklinik, 1993.
[26] Bönninghausen C v. Bönninghausens therapeutisches Taschenbuch, Revidierte Ausgabe, Hrsg. K-H. Gypser. Stuttgart: Sonntag, 2000.
[27] Lattmann P, Schneider A. Informationen für den Prüfer zur Durchführung klinischer Versuche mit Heilmitteln in der Schweiz. Zürich: SGCI, 1995.
[28] World Medical Association, Declaration of Helsinki. Washington, 2002.
[29] Grizzle JE. The two-period change-over design and its use in clinical trials. *Biometrics* 1965; 21: 467-480.
[30] Senn S. Cross-over Trials in Clinical Research. Chichester: John Wiley and Sons, 1993: 12-13.
[31] Brown H, Prescott R. Applied Mixed Models in Medicine. Chichester: John Wiley and Sons, 1999: 261-294.
[32] Verbeke G, Molenberghs G. (Editors) Linear Mixed Models in Practice. New York: Springer, 1997.
[33] Allen TF. The Encyclopaedia of Pure Materia Medica, Volume 1-12, reprint New Delhi: Jain, 1990.
[34] Mehta MA, Goodyer IM, Sahakian BJ. Methylphenidate improves working memory and set shifting in AD/HD: relationships to baseline memory capacity. *J Child Psychol and Psychiatr* 2004; 45: 293-305.
[35] Snyder SM, John F, Xenakis SN. Validation of ADHD rating scales. *J Am Acad Child Adolesc Psychiatry* 2004; 43:1189-90.

In: Attention Deficit Hyperactivity Disorder (ADHD)
Editors: Stuart M. Gordon and Aileen E. Mitchell
ISBN 978-1-60741-581-7

Chapter 8

ADHD and Sleep

Ahmad Ghanizadeh *
Child and Adolescent Psychiatry, Research Center for Psychiatry and Behavioral Sciences, Department of Psychiatry, Shiraz University of Medical Sciences, Shiraz, Iran
Academic Child Psychiatry Unit, Royal Children's Hospital, University of Melbourne, Melbourne, Australia

Introduction

ADHD symptoms are one of the most common psychiatric problems in children and adolescents [1]. On other hand, the magnitude of sleep problems in children and adolescents is high and it is a major public health concern [2]. The association of sleep and ADHD is still poorly recognized [3].

Prevalence and Importance

Sleep problems are common in children with ADHD [4] and usually continue from childhood to adulthood and these children's objective sleep characteristics is similar to their adulthood sleep characteristics [5]. Sleep problems in clinical samples of children and adolescents with ADHD is reported to be about 25% to 50% [6].

There is a high percentage of symptom overlap between primary hypersomnia and ADHD, indicating possible misdiagnosis of both conditions [7]. Sleep deprivation is related with ADHD-like behavior [8]. In addition, there is an increased instability in sleep onset, sleep duration, and true sleep in children with ADHD compared with the control group. This instability of the sleep-wake system is supposed to be a characteristic of children with ADHD [9]. Assessment of sleep problems in evaluating of children with potential ADHD is required

* Research Center for Psychiatry and Behavioral Sciences, Hafez Hospital, Shiraz, Iran.
Tel: +98 711 627 30 70, Email: ghanizad@sina.tums.ac.ir
Tel: +61 3 9345 4666

[10]. It is recommended that sleep problems should be evaluated before starting drug treatment for ADHD [11].

Sleep problems in children with ADHD are associated with poorer child, caregiver, and family outcomes [12]. The level of sleep efficiency of children with ADHD moderates their performance on the cognitive function [13]. Insufficient and poor-quality sleep leads to daytime sleepiness, and behavioral problems. Also, sleep insufficiency affects on attention, working memory, and other executive functions of the prefrontal cortex [8, 14]. Daytime sleepiness results in a decline of verbal creativity, poor abstract reasoning, impaired motor skills, impairment of attention, vigilance, and memory functions [15, 16].

There is a possibility that sleep problems in children with ADHD are primary conditions that lead to other symptoms such as hyperactivity and inattentiveness. So, some studies reported that sleep disorders might be misdiagnosed as ADHD [17]. Another possibility is that ADHD is the primary condition and sleep problems are its consequenmces [18]. There is a bidirectional way between sleep problems and ADHD. ADHD symptoms may be mimicked by sleep problems and sleep problems may be mimicked or exacerbated by ADHD symptoms [19].

Association of Sleep and ADHD

There are controversies about the sleep pattern and problems in children with ADHD [4, 20]. Restless sleep was a part of diagnostic criteria of ADHD in DSM-III [21]. It was not a diagnostic criterion in DSM-III-R and IV. Probably, studies using DSM-III have been confounded by this criterion. Some screening instruments such as the Conners Parent Rating Scale included sleep problems as a part of the diagnostic procedures for ADHD [22].

A study reported decreased REM sleep in children with ADHD [23]. Another study did not report decreased REM-sleep in ADHD [24].

A systematic review study indicated that sleep onset latency and sleep-architecture parameters including the number of stage changes; percentages of stage 1, 2, slow wave, and REM sleep; REM latency; and sleep efficiency in children with ADHD were not different from those of controls [4]. This study considered confounding factors such as co-morbid psychiatric disorders and medication status. Some studies reported normal sleep architecture in children with ADHD and it was concluded that sleep problems and ADHD are two different clinical conditions with similarity symptoms [18].

Sleep problems in ADHD children taking medications are part of behavioral phenotype of ADHD rather than the side effects of treatment [25] and the problems are probably related to the underlying pathophysiology of the disorder [26].

So, prevalence of sleep problems in children with ADHD is frequent and the association of ADHD and sleep is complicated. It is a great challenge for clinicians that should be addressed.

ADHD Subtypes

While some studies emphasize the importance of distinguishing between inattentive type and hyperactive /impulsive type of ADHD and their association with sleep problems in children with ADHD[27], others have reported lack of a significant difference related to ADHD subtype or severity of ADHD [28].

A recently published study concluded that increased parent-reported sleep problems is associated with severe ADHD as opposed to mild/moderate, and primarily mixed ADHD subtype as opposed to inattentive subtype, and with co-morbidity of oppositional defiant disorder [29]. Inattentive type of ADHD is related to daytime sleepiness more than that of hyperactive/impulsive type [27]. Children with ADHD-Inattentive alone are not different from controls regarding sleep problems except daytime sleepiness [30]. Daytime sleepiness is primarily associated with IN subtype, while sleep- disordered breathing and movement during sleep are primarily related to HI subtype [31, 32]. A recent study that considered other co-morbid psychiatric disorders in preschool children with ADHD showed that neither hyperactive-impulsive nor inattentive ADHD symptomatology was uniquely related to parent-reported problems involving sleep assistance, parasomnias, or dyssomnias. Just, inattentive symptomatology was uniquely related to daytime sleepiness [27].

ADHD and Co-Morbidity with Other Psychiatric Problems

More than 75% of the children with ADHD in clinical sample have one or more other co-morbid psychiatric disorder [33]. Anxiety and depression in ADHD children increase the risk of sleep problems [30, 34]. Sleep problems are common in ADHD even than in controls with other psychiatric diagnoses [35]. A lack of morning refreshment is very closely associated with ADHD and insomnia is related to the presence of depressive symptoms in ADHD [36]. Sleep problems such as bedtime resistance, problems with staying asleep, and excessive daytime sleepiness are associated with depressive disorders [37]. Sleep onset delay is associated with anxiety disorder [37].

Moreover, co-morbid disorder of oppositional defiant disorder is frequent in children with ADHD [33]. This disorder may be associated with sleep problems in the ADHD children. For example, oppositional defiant disorder is related to bedtime resistance [38]. However, an objective study reported that there was no relationship between sleep problems and oppositional defiant disorder in children with ADHD [39].

Children with tic disorder and ADHD have shorter REM sleep latency or an elevated REM sleep drive, and their REM sleep duration is increased in comparison to healthy controls in polysomnography [40]. Co-morbidity of tic disorder with ADHD increases sleep problems of the ADHD children [41].

A recent objective study suggests that children with ADHD and without any other co-morbidity or primary sleep disorders and those who are not taking any psychotropic medications have not a prolonged sleep onset latency in comparison to the controls [29].

Medical Condition

General medical conditions are associated with sleep problems. Obese adolescents with excessive sleep may be at a higher risk of ADHD symptoms. This association is independent from symptoms of anxiety/depression [42]. ADHD symptoms should be searched in obese patients with sleepiness [43].

Circadian Rhythm

A deviant circadian rhythm pattern is suggested in children with ADHD [44]. A polymorphism of a gene within the circadian "clock" mechanism is a contributing factor in adults with ADHD [45]. There is a delayed melatonin onset phase in children with ADHD and early insomnia [46]. The symptoms of increased sleep onset latency, subjective complaints on getting to bed at night and wake up in the morning may be related to this delayed phase in the circadian rhythm of sleep and wakefulness. Of course, it is unclear if children with ADHD go to bed later due to a phase delay in their circadian rhythm [47]. Light therapy in the fall/winter period may be a useful adjunct in some adults with ADHD. This improvement is more than alleviation of co-morbid seasonal affective disorder [48].

Hypoarousal States

The day sleepiness in children with ADHD is throughout the day and not only at a particular time [49]. Hypoarousal condition has been related to the etiology of ADHD and hyperactivity is supposed to be a reaction to the hypoarousal condition to counteract somnolence [3, 50, 51].

Restless Legs Syndrome (RLS) and Periodic Leg Movements During Sleep (PLMS)

The PLMS and RLS are probably more frequent in children with ADHD than among controls [52-54] and many children with PLMS have ADHD [55]. In addition, treating of RLS with dpaminerigic medications improves ADHD [56]. The rate of PLMS in children with RLS is about 80% [57]. In a clinical study, 44% of the children with ADHD met definite or probable RLS criteria [58] and about one fifth of those with RLS had co-morbidity with ADHD [59].

Growing Pain

Growing pain is limb discomfort that does not meet criteria for other diagnoses [60]. Some of the clinical samples of children with growing pain meet criteria for RLS [60, 61]. It is interesting that a study reported that neither childhood growing pains nor ADHD is associated to RLS [62].

Sleep-Disordered Breathing

Some studies reported possible association of ADHD and sleep-disordered breathing [53, 63]. Recognition and treatment of underlying sleep-disordered breathing may prevent unnecessary long-term medication usage [64].

Quite a few studies reported that the prevalence of obstructive sleep apnea syndrome in children with ADHD symptoms is not increased [3, 65]. There is no association between anxiety disorder and presence of teeth grinding in ADHD [66]. So, inattention or hyperactivity is not probably due to obstructive sleep apnea syndrome.

In addition, sleep-disordered breathing in children with significant symptoms of ADHD is not different from that of the general pediatric population and it can be readily misperceived and can potentially delay the diagnosis and appropriate treatment [23].

Bruxism

The rate of major depression in the mothers of children with ADHD and teeth grinding is more than those ADHD children without teeth grinding. In addition, the rate of oppositional defiant disorder in ADHD children with teeth grinding is higher. The study did not confirm that anxiety is associated with teeth grinding in ADHD children [66].

Medications

Stimulants

The most common medications for treatment of children with ADHD are stimulants. The effect of these medications on ADHD is also controversial. While, beneficial effects of them on sleep parameters in ADHD have been reported [5, 67], others reported that sleep disturbance is a known adverse effects of stimulant in ADHD [68, 69]. A parental reported study indicated that 61.5% of the 13 ADHD children experienced sleep disturbances [70]. The parental reported problems include long sleep onset latency and frequent nighttime wakening [71]. Relative to baseline, sleep-onset latency is significantly increased in children on thrice-daily methylphenidate [67]. One of the frequent side effects of stimulants is insomnia [72]. Sleep disturbance is the most frequent adverse event reported after taking methylphenidate transdermal system [73].

Stimulants stimulate the central nervous system. Behavioral effects of amphetamine are mediated primarily through dopamine and depend on the dopamine transporter [74]. It is speculated that these increases in extracellular dopamine increases the performance on tasks requiring vigilance and mental awareness, as well as decreased need for sleep which causes insomnia [75]. Sleep architecture of children with ADHD who are on stimulant therapy is different from those children with ADHD who are not on stimulant therapy [65].

Stimulants affect sleep directly and indirectly. Its direct effect is due to its effect on neurotransmitters such as dopamine. The indirect effect is through their rebound effect when the medications level decreases to wear off. So, in addition to the dosage of medication, half life of medication (short acting and longer acting stimulants), dosing-schedule effect, timing of taking medication (in the morning or later) may affect sleep in children with ADHD. Of course, there are not unwanted effects of MPH on sleep, if Mph is administered late in the afternoon in children with ADHD [76].

More recent studies reported that stimulant treatment neither causes nor worsens sleep problems but improves the quality of sleep in adults with ADHD [47]. It is interesting that treatment of initial insomnia has no significant effect on ADHD symptoms [77]. It seems that the main predictor of sleep problems is baseline preexisting sleep problems rather than medication [78]. Actigraphy data indicate that methylphenidate decreases nighttime awakenings in children with ADHD [67]. Analyses of actigraphy indicated significant changes in the children's total sleep time and sleep onset latency in the children with medication compared to the no medication conditions. Nevertheless, the sleep questionnaire did not show it [79].

It is worth noticing that children and adults with ADHD have increased nighttime activity [18, 80]. It is suggested that at least in some of the children with ADHD, ADHD is a disorder with 24-hour duration [4].

Atomoxetine

It is another medication for treatment of ADHD [81]. However, it is a non-stimulant treatment with mechanism of a highly specific norepinephrine reuptake inhibitor effect. It does not increase extracellular dopamine [82]. Atomoxetine may be administered for children with ADHD who have sleep disturbances [83].

Comparing of Atomoxetine and Methylphenidate

Children taking atomoxetine in comparison with methylphenidate report that it is easier to get up in the morning, take less time to fall asleep, and sleep better [67]. Furthermore, parents reported that children who were treated with atomoxetine as compared to methylphenidate were less irritable and less quick to lose their tempers in the morning. Their settling down and getting ready to bed is easier. In contrast to methylphenidate, atomoxetine decreases sleep-onset latency based on both objectives (actigraphy, polysomnography) and subjective (child and parent diaries) measures of sleep. However, methylphenidate decreases sleep interruptions or awakenings more than atomoxetine [67].

Melatonin

An effective treatment for initial insomnia in children with ADHD taking stimulant medication is combined sleep hygiene and melatonin [84]. Melatonin has no significant effect on behavior and cognition of children with ADHD. However, it advances circadian rhythms of sleep-wake and endogenous melatonin. Moreover, melatonin enhances the total time asleep in children with ADHD and chronic sleep onset insomnia [85].

Objective and Subjective Methods

Subjective parent reports of their children with ADHD display a higher rate of sleep problems than the control group children [29]. Some of the most common reported problems are bedtime resistance [86], delayed sleep onset [71], and higher motor movements in sleep[6].

It is possible that the sleep problems are parents' perception rather than the child's actual problems. In fact, there are discrepancies between the objectively measured actigraphy and parent-reported sleep problems [29, 39, 87].

Objective methods are as polysomnography, infrared video camera, actigraphy, and the Multiple Sleep Latency Test (MSLT) [4]. Actigrah is an instrument that detects and stores movement, pattern of sleep and wake and circadian rhythm indexes. This computerized instrument quantifies movement during sleep. So, it distinguishes sleep and wake stages. It is usually worn around the wrist [88]. Actigraphy study indicates a decrease in activity during the day with stimulant treatment in children with ADHD [89].

Video recordings are also used to objectively study movement disorder in sleep. None of the actigraphy and video recordings measure EEG sleep stages or architecture.

Sleep architecture and the stages of EEG sleep can be studied by polysomnography which records some of physiological indexes in laboratory settings [20]. Of course, the correlation of actigraphy data on sleep characteristics with data gathered using polysomnography is well [90].

Multiple sleep latency test (MSLT) is an objective and standardized physiologic measure of sleepiness in children [91]. It is a series of 20-minute daytime nap opportunities with a polysomnographic assessment of sleep onset in a quiet and dark room. Sleep periods and shorter sleep onset latency during the nap opportunities indicates higher levels of physiologic sleepiness.

Most of the studies of sleep using overnight polysomnography (PSG) or actigraphy did not report consistent differences in sleep architecture and patterns between children with ADHD and those without ADHD [4, 92] except for more nocturnal movements[24]. Higher rate of daytime sleepiness and faster falling asleep were consistently reported in objective studies using multiple sleep latency test (MSLT)[49, 93].

Management of Sleep Problems in Children with ADHD

Co-morbid psychiatric disorders and sleep problems should be screened in children with ADHD. Education of parents for sleep hygiene and prescription of medication might be helpful. There are scanty data about the efficacy and safety of different medications on sleep problems in children with ADHD. However, some medications such as some types of antidepressants, hypnotices, and antihistamines might be helpful [19]. It is interesting that symptoms of insomnia in children with ADHD are usually treated by clinicians with medications without enough evidence of their efficacy or safety [94].

Future Direction with Consideration of the Limitations of Previous Studies

There are many methodological problems that prevent us from reaching any firm conclusion about the association of ADHD and sleep [6]. Many of previous stdies have had small sample size from clinical samples with possible referral bias that cannot lead to a reliable conclusion [69, 76]. So, epidemiological studies from general population are required to evaluate the association between sleep problems and ADHD.

There are a few studies that include confounding factors. Sometimes, learning problems or educational problems are not separated from ADHD. The study that included these limitations concluded that sleep disorders and problems are not more common in ADHD children than control group [4]. Association of sleep problems in children with ADHD and developmental and pubertal phases is an ignored research area.

Gold-standard evaluations of ADHD including gathering information from multiple informants such as teachers should be used. A diagnostic criterion of ADHD has been changed from the DSM-III-R. So, a possible bias in diagnosis is possible in studies using DSM-III.

ADHD is not a homogenous disorder. It has different subtypes that should be considered in future studies. Severity of ADHD is usually ignored. Distinction between attention and behavioral problems and disorders should be addressed. Another important factor is considering the chronicity of behavior and sleep pattern and problems.

Future studies should be directed to neuroanatomic, neurophysiologic, and neurochemistric basis of sleep problems in children with ADHD which are under-studied at present.

Some terms such as sleep-disordered breathing and obstructive sleep apnea are not completely defined. There is a spectrum of disorders that vary in severity such as obstructive sleep apnea hypopnea syndrome to snoring without ventilatory abnormalities [19]. Studies using of thermistors and nasal cannulas are required to survey the association of obstructive sleep apnea syndrome and ADHD [3]. Also, body mass index is not usually considered.

There is a paucity of randomized, controlled, double-blinded, placebo-controlled studies about the effects of medication on sleep in children with ADHD [51]. Therefore, further methodologically sound studies are required. Different treatment modalities such as pharmacotherapy and psychotherapy and their efficacy on sleep problems in ADHD in long term have not been studied well.

The instability of the sleep-wake system in children with ADHD is a confounding factor that should be considered [9]. The majority of these sleep differences reported by their parents are not verified by actigraphy [86].

There are some sleep problems that are usually ignored in research in sleep problems such as narcolepsy [86].

Further studies using objective methods to assess sleep/alertness disturbances are needed to gain insight into the relationship between sleep/alertness disturbances and ADHD in obese individuals. However, some of measures of objective evaluation of sleep problems in children have not been standardized [49]. However, recording of the sleep characters in an unfamiliar environment, laboratory setting, may cause an unnatural sleep-wake cycle [95].

Most of the current literature is from clinical samples of ADHD. Although half-life of methylphenidate is very short and 3 days off medication eliminates potential withdrawal effects. However, it should be considered in future studies [96].

Conclusion

The findings of different studies are not consistent. However, most of the studies that considered covariant factors and objective studies such as actigraphy studies have not reported consistent significant differences in sleep architecture and patterns in children with ADHD and controls. Moreover, ADHD is associated with hypoarousal. Hyperactivity is considered as an adaptive behavior that works against the effects of underlying sleepiness during day [19].

References

[1] Ghanizadeh A, Distribution of symptoms of attention deficite hyperactivity disorder in school children of Shiraz, South of Iran. . *Arch Iranian Med* 2008; 11(6); 618-624

[2] Ghanizadeh A, Kianpoor M, Rezaei M, Rezaei H, Moini R, Aghakhani K, Ahmadi J, and Moeini S R, Sleep patterns and habits in high school students in Iran. *Ann. Gen. Psychiatry* 2008; 7: 5.

[3] Miano S, Donfrancesco R, Bruni O, Ferri R, Galiffa S, Pagani J, Montemitro E, Kheirandish L, Gozal D, and Pia Villa M, NREM sleep instability is reduced in children with attention-deficit/hyperactivity disorder. *Sleep* 2006; 29(6): 797-803.

[4] Cortese S, Konofal E, Yateman N, Mouren M C, and Lecendreux M, Sleep and alertness in children with attention-deficit/hyperactivity disorder: a systematic review of the literature. *Sleep* 2006; 29(4): 504-11.

[5] Sobanski E, Schredl M, Kettler N, and Alm B, Sleep in adults with attention deficit hyperactivity disorder (ADHD) before and during treatment with methylphenidate: a controlled polysomnographic study. *Sleep* 2008; 31(3): 375-81.

[6] Corkum P, Tannock R, and Moldofsky H, Sleep disturbances in children with attention-deficit/hyperactivity disorder. *J. Am. Acad.Child Adolesc. Psychiatry* 1998; 37(6): 637-46.

[7] Oosterloo M, Lammers G J, Overeem S, de Noord I, and Kooij J J, Possible confusion between primary hypersomnia and adult attention-deficit/hyperactivity disorder. *Psychiatry Res* 2006; 143(2-3): 293-7.

[8] Fallone G, Acebo C, Arnedt J T, Seifer R, and Carskadon M A, Effects of acute sleep restriction on behavior, sustained attention, and response inhibition in children. *Percept. Mot Skills* 2001; 93(1): 213-29.

[9] Gruber R, Sadeh A, and Raviv A, Instability of sleep patterns in children with attention-deficit/hyperactivity disorder. *J. Am. Acad. Child Adolesc. Psychiatry* 2000; 39(4): 495-501.

[10] Lam L T and Yang L, Duration of sleep and ADHD tendency among adolescents in China. *J. Atten. Disord.* 2008; 11(4): 437-44.

[11] Huang Y S, Chen N H, Li H Y, Wu Y Y, Chao C C, and Guilleminault C, Sleep disorders in Taiwanese children with attention deficit/hyperactivity disorder. *J. Sleep Res.* 2004; 13(3): 269-77.

[12] Sung V, Hiscock H, Sciberras E, and Efron D, Sleep problems in children with attention-deficit/hyperactivity disorder: prevalence and the effect on the child and family. *Arch. Pediatr. Adolesc. Med.* 2008; 162(4): 336-42.

[13] Gruber R, Grizenko N, Schwartz G, Ben Amor L, Gauthier J, de Guzman R, and Joober R, Sleep and COMT polymorphism in ADHD children: preliminary actigraphic data. *J. Am. Acad. Child Adolesc. Psychiatry* 2006; 45(8): 982-989.

[14] Fallone G, Owens J A, and Deane J, Sleepiness in children and adolescents: clinical implications. *Sleep Med. Rev.* 2002; 6(4): 287-306.

[15] Randazzo A C, Muehlbach M J, Schweitzer P K, and Walsh J K, Cognitive function following acute sleep restriction in children ages 10-14. Sleep 1998; 21(8): 861-8.

[16] Fallone G, Seifer R, Acebo C, and Carskadon M A, Prolonged sleep restriction in 11- and 12-year-old children: effects on behavior, sleepiness, and mood. *Sleep* 2000; 23: 28.

[17] Naseem S, Chaudhary B, and Collop N, Attention deficit hyperactivity disorder in adults and obstructive sleep apnea. *Chest* 2001; 119(1): 294-6.

[18] Cohen-Zion M and Ancoli-Israel S, Sleep in children with attention-deficit hyperactivity disorder (ADHD): a review of naturalistic and stimulant intervention studies. *Sleep Med. Rev.* 2004; 8(5): 379-402.

[19] Owens J A, The ADHD and sleep conundrum: a review. *J. Dev. Behav. Pediatr.* 2005; 26(4): 312-22.

[20] Kirov R, Kinkelbur J, Heipke S, Kostanecka-Endress T, Westhoff M, Cohrs S, Ruther E, Hajak G, Banaschewski T, and Rothenberger A, Is there a specific polysomnographic sleep pattern in children with attention deficit/hyperactivity disorder? *J. Sleep Res.* 2004; 13(1): 87-93.

[21] *American Psychiatric Association. Diagnostic and Statistical Manual of Mental Disorders* Third Edition (DSM-III) ed. 1980, Washington, DC: *American Psychiatric Association.*

[22] Conners C K, *Conners' Rating Scales—Revised. Technical Manual.* 1997, Toronto: Multi-Health System.

[23] O'Brien L M, Holbrook C R, Mervis C B, Klaus C J, Bruner J L, Raffield T J, Rutherford J, Mehl R C, Wang M, Tuell A, Hume B C, and Gozal D, Sleep and neurobehavioral characteristics of 5- to 7-year-old children with parentally reported symptoms of attention-deficit/hyperactivity disorder. *Pediatrics* 2003; 111(3): 554-63.
[24] Konofal E, Lecendreux M, Bouvard M P, and Mouren-Simeoni M C, High levels of nocturnal activity in children with attention-deficit hyperactivity disorder: a video analysis. *Psychiatry Clin. Neurosci.* 2001; 55(2): 97-103.
[25] Crabtree V M, Ivanenko A, O'Brien L M, and Gozal D, Periodic limb movement disorder of sleep in children. *J. Sleep Res.* 2003; 12(1): 73-81.
[26] Gruber R, Grizenko N, Schwartz G, Ben Amor L, Gauthier J, de Guzman R, and Joober R, Sleep and COMT polymorphism in ADHD children: preliminary actigraphic data. *J. Am. Acad. Child Adolesc. Psychiatry* 2006; 45(8): 982-9.
[27] Willoughby M T, Angold A, and Egger H L, Parent-reported attention-deficit/hyperactivity disorder symptomatology and sleep problems in a preschool-age pediatric clinic sample. *J. Am. Acad. Child Adolesc. Psychiatry* 2008; 47(9): 1086-94.
[28] Wiggs L, Montgomery P, and Stores G, Actigraphic and parent reports of sleep patterns and sleep disorders in children with subtypes of attention-deficit hyperactivity disorder. *Sleep* 2005; 28(11): 1437-45.
[29] Owens J, Sangal R B, Sutton V K, Bakken R, Allen A J, and Kelsey D, Subjective and objective measures of sleep in children with attention-deficit/hyperactivity disorder. *Sleep Med.* 2008.
[30] Mayes S D, Calhoun S L, Bixler E O, Vgontzas A N, Mahr F, Hillwig-Garcia J, Elamir B, Edhere-Ekezie L, and Parvin M, ADHD Subtypes and Comorbid Anxiety, Depression, and Oppositional-Defiant Disorder: Differences in Sleep Problems. *J. Pediatr Psychol.* 2008.
[31] LeBourgeois M K, Avis K, Mixon M, Olmi J, and Harsh J, Snoring, sleep quality, and sleepiness across attention-deficit/hyperactivity disorder subtypes. *Sleep* 2004; 27(3): 520-5.
[32] Brown T E and McMullen W J, Attention deficit disorders and sleep/arousal disturbance. *Ann. N Y Acad. Sci.* 2001; 931: 520-525.
[33] Ghanizadeh A, Mohammadi M R, and Moini R, Comorbidity of psychiatric disorders and parental psychiatric disorders in a sample of Iranian children with ADHD. *J. Atten. Disord* 2008; 12(2): 149-55.
[34] Ivanenko A, Crabtree V M, Obrien L M, and Gozal D, Sleep complaints and psychiatric symptoms in children evaluated at a pediatric mental health clinic. *J. Clin. Sleep Med.* 2006; 2(1): 42-8.
[35] Day H D and Abmayr S B, Parent reports of sleep disturbances in stimulant-medicated children with attention-deficit hyperactivity disorder. *J. Clin. Psychol* 1998; 54(5): 701-16.
[36] Schredl M, Alm B, and Sobanski E, Sleep quality in adult patients with attention deficit hyperactivity disorder (ADHD). *Eur. Arch. Psychiatry Clin. Neurosci.* 2007; 257(3): 164-8.
[37] Ivanenko A, Crabtree V M, and Gozal D, Sleep and depression in children and adolescents. *Sleep Med. Rev.* 2005; 9(2): 115-29.

[38] O'Brien L M and Gozal D, Sleep in children with attention deficit/hyperactivity disorder. *Minerva Pediatr.* 2004; 56(6): 585-601.

[39] Hvolby A, Jorgensen J, and Bilenberg N, Actigraphic and parental reports of sleep difficulties in children with attention-deficit/hyperactivity disorder. *Arch. Pediatr. Adolesc. Med.* 2008; 162(4): 323-9.

[40] Kirov R, Banaschewski T, Uebel H, Kinkelbur J, and Rothenberger A, REM-sleep alterations in children with co-existence of tic disorders and attention-deficit/hyperactivity disorder: impact of hypermotor symptoms. *Eur. Child Adolesc. Psychiatry* 2007; 16 Suppl 1: 45-50.

[41] Kirov R, Kinkelbur J, Banaschewski T, and Rothenberger A, Sleep patterns in children with attention-deficit/hyperactivity disorder, tic disorder, and comorbidity. *J. Child Psychol. Psychiatry* 2007; 48(6): 561-70.

[42] Cortese S, Maffeis C, Konofal E, Lecendreux M, Comencini E, Angriman M, Vincenzi B, Pajno-Ferrara F, Mouren M C, and Dalla Bernardina B, Parent reports of sleep/alertness problems and ADHD symptoms in a sample of obese adolescents. *J. Psychosom. Res.*2007; 63(6): 587-90.

[43] Cortese S, Konofal E, Dalla Bernardina B, Mouren M C, and Lecendreux M, Does excessive daytime sleepiness contribute to explaining the association between obesity and ADHD symptoms? *Med. Hypotheses* 2008; 70(1): 12-6.

[44] van der Heijden K B, Smits M G, and Gunning W B, Sleep-related disorders in ADHD: a review. *Clin. Pediatr. (Phila)* 2005; 44(3): 201-10.

[45] Kissling C, Retz W, Wiemann S, Coogan A N, Clement R M, Hunnerkopf R, Conner A C, Freitag C M, Rosler M, and Thome J, A polymorphism at the 3'-untranslated region of the CLOCK gene is associated with adult attention-deficit hyperactivity disorder. *Am. J. Med. Genet. B Neuropsychiatr Genet* 2008; 147(3): 333-8.

[46] Van der Heijden K B, Smits M G, Van Someren E J, and Gunning W B, Idiopathic chronic sleep onset insomnia in attention-deficit/hyperactivity disorder: a circadian rhythm sleep disorder. *Chronobiol. Int.* 2005; 22(3): 559-70.

[47] Boonstra A M, Kooij J J, Oosterlaan J, Sergeant J A, Buitelaar J K, and Van Someren E J, Hyperactive night and day? Actigraphy studies in adult ADHD: a baseline comparison and the effect of methylphenidate. *Sleep* 2007; 30(4): 433-42.

[48] Rybak Y E, McNeely H E, Mackenzie B E, Jain U R, and Levitan R D, An open trial of light therapy in adult attention-deficit/hyperactivity disorder. *J. Clin. Psychiatry* 2006; 67(10): 1527-35.

[49] Golan N, Shahar E, Ravid S, and Pillar G, Sleep disorders and daytime sleepiness in children with attention-deficit/hyperactive disorder. *Sleep* 2004; 27(2): 261-6.

[50] Weinberg W A and Harper C R, Vigilance and its disorders. Neurol Clin 1993; 11(1): 59-78.

[51] Lecendreux M and Cortese S, Sleep problems associated with ADHD: a review of current therapeutic options and recommendations for the future. *Expert Rev. Neurother.* 2007; 7(12): 1799-806.

[52] Crabtree V M, Ivanenko A, and Gozal D, Clinical and parental assessment of sleep in children with attention-deficit/hyperactivity disorder referred to a pediatric sleep medicine center. *Clin. Pediatr (Phila)* 2003; 42(9): 807-13.

[53] Chervin R D, Archbold K H, Dillon J E, Pituch K J, Panahi P, Dahl R E, and Guilleminault C, Associations between symptoms of inattention, hyperactivity, restless legs, and periodic leg movements. *Sleep* 2002; 25(2): 213-8.

[54] Picchietti D L, England S J, Walters A S, Willis K, and Verrico T, Periodic limb movement disorder and restless legs syndrome in children with attention-deficit hyperactivity disorder. *J. Child Neurol.* 1998; 13(12): 588-94.

[55] Picchietti D L and Walters A S, Moderate to severe periodic limb movement disorder in childhood and adolescence. *Sleep* 1999; 22(3): 297-300.

[56] Walters A S, Mandelbaum D E, Lewin D S, Kugler S, England S J, and Miller M, Dopaminergic therapy in children with restless legs/periodic limb movements in sleep and ADHD. Dopaminergic Therapy Study Group. *Pediatr. Neurol* .2000; 22(3): 182-6.

[57] Montplaisir J, Boucher S, Poirier G, Lavigne G, Lapierre O, and Lesperance P, Clinical, polysomnographic, and genetic characteristics of restless legs syndrome: a study of 133 patients diagnosed with new standard criteria. *Mov. Disord.* 1997; 12(1): 61-5.

[58] Konofal E, Lecendreux M, Arnulf I, and Mouren M C, Restless legs syndrome and serum ferritin levels in ADHD children. *Sleep* 2003; 26: A136.

[59] Picchietti D L and Stevens H E, Early manifestations of restless legs syndrome in childhood and adolescence. *Sleep* Med 2007.

[60] Walters A S, Is there a subpopulation of children with growing pains who really have Restless Legs Syndrome? A review of the literature. *Sleep Med.* 2002; 3(2): 93-8.

[61] Rajaram S S, Walters A S, England S J, Mehta D, and Nizam F, Some children with growing pains may actually have restless legs syndrome. Sleep 2004; 27(4): 767-73.

[62] Gamaldo C E, Benbrook A R, Allen R P, Scott J A, Henning W A, and Earley C J, Childhood and adult factors associated with restless legs syndrome (RLS) diagnosis. *Sleep Med.* 2007; 8(7-8): 716-22.

[63] Guilleminault C, Ariagno R, Korobkin R, Coons S, Owen-Boeddiker M, and Baldwin R, Sleep parameters and respiratory variables in "near miss' sudden infant death syndrome infants. *Pediatrics* 1981; 68(3): 354-60.

[64] Huang Y S, Guilleminault C, Li H Y, Yang C M, Wu Y Y, and Chen N H, Attention-deficit/hyperactivity disorder with obstructive sleep apnea: a treatment outcome study. *Sleep Med.* 2007; 8(1): 18-30.

[65] O'Brien L M, Ivanenko A, Crabtree V M, Holbrook C R, Bruner J L, Klaus C J, and Gozal D, The effect of stimulants on sleep characteristics in children with attention deficit/hyperactivity disorder. *Sleep Med.* 2003; 4(4): 309-16.

[66] Ghanizadeh A, ADHD, bruxism and psychiatric disorders: does bruxism increase the chance of a comorbid psychiatric disorder in children with ADHD and their parents? *Sleep Breath* 2008; 12(4):375-80.

[67] Sangal R B, Owens J, Allen A J, Sutton V, Schuh K, and Kelsey D, Effects of atomoxetine and methylphenidate on sleep in children with ADHD. *Sleep* 2006; 29(12): 1573-85.

[68] Manos M J, Pharmacologic treatment of ADHD: road conditions in driving patients to successful outcomes. *Medscape J. Med.* 2008; 10(1): 5.

[69] Stein M A, Blondis T A, Schnitzler E R, O'Brien T, Fishkin J, Blackwell B, Szumowski E, and Roizen N J, Methylphenidate dosing: twice daily versus three times daily. *Pediatrics* 1996; 98(4 Pt 1): 748-56.

[70] Ring A, Stein D, Barak Y, Teicher A, Hadjez J, Elizur A, and Weizman A, Sleep disturbances in children with attention-deficit/hyperactivity disorder: a comparative study with healthy siblings. *J. Learn Disabil.* 1998; 31(6): 572-8.

[71] Stein M A, Unravelling sleep problems in treated and untreated children with ADHD. *J. Child Adolesc Psychopharmacol.* 1999; 9(3): 157-68.

[72] Stein M A, Sarampote C S, Waldman I D, Robb A S, Conlon C, Pearl P L, Black D O, Seymour K E, and Newcorn J H, A dose-response study of OROS methylphenidate in children with attention-deficit/hyperactivity disorder. *Pediatrics* 2003; 112(5): e404.

[73] Kowalik S, Minami H, and Silva R R, Critical assessment of the methylphenidate transdermal system. *Drugs Today* (Barc) 2007; 43(8): 515-27.

[74] Boutrel B and Koob G F, What keeps us awake: the neuropharmacology of stimulants and wakefulness-promoting medications. *Sleep* 2004; 27(6): 1181-94.

[75] Bricard C and Boidein F, [Prescribing ritalin in combined modality management of hyperactivity with attention deficit]. *Encephale* 2001; 27(5): 435-43.

[76] Kent J D, Blader J C, Koplewicz H S, Abikoff H, and Foley C A, Effects of late-afternoon methylphenidate administration on behavior and sleep in attention-deficit hyperactivity disorder. *Pediatrics* 1995; 96(2 Pt 1): 320-5.

[77] Weiss M, Wasdell M, Bomben M, Rea K, and Freeman R, Sleep Hygiene and Melatonin Treatment for Children and Adolescents With ADHD and Initial Insomnia. *J. Am. Acad. Child Adolesc. Psychiatry* 2006.

[78] Faraone S V, Glatt S J, Bukstein O G, Lopez F A, Arnold L E, and Findling R L, Effects of Once-Daily Oral and Transdermal Methylphenidate on Sleep Behavior of Children With ADHD. *J Atten. Disord.* 2008.

[79] Corkum P, Panton R, Ironside S, Macpherson M, and Williams T, Acute impact of immediate release methylphenidate administered three times a day on sleep in children with attention-deficit/hyperactivity disorder. *J. Pediatr. Psychol* .2008; 33(4): 368-79.

[80] Philipsen A, Feige B, Hesslinger B, Ebert D, Carl C, Hornyak M, Lieb K, Voderholzer U, and Riemann D, Sleep in adults with attention-deficit/hyperactivity disorder: a controlled polysomnographic study including spectral analysis of the sleep EEG. *Sleep* 2005; 28(7): 877-84.

[81] Cheng J Y, Chen R Y, Ko J S, and Ng E M, Efficacy and safety of atomoxetine for attention-deficit/hyperactivity disorder in children and adolescents-meta-analysis and meta-regression analysis. *Psychopharmacology* (Berl) 2007; 194(2): 197-209.

[82] Bymaster F P, Katner J S, Nelson D L, Hemrick-Luecke S K, Threlkeld P G, Heiligenstein J H, Morin S M, Gehlert D R, and Perry K W, Atomoxetine increases extracellular levels of norepinephrine and dopamine in prefrontal cortex of rat: a potential mechanism for efficacy in attention deficit/hyperactivity disorder. *Neuropsychopharmacology* 2002; 27(5): 699-711.

[83] Prasad S and Steer C, Switching from neurostimulant therapy to atomoxetine in children and adolescents with attention-deficit hyperactivity disorder : clinical

approaches and review of current available evidence. *Paediatr. Drugs*. 2008; 10(1): 39-47.

[84] Weiss M D, Wasdell M B, Bomben M M, Rea K J, and Freeman R D, Sleep hygiene and melatonin treatment for children and adolescents with ADHD and initial insomnia. *J. Am.Acad. Child Adolesc. Psychiatry* 2006; 45(5): 512-9.

[85] Van der Heijden K B, Smits M G, Van Someren E J, Ridderinkhof K R, and Gunning W B, Effect of melatonin on sleep, behavior, and cognition in ADHD and chronic sleep-onset insomnia. *J. Am. Acad. Child Adolesc. Psychiatry* 2007; 46(2): 233-41.

[86] Corkum P, Tannock R, Moldofsky H, Hogg-Johnson S, and Humphries T, Actigraphy and parental ratings of sleep in children with attention-deficit/hyperactivity disorder (ADHD). *Sleep* 2001; 24(3): 303-12.

[87] Owens J A, Maxim R, Nobile C, McGuinn M, and Msall M, Parental and self-report of sleep in children with attention-deficit/hyperactivity disorder. *Arch. Pediatr. Adolesc. Med.* 2000; 154(6): 549-55.

[88] Ancoli-Israel S, Cole R, Alessi C, Chambers M, Moorcroft W, and Pollak C P, The role of actigraphy in the study of sleep and circadian rhythms. *Sleep* 2003; 26(3): 342-92.

[89] Konrad K, Gunther T, Heinzel-Gutenbrunner M, and Herpertz-Dahlmann B, Clinical evaluation of subjective and objective changes in motor activity and attention in children with attention-deficit/hyperactivity disorder in a double-blind methylphenidate trial. *J. Child Adolesc. Psychopharmacol.* 2005; 15(2): 180-90.

[90] Sadeh A, Hauri P J, Kripke D F, and Lavie P, The role of actigraphy in the evaluation of sleep disorders. *Sleep* 1995; 18(4): 288-302.

[91] Hoban T F and Chervin R D, Assessment of sleepiness in children. *Semin. Pediatr. Neurol* 2001; 8(4): 216-28.

[92] Sadeh A, Pergamin L, and Bar-Haim Y, Sleep in children with attention-deficit hyperactivity disorder: a meta-analysis of polysomnographic studies. *Sleep Med. Rev.* 2006; 10(6): 381-98.

[93] Lecendreux M, Konofal E, Bouvard M, Falissard B, and Mouren-Simeoni M C, Sleep and alertness in children with ADHD. *J. Child Psychol. Psychiatry* 2000; 41(6): 803-12.

[94] Owens J A, Rosen C L, and Mindell J A, Medication use in the treatment of pediatric insomnia: results of a survey of community-based pediatricians. *Pediatrics* 2003; 111(5 Pt 1): e628-35.

[95] Wiggs L and Stores G, Children's sleep: how should it be assessed? . ACPP Review *Newsletter* 1995; 17: 153-157.

[96] Nahas A D and Krynicki V, Effect of methylphenidate on sleep stages and ultradian rhythms in hyperactive children. *J. Nerv. Ment. Dis.* 1977; 164(1): 66-9.

In: Attention Deficit Hyperactivity Disorder (ADHD)
Editors: Stuart M. Gordon and Aileen E. Mitchell
ISBN 978-1-60741-581-7

Chapter 9

Environmental Contributions to Attention Deficit Hyperactivity Disorders

Masami Ishido
Environmental Risk Research Programme, National Institute for Environmental Studies, 16-2 Onogawa, Tsukuba 305-8506, Japan

Abstract

Since an emerging body of evidence is accumulating that endocrine disrupting chemicals exert their effects on the central nervous system, their neuronal risk assessment is now required. A previous study showed that a single intracisternal administration of bisphenol A, an endocrine disrupting chemical, into neonatal rats caused hyperactivity, seen in patients with attention deficit hyperactivity disorders(ADHD). To evaluate environmental contributions of bisphenol A to ADHD, it is very important to test the potential of the chemical via an environmental exposure route. In this study, we tested the hypothesis that oral exposure to bisphenol A would exhibit effects observed previously with direct instillation in the rat. Oral administration of 600 μg/pup/day bisphenol A into male Wistar rats aged 5 days to 3 weeks caused significant hyperactivity at 4-5 weeks of age. Treated rats were about 1.3 times as active in the nocturnal phase as were vehicle-treated control rats ($p < 0.005$). The long-term effects of the chemical resulted in a large reduction of immunoreactivity for tyrosine hydroxylase in the midbrain at 7 weeks of age, where terminal deoxynucleotidyl transferase-mediated dUTP nick end-labeling (TUNEL)-positive cells were detected. Furthermore, bisphenol A decreased gene expression levels of dopamine transporter in adult rats.

Introduction

Environmental estrogens are originally defined as a diverse group of synthetic and naturally occurring compounds that mimic the action of steroidal estrogens. These chemicals are called *endocrine disruptors* or *endocrine disrupting chemicals*.

Bisphenol A is one of the well-known endocrine disrupting chemicals (Figure1). Bisphenol A [2,2-bis(4-hydroxyphenyl)propane] is used as a monomer in the manufacture of polycarbonate plastics, epoxy resins, and composites and consequently has extensive applications in the food packaging industry and dentistry [1]. Bisphenol A is released from polycarbonate flasks during autoclaving or from lacquer coatings in food cans, showing estrogenicity for human breast cancer MCF-7 cells [2, 3]. The reproductive effects of this endocrine disruptor have thus been examined.

An emerging body of evidence is accumulating that endocrine disrupting chemcials exert their effects on the central nervous system in rodents. We demonstrated that intracisternal administration of bisphenol A causes hyperactivity in the Wistar male rat [4], following the protocol by Shaywitz *et al.* (1976) who reported that rat pups treated with 6-hydroxydopamine (6-OHDA) by intracisteral administration at 5 days of age exhibited increased motor activity, leading to cognitive difficulties in shuttle-box learning between 2 and 4 weeks of age [5]. Thus, bisphenol A seems to have neurotoxicity in the developing rat brain, although it is still unknown if the chemicals exert their neuronal effects on the developing brain through the action of endocrine disruption or through yet uncharacterized processes.

In addition, the effects of perinatal exposure to bisphenol A have been shown to affect various aspects of behavior such as exploratory, sociosexual [6], and aggressive behaviors [7], as well as anxiety level [8], and nociception [9], and the response to *D*-amphetamin [10]. Impairment by bisphenol A of the sexual differentiation of the exploratory behavior and the size of the locus coeruleus was also observed [11], and depression-like behavior was increased by the chemical [12]. Furthermore, neocortical hisogenesis was perturbed by bisphenol A [13].

Thus, these studies strongly suggested that bisphenol A could pass through the placental and blood-brain barriers and that the developing brain seems to be extremely vulnerable to exposure to the chemical. Although we previously demonstrated that bisphenol A in the neonatal brain by direct instillation caused hyperactivity, it is unknown if bisphenol A via an environmental exposure route such as oral administration might cause hyperactivity. Therefore, it is very important to demonstrate that the chemical might induce hyperactivity under exposure scenarios of daily life. Since it is hard to estimate the human exposure levels of bisphenol A, various *in vivo* toxicity studies of bisphenol A evaluated its No-Observed-Adverse-Effect-Level (NOAEL) as 50 mg/kg/day [14]. The exposure scenario consists of its source, route, and the amount of the chemical exposed. Thus, in this study, we tested the hypothesis that oral exposure to bisphenol A would exhibit effects observed previously with direct intracisternal administration as the first step to evaluate environmental contributions of the chemical to the psychiatric disorder.

Materials and Methods

Chemicals

Bisphenol A was purchased from Wako Pure Chemical Industries Ltd. (Osaka, Japan). The 30% (w/w) milk-oil solution was composed of nonfat milk (Meiji. Tokyo, Japan) and olive oil (nacalai tesque, Kyoto, Japan).

Animals and Treatments with Chemicals

Pregnant Wistar rats were obtained from Clea Japan (Tokyo).They were maintained in home cages and fed with a standard laboratory chow (MF diet, Oriental Yeast, Tokyo, Japan) and distilled water *ad libitum* at 22°C on a light-dark cycle (12 h/12 h) for at least 1 week. Approximately 50 male pups were born from 10 pregnant females, 5-7 of which were randomly housed and weaned at 3 weeks of age. Bisphenol A was suspended in an olive oil alone and then mixed with the 30% (w/w) milk-oil solution at a 1:2 ratio. The chemical (600 μg/30 μl/pup/day) was orally administered with a microman (Figure2; Gilson SAS, Villiers-le-Bel, France) daily from 5 days to 3 weeks of age, when they were weaned. Control rats were injected with vehicle alone (30 μl) in the same way. All animals were treated humanely in accordance with the guidelines of the National Institute for Environmental Studies,Japan.

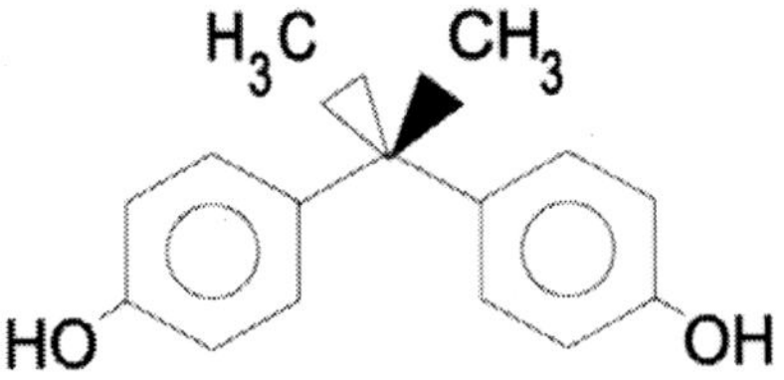

Figure 1. Chemical structure of bisphenol A.

Measurements of Spontaneous Motor Activity

Spontaneous motor activity was measured at 4-5 weeks of age, using the Supermex system (Figure3; Muromachi Kikai, Tokyo, Japan), as described previously [15]. Briefly, a Supermex sensor head comprising paired infrared pyroelectric detectors was used to measure the radiated body heat of each animal. The system detected any object with a temperature at least 5°C higher than that of background within a cone-shaped area (6-m diameter. 110° vertex). Motion was monitored in several directions using an array of Fresnel lenses placed above the cage, so movement in the *x*-, *y*-, and *z*-axes could be determined. Activity was measured at 15-min intervals for 22-24 h under a 12-h light-dark cycle. Food and water were fully given at the beginning of counting and the rats were not disturbed during the assessment period. Measurements from 12 animals were recorded concurrently.

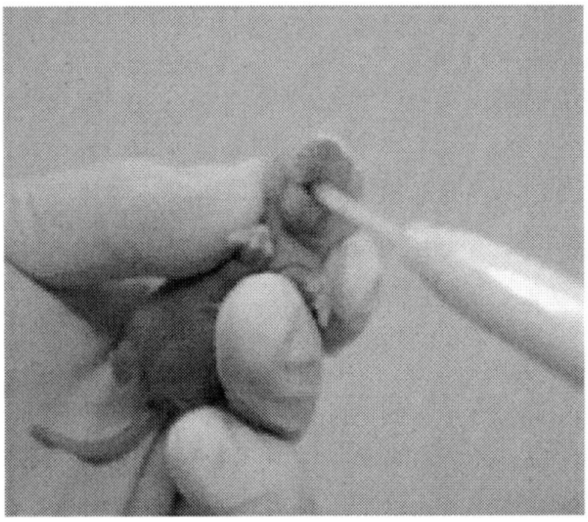

Figure 2. Oral administration of bisphenol A into a rat pup with a microman. Bisphenol A was suspended in 30% (w/w) milk-oil solution at a 1:2 ratio and was orally administered with a microman daily from 5 days to 3 weeks of age.

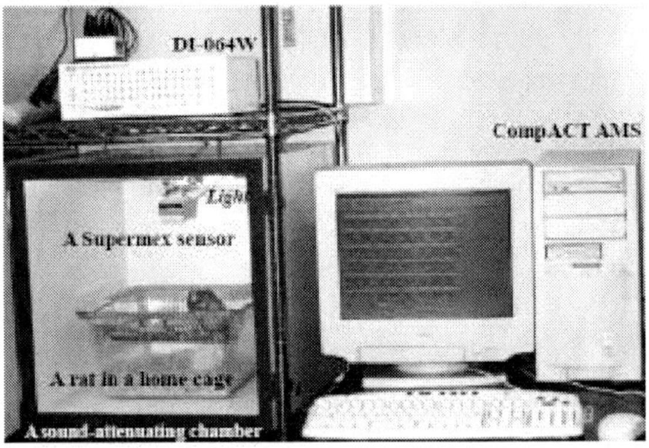

Figure. 3. The Supermex system. The general view of the system consisting of a sound-attenuating chamber, a Supermex sensor, a rat in the home cage, a 64-channel interface (DI-064W), and a personal computer with CompACT AMS software.

Immunohistochemistry and in situ terminal deoxynucleotidyl transferase-mediated dUTP nick-end labeling

Immunohistochemistry and *in situ* terminal deoxynucleotidyl transferase-mediated dUTP nick-end labeling Immunostaining and *in situ* terminal deoxunucleotidyl transferase-mediated dUTP nick end-labeling (TUNEL) were carried out as described previously [16-19]. Rats were sacrificed by decapitation at 7 weeks of age. Whole brain samples were fixed in 10% phosphate-buffered formalin (pH 7.2) and embedded in paraffin. Coronal sections (30 μm) were mounted on the slides coated with BioBond (British BioCell International, Cardiff, U.K.), deparaffinized in xylene, and hydrated through a series of graded ethanols.

For immunostaining, the section was then permeabilized with 0.5% Triton X-100 in phosphate-buffered saline (PBS), and blocked with 10% normal horse serum plus 1% bovine serum albumin for 30 min at 4°C. The sample was incubated with primary monoclonal anti-tyrosine hydroxylase antibody (1:100; Sigma-Aldrich, St. Louis, MO) or with anti-glutamic-acid decarboxylase (1:100; Sigma-Aldrich) in the presence of 4% bovine serum albumin and 0.05% Triton X-100. After three washes with PBS containing 0.1% Tween 20, each sample was incubated with appropriate secondary antibodies conjugated to FITC (1:200; Sigma-Aldrich) or to TRITC (1:200; Sigma-Aldrich) for 60 min at room temperature. Each fluorescence-labelled specimen was washed twice with PBS and observed under a microscope.

For *in situ* TUNEL labeling, the sample was treated with 20 μg/mL of proteinase K for 15 min at room temperature. After washing twice with PBS, H_2O_2 (2%) was used to quench the endogenous peroxidase. The sample was then incubated with equilibration buffer for 15 seconds, followed by terminal deoxynucleotidyl transferase reaction solution for 1 h at 37°C in the presence of 5 mM digoxigenin-conjugated dUTP and Reaction Stop buffer for 10 min. It was then blocked in 4% serum and 0.1% Triton X-100 in PBS for 30 min with intermittent washes in PBS. The sample was incubated with a peroxidase-conjugated sheep anti-digoxigenin antibody overnight at 4°C. Finally, it was processed for the visualization of immunoreactive protein using 3,3′-diaminobenzidine as the substrate for the colour reaction and methylgreen for counterstaining.

Images were captured using Viewfinder Lite version 1.0 camera software and a DP-50 digital camera equipped with an inverted microscope (IX-70; Olympus) or a Leica TCS SP5 conforcal microscope system equipped with an inverted microscope (AF6000). Four independent experiments were performed for comparative analyses.

Reverse Transcription Polymerase Chain Reaction (RT-PCR)

Whole brains of control rats or rats treated with bisphenol A were removed at 7 weeks of age. Total RNA was isolated from the midbrain using an RNeasy kit (QIAGEN KK, Tokyo, Japan). Reverse transcription polymerase chain reaction (RT-PCR) was carried out with a OneStep RT-PCR kit (QIAGEN KK), which contained Omniscript™ reverse transcriptase, Sensiscript™ reverse transcriptase, HotStartTaq, DNA polymerase, 12.5-mM $MgCl_2$, and 10-mM dNTP. Forty cycles of a thermal cycler program were carried out, setting to 94°C for 1 min, 50°C for 1 min, and 72°C for 1 min. Dopamine transporter primers were 5'-CTT GGC ATT GTC CTG GCT ACT TTC C-3' and 5'-CAG CAT AGC CGC CAG TAC AGG TTG-3'. PCR products were separated by electrophoresis on a 1.5% agarose gel. A photograph was taken with the bioimaging system CHEMI GENIUS^2 (Syngene, Cambridge, U.K.).

Statistics

Statistical analyses were carried out using the StatView version 5.0 software (SAS Institute, Cary, NC). Total activity in the nocturnal phase was analyzed by Student's *t*-test.

Results

Since direct instillation of bisphenol A into neonatal brain caused rat hyperactivity during the juvenile developmental stage [4], for its neural risk assessment, it is important to examine whether or not the chemical could pass through the blood-brain barrier in the rat via an exposure route of daily life. Bisphenol A (600 µg/pup/day) was orally administered to pups daily from 5 days to 3 weeks of age, and their spontaneous motor activity was measured at 4-5 weeks of age. Figure 4A shows that bisphenol A increased motor activity through the nocturnal phase of the light-dark cycle. In the dark periods (12h), total spontaneous motor activity in the bisphenol A-treated rats was 1.3 times as active as were vehicle-treated control rats ($p < 0.005$). In the light phases, there was no significant difference in motor activity between control and treated rats. The pattern of rhythmic curves of each rat was identical, indicating that the day-night cycle was retained (data not shown).

Body weights of the chemical-treated rats were indistinguishable from those of the solvent-treated rats (Figure 4B).

To investigate the long-term effects of the chemical at protein levels, brain tissues at 7 weeks old were processed for immunoreactivity to tyrosine hydroxylase, a rate-limiting enzyme for catecholamine synthesis. The substantia nigra in the control tissue was strongly stained with the anti-tyrosine hydroxylase antibody used (Figure 5. A and B). Oral administration of bisphenol A into rat pups resulted in a large reduction of tyrosine hydroxylase immunoreactivity in the substantia nigra pars compacts, suggesting degeneration in dopaminergic neurons (Figure 5. C and D *triangles*). The reduction of immunoreactivity of tyrosine hydroxylase was also seen in ventral tegmental areas (Figure 5. B and D *rhombus*). In contrast, immunostaining for glutamic-acid decarboxylase, which is involved in γ-aminobutyric-acid synthesis, revealed the immunoreactive enzyme in the substantia nigra pars reticulate of the specimen (Figure 5F). This confirms that the effects of bisphenol A are specific to the dopaminergic neurons.

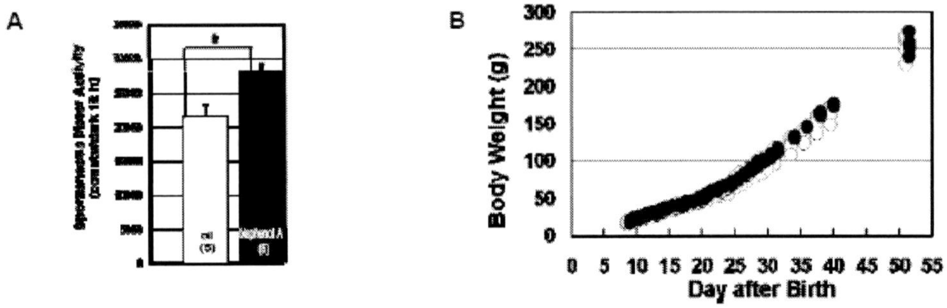

Figure 4. Effects of oral administration of bisphenol A on Spontaneous motor activity (A) and growth (B) in the rats. A; Spontaneous motor activity of vehicle- or bisphenol A-treated rats was measured by the Supermex system, as indicated. Spontaneous motor activity during nighttime was integrated. Data are indicated as mean ± S.E. *Significantly different from control rats ($p<0.005$, Student's t test). Reproduced with permission from Toxicl. Lett. (Elsevier)B; The pups were orally administrated without (O) or with 600 µg (●) of bisphenol A during suckling periods, followed by measuring their body weight.

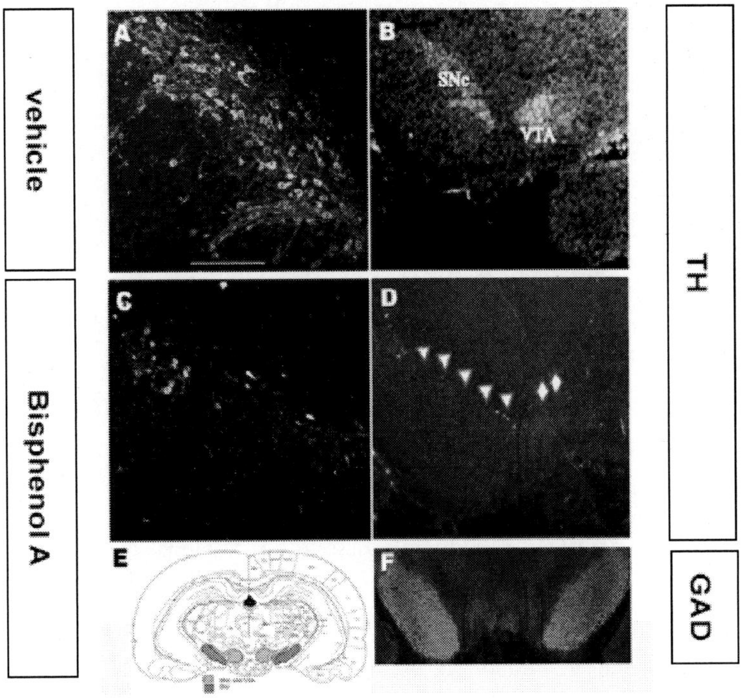

Figure 5. Impairment of tyrosine hydroxylase immunoreactivity. After oral administration of vehicle (A and B) or bisphenol A (C , D and F), coronal sections of brain tissues at 7 weeks of age were stained with anti- tyrosine hydroxylase antibody (A-D) or anti-glutamic-acid decarboxylase 65/67 (F). The specimens were observed under a fluorescence microscope. A and C are magnifications of the substantia nigra pars compacts (SNc) of B and C. A schematic drawing of dissection was shown in E. The substantia nigra pars compacta (SNc) and the ventral tegmental area (VTA) are indicated by triangles and rhombus, respectively. TH, tyrosine hydroxylase; GAD, glutamic-acid decarboxylase. Scale bar = 100 μm.

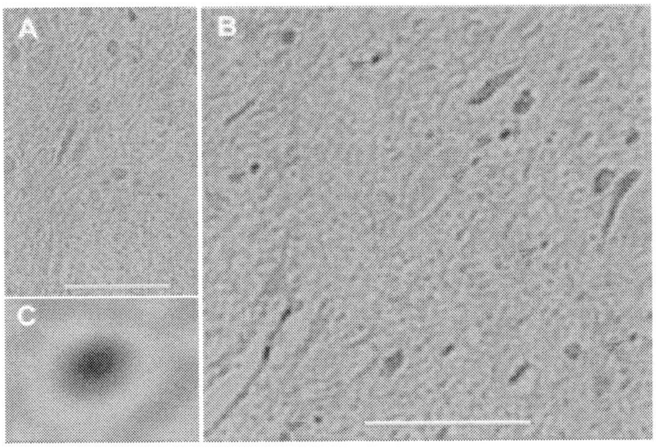

Figure 6. In situ transferase-mediated dUTP nick end-labeling. Sections of brain from control (A) and bisphenol A-treated rats (B) at 7 weeks of age were labeled with 5 mM digoxigenin-conjugated dUTP in the presence of 10 U terminal deoxynucleotidyl transferase, as described in Materials and Methods. A higher-resolution image of the apoptotic nuclei induced by the chemical is shown (C). Scale bar= 50 μm. Reproduced with permission from Toxicol. Lett (Elsevier).

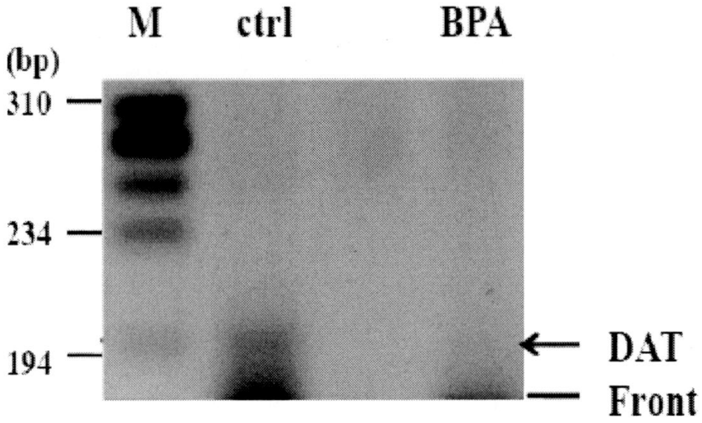

Figure 7. Reverse transcription polymerase chain reaction of dopamine transporter in the midbrain. Total cellular RNA was isolated from control (*ctrl*) and bisphenol A-treated rats (*BPA*) at 7 weeks of age. Dopamine transporter (DAT) was amplified as described in 'Material and Methods'. Size markers are given in the left lane (M) and on the left margin (bp; base pairs). Reproduced with permission from Toxicol. Lett (Elsevier).

To examine if the large reduction by bisphenol A of immunoreactivity for tyrosine hydroxylase reflects a neurodegeneration in the midbrain, we carried out TUNEL using brain sections from 7 week-old rats. No labeling was found in the control substantia nigra (Figure 6A). In contrast, as seen in Figure 6B, the TUNEL-positive cells were detected with nuclear condensation (Figure 6C) in the bisphenol A-treated brains, demonstrating that the chemical caused apoptotic cell death in the substantia nigra.

To further examine the effect of bisphenol A on gene expression levels of dopaminergic tone, brain tissues at 7 weeks old were subjected to RT-PCR. As shown in Fig 7, the gene expression of dopamine transporter in the midbrain at 7 weeks of age was completely inhibited by bisphenol A, indicating that orally administered bisphenol A affected the dopaminergic system at gene expression levels, as well.

Discussion

The etiology of multifactorial disorders such as a neurodevelopmental disorder of attention-deficit/hyperactivity disorder (ADHD) has been considered to be the interaction between a range of intrinsic (gene) and extrinsic (environment) factors. The symptoms of ADHD are inattention, excess impulsivity, uncontrolled hyperactivity, and the deficit in social communication, affecting ~5% of children and adolescents and ~3% of adults [20]. ADHD is more frequently diagnosed in boys, with male: female ratios between 3:1 and 4:1. ADHD is defined by the presence of six or more symptoms of inattention and/or hyperactivity-impulsivity that lead to significant impairment in at least two settings and have their onset by age 7 years. Comorbidity is common in ADHD, with oppositional disorders, mood disorders, anxiety, and learning disabilities being the most prevalent conditions, likely reflecting the complexity of the biological etiology. ADHD has a significant genetic component. Data from clinical studies consistently support the familial nature of ADHD. Twin studies of categorically defined ADHD and/or continuous rating scales of hyperactivity, impulsivity, and inattention lead to estimates of heritability of ~60%-90% and reported sibling relative risk ratios of 4.0-8.0.

Thus, this disorder seems to be inheritable neurodevelopmental disorders. However, recent evidence in animal models has shown that environmental chemicals *per se*, including endocrine disrupting chemicals [4, 15, 21-23] and a pesticide rotenone, cause hyperactivity, seen in patients with ADHD. There have been reports that environmental chemicals cause neurodevelopmental disorders in human: polychlorinated biphenyls (PCBs) distributed in the environment cross the placenta to cause *in utero* injury to the developing brain, correlating with a decrease in intelligence quotient [24, 25]. Second, many chemicals such as dioxins, PCBs, bisphenol A, and heavy metals have been detected in human umbilical cords and cord serum, suggesting that they transfer transplacentally from mother to fetus and that the chemicals might exert their effects on the developing brain [26]. These circumstances made us hypothesize that environmental chemicals including endocrine disrupting chemicals might contribute to the incidence of neurodevelopmental disorders such as ADHD.

The pioneer work of the animal model for hyperactivity was carried out by Shaywitz *et al.* (1976), who demonstrated that rat pups treated with 6-OHDA via intracisternal administration at 5 days of age developed increased motor activity, leading to cognitive difficulties in shuttle-box learning between 2-4 weeks of age [5]. These observations were strikingly similar to the clinical syndrome of minimal brain dysfunction, called ADHD at present, found in children. In 6-OHDA-treated rat pups, brain dopamine was depleted, suggesting that brain dopamine may be involved in the pathogenesis of the disorder [5].

Following the protocol by Shaywitz, in the previous study we intracisternally administered an endocrine disrupting chemical into the 5-day-old rat [4]. Single intracisternal administration of bisphenol A (0.2-20 μg) into 5-day-old male Wistar rats caused significant hyperactivity at 4-5 weeks of age. It was about 1.6 fold more active in the nocturnal phase after administration of 2 μg of bisphenol A than control rats. The response was dose-dependent; while 20 ng of bisphenol A failed to cause hyperactivity, it was significantly detectable by injection of 200 ng of the chemical, as assessed by the Supermex system. A dose of 2 μg bisphenol A was as effective as 20 μg of the chemical. Based on DNA array analyses of the midbrain, bisphenol A decreased the levels of gene expression of dopamine D4 receptor at 4 weeks old and dopamine transporter at 8 weeks old more than 2 fold. Furthermore, bisphenol A completely abolished immunoreactivity for tyrosine hydroxylase in the substantia nigra at 8 weeks of age.

Thus, the neural risk assessment of bisphenol A is next required at the endpoint of juvenile hyperactivity. The current methodology for risk assessment is focused on its source, route, and the amount of those factors exposed. The risk assessment process is divided into four distinct steps: hazard identification, exposure assessment, exposure-response assessment and risk characterization [27].

The purpose of hazard identification is to evaluate qualitatively the weight of evidence for adverse effects in humans based on the assessment of all the available data on toxicology and modes of action. Exposure assessment is the determination of the nature and extent of exposure to the environmental factors. Exposure-response assessment is the process of quantitatively characterizing the relationship between the exposure received and the occurrence of an effect. Risk characterization is the final step in the risk assessment process. Its purpose is to support risk managers by providing the essential scientific evidence and rationale about risk that they need for decision-making. In risk characterization, estimates of the risk to human health under relevant exposure scenarios are provided.

For bisphenol A the lowest dose previously examined for risk assessment purposes was 50 mg/kg/day in studies of reproductive toxicity with rats and mice. The reference dose (RfD) of bisphenol A is calculated by the US Environmental Protection Agency as 50 μg/kg/day by dividing the Lowest-Observed Adverse-Effect-Level (LOAEL) by an uncertainty factor of 1,000. This current reference dose is based on traditional toxicological experiments conducted in the 1980's [28]. However, recent reports show adverse effects of bisphenol A at lower doses than the RfD, called 'low-doses' issue of endocrine disruptors [29, 30]. One can't accept this fact when considering that estrogenic bisphenol A binds to classical nuclear estrogen receptors with affinity of 10,000-100,000-fold less potential than that of estradiol. Recent findings show that bisphenol A has equal potentials with changes in cell function at a dose of 1 pM through mechanisms that are thought to be membrane-associated forms of the estrogen receptors [31, 32]. The finding of specific receptor for bisphenol A, estrogen-related receptor γ would be also expected to settle the 'low doses' issue [33].

Timing of exposure to bisphenol A should be also considered for its risk assessment [34]. Exposures to bisphenol A have different effects depending on the life stage of the exposed animals. Effects resulting from adult exposure are generally reversible. Effects resulting from exposure during organ development may result in persistent alterations of the affected systems. Thus, vulnerable windows for exposure are evident during prenatal development and continuing in postnatal life through puberty.

In this study, we tested the hypothesis that oral exposure to bisphenol A would exhibit effects observed previously with direct intracisternal administration. Bisphenol A (600 μg/pup/day) was orally administered into a pup daily from 5 days to 3 weeks of age; this was equivalent to 12 mg~60 mg/kg body weight. Weight and growth characteristics of the chemical-treated rats were indistinguishable (Figure 4B). Exposure through the oral route led to hyperactivity in the rat, concomitantly with impairment of tyrosine hydroxylase immunoreactivity (Figure 5). The large reduction of the immunoreactivity by the chemical would be a reflection of neurodegeneration in the substantia nigra since TUNEL-positive cells were detectable (Figure 6). Furthermore, the gene expression of mesencephalic dopamine transporter was largely decreased by the chemical (Figure 7). These observations suggest the etiology of rat hyperkinesias might be explained by multiple-hit hypothesis in dopaminergic neurons. The brain may readily be able to compensate for the effects of a chemical alone acting on a particular system of the brain. However, when multiple targets or functional sites within that particular system are attacked by multiple actions, the system may no longer be able to homeostatically reregulate itself, thereby leading to sustained or cumulative damage of the dopaminergic neurons.

Dopamine is a highly conserved neurotransmitter [35]. The central and peripheral dopamine systems are involved in a number of complex functions such as regulation of blood pressure, movements, goal-directed behavior, cognition, attention and reward. From anatomical studies of the dopamine system, there are three major categories based on the length of the efferent dopamine fibers: ultrashort systems, intermediate-length systems, and long systems. The long systems are the long projections linking the ventral tegmental area (A10) and substantia nigra pars compacta (A9) dopamine cells with three principal sets of targets: the neostriatum, the limbic cortex (mesocortical projection), and other limbic structure (mesolimbic projection).

Dopamine synthesis originates from tyrosine, and its rate-limiting step is the conversion of L-dihydroxyphenylalanine (L-DOPA) by tyrosine hydroxylase. DOPA is subsequently converted to dopamine by L-aromatic amino acid decarboxylase at rate so rapid that DOPA levels in the brain are negligible. Endogenous mechanisms for regulating the rate of dopamine synthesis in dopamine neurons primarily involve modulation of tyrosine hydroxylase activity.

Ontogenetic studies in the rat showed that midbrain dopamine neurons appear between embryonic days E12-15, near the midbrain-hindbrain junction (rhombic isthmus) [36]. These neurons begin to express tyrosine hydroxylase by E12.5, and then extensively migrate from the rhombic isthmus in a rostro-ventral direction to the ventral midbrain. Development of the ventral midbrain requires the orchestration of a number of genes, such as Engrailed1, 2, Pax2, Pax5, Wnt1, Sonic hedgehog, and Fgf8. Also, Ptx3 and Nurr1 are implicated in specification of the mesencephalic dopamine system. Nurr1 are required for induction of the tyrosine hydroxylase. A recent study identified two genes, Lmx1a and Msx1, as major upstream regulators of the dopaminergic neural subtype specification [37]. Developmental processes such as differentiation and synaptogenesis are still incomplete in the 5-day old rat [38] when we exposed to bisphenol A. Thus, it is highly expected that exposure during critical periods of neural development to environmental chemicals cause deficit in neural networks.

Dysfunction of dopamine systems has been associated to several neurodegenerative disorders. Tyrosine hydroxylase has been reported to be an oxidatively labile enzyme [39]. Animal models of dopaminergic neurodegeneration have been reported for Parkinson's disease through treatment with 1-methyl-4-phenyl-1,2,3,6-tetrahydropyridine (MPTP) [40] and some pesticides such as rotenone [41], maneb, and paraquat [42], suggesting that oxidative stress is a primary mediator of the dopaminergic neurodegeneration. Furthermore, it has been reported that bisphenol A stimulates ·OH generation in rat striatum [43] and that the chemical facilitates MPTP-induced ·OH generation [44]. Thus, it is most likely that the toxicity of bisphenol A may be attributed to the degeneration of dopaminergic neurons. Whether this would attribute to hyperactivity remains unclear. We could not still eliminate the possibility that the estrogenicity of bisphenol A might, at least in part, be involved.

Gene manipulation techniques have developed many models of animals for a study of dopamine systems. The mice lacking the genes for dopamine type 3 receptor [45] or the dopamine transporter were hyperactive [46]. In the other hands, the mice lacking the genes for dopamine type 1, 2, or 4 types receptors show hypoactivity [47-49]. Thus, locomotor hyperactivity has been associated with not only hypodopaminergic [5] but also hyperdopaminergic animal models, indicating that imbalance in dopamine systems can produce behavioral and cognitive dysregulation [50]. Hyperactivity in our animal model might be due to hypofunctioning of dopamine since immunoreactivity of tyrosine hydroxylase was largely decreased, reflecting a dysfunction of the enzyme. Tyrosine hydroxylase may play a crucial role in rat hyperkinesia.

Hyperactivity among children was first described by von Economo (1931) in cases of encephalic lethargica. Hyperactivity, sleep disorders and antisocial personality disorder are all associated with this disease in childhood and Parkinsonism was observed in adult cases [51]. This suggests that the etiology of hyperactivity in children could involve the potentially irreversible degeneration of dopaminergic neurons since Parkinson disease is caused by the selective loss of dopaminergic neurons.

Currently, hyperactivity is associated with ADHD or autism. The etiology seems to be, in part, associated with dopaminergic tone. Dopamine transporter may be involved in the pathogenesis of ADHD, as methylphenidate, which increases the synaptic concentration of dopamine by blocking the dopamine transporters, has been used for the treatment of ADHD [52]. The present study showed that the gene expression of dopamine transporter was largely decreased in bisphenol A-treated rats (Figure 7). Genetic studies have associated certain alleles of the human D4 receptor gene with the occurrence of ADHD [53].

Thus, although the molecular mechanism is unknown, the developmental deficit of several components of the dopaminergic system may underlie motor hyperactivity, most likely due to chemical-induced neurodegeneration.

References

[1] Ben-Jonathan N, Steinmetz R. (1998) Xenoestrogens: The emerging story of bisphenol A. *Trends Endocrinol. Metabol.* 9:124-128.

[2] Brotons JA, Serrano FO, Villalobos M, Pedraza V, Olea N. (1995) Xenoestrogens released from lacquer coatings in food cans.*Environ. Health Perspect.* 103: 608-612.

[3] Krishman AV, Stathis P, Permuth SF, Tokes L, Feldman D. (1993) Bisphenol A: An estrogenic substance is released from polycarbonate flasks during autoclaving. *Endocrinology* 132: 2279-2286.

[4] Ishido M, Masuo Y, Kunimoto M, Oka S, Morita M. (2004) Bisphenol A causes hyperactivity in the rat concomitantly with impairment of tyrosine hydroxylase immunoreactivity. *J. Neurosci. Res.* 76: 423-433.

[5] Shaywitz BA, Yager RD, Klopper JH. (1976) Selective brain dopamine depletion in developing rats: an experimental model of minimal brain dysfunction. *Science* 191: 305-308.

[6] Farabollini F, Porrini S, Della Seta D, Bianchi F, Dessi-Fulgheri F. (2002) Effects of perinatal exposure to bisphenol A on sociosexual behavior of female and male rats *Environ. Health Perspect.* 110(Suppl. 3): 409-414.

[7] Kawai K, Nozaki T, Nishikata H, Aou S, Takai M, Kubo C. (2003) Aggressive behavior and serum testosterone concentration during the maturation process of male mice: The effects of fetal exposure to bisphenol A. *Environ. Health Perspect.* 111: 175-178.

[8] Farabollini F, Porrini S, Dessi-Fulgheri F. (1999) Perinatal exposure to the estrogenic pollutant bisphenol A affects behavior in male and female rats. *Pharmacol. Biochem. Behav.* 64: 687-694.

[9] Aloisi AM, Della Seta D, Rendo C, Ceccarelli I, Scaramuzzino A, Farabollini F. (2002) Exposure to the estrogenic pollutant bisphenol A affects pain behavior induced by subcutaneous formalin injection in male and female rats. *Brain Res.* 937: 1-7.

[10] Adriani W, Della-Seta D, Dessi-Fulgheri F, Farabollini F, Laviola G. (2003) Altered profiles of spontaneous novelty seeking, impulsive behavior, and response to D-amphetamine in rats perinatally exposed to bisphenol A. *Environ. Health Perspect.* 111: 395-401.

[11] Kubo K, Arai O, Omura M, Watanabe R, Ogata R, Aou S. (2003) Low dose effects of bisphenol A on sexual differentiation of the brain and behavior in rats. *Neurosci. Res.* 45: 345-356.

[12] Fujimoto T, Kubo K, Aou S. (2006) Prenatal exposure to bisphenol A impairs sexual differentiation of exploratory behavior and increases depression-like behavior in rats. *Brain Res.* 1068: 49-55.

[13] Nakamura K, Itoh K, Yaoi T, Fujiwara Y, Sugimoto T, Fushiki S. (2006) Murine neocortical histogenesis is perturbed by prenatal exposure to low doses of bisphenol A. *J. Neurosci. Res.* 84: 1197-1205.

[14] Tyl RW, Myers CB, Marr CM, Thomas BF, Keimowitz AR, Brine DR, Veselica MM, Fail PA, Chang TY, Seely JC, Joiner RL, Butala JH, Dimond SS, Cagen SZ, Shiotsuka RN, Stropp G.D, Waechter JM.(2002) Three-generation reproductive toxicity study of dietary bisphenol A in CD Sprague-Dawley rats. *Toxicol. Sci.* 68: 121-146.

[15] Ishido M, Masuo Y, Oka S, Kunimoto M, Morita M. (2002) Application of Supermex system to screen behavioral traits produced by tributyltin in the rat. *J. Health Sci.* 48: 451-454.

[16] Ishido M, Takeda S, Tohyama C, Suzuki T. (1998) Apoptosis in renal proximal tubular cells induced by cadmium. *J. Toxicol. Environ. Health* 55: 101-112.

[17] Ishido M, Suzuki T, Adachi T, Kunimoto M. (1999) Zinc stimulates DNA synthesis during its antiapoptotic action, independently with increments of an antiapoptotic protein, Bcl-2, in porcine kidney LLC-PK_1 cells. *J. Pharmacol. Exp. Ther.* 290: 923-928.

[18] Ishido M. (2005) Overexpression of Bcl-2 inhibits nuclear localization of annexin I during tumor necrosis factor-alpha-mediated apoptosis in porcine renal LLC-PK_1 cells. *Regul. Peptides* 124: 45-51.

[19] Ishido M. (2007) Melatonin inhibits maneb-induced aggregation of alpha-synuclein in rat pheochromocytoma cells. *J. Pineal Res.* 42: 125-130.

[20] Goldman LS, Genel M, Bezman RJ, Slanetz PJ. (1998) Diagnosis and treatment of attention-deficit/hyperactivity disorder in children and adolescents. *JAMA* 279: 1100-1107.

[21] Ishido M, Masuo Y, Oka S, Niki E, Morita M. (2004) *p*-Nitrotoluene causes hyperactivity in the rat. *Neurosci. Lett.* 366: 1-5.

[22] Ishido M, Masuo Y, Suzuki J, Oka S, Niki E, Morita M. (2004) Dicyclohexylphthalate causes hyperactivity in the rat concomitantly with impairment of tyrosine hydroxylase immunoreactivity. *J. Neurochem.* 91: 69-76.

[23] Ishido M, Masuo Y, Oka S, Niki E, Morita M. (2004) Intracisternal administration of *p*-n-octylphenol into neonatal rats causes hyperactivity concomitantly with terminal deoxynucleotidyl transferase-mediated dUTP nick end-labelling (TUNEL)-positive cells in the mesencephalon where immunoreactivity for tyrosine hydroxylase is reduced by the chemical. *J. Health Sci.* 50: 407-412.

[24] Jacobson JL, Jacobson SW. (1996) Intellectual impairment in children exposed to polychlorinated bisphenyls *in utero*. *N. Engl. J. Med.* 335: 783-789.

[25] Patandin S, Lanting CI, Mulder PG, Boersma ER, Sauer PJ, Weisglas-Kuperus N. (2003) Effects of environmental exposure to polychlorinated biphenyls and dioxins on cognitive abilities in Dutch children at 42 months of age. *J. Pediar.* 134: 33-41.

[26] Schnonfelder G, Wittfoht W, Hopp H, Talsness CE, Paul M, Chaoud I. (2003) Parental bisphenol A accumulation in human maternal-fetal-placental unit. *Environ. Health Perspect.* 110:A703-A707.

[27] Van Leeuwen CJ. (2007) General Introduction. In: *Risk assessment of chemicals: an introduction,* Van Leeuwen CJ and Vermeire TG. (eds), Springer, Netherlands. 1-36.

[28] Integrated Risk Information System (IRIS). (1988) *USA-EPA Integrated Risk Information System Substance File.*

[29] Colerangle JB, Roy D. (1997) Profound effects of the weak environmental estrogen-like chemical bisphenol A on the mammary gland of noble rats. *J. Steroid Biochem. Mol. Biol.* 60: 153-160.

[30] Steinmmetz R, Brown NG, Allen DL, Bigsby RM, Ben-Jonathan N. (1997) The environmental estrogen bisphenol A stimulates prolactin release *in vitro* and *in vivo*. *Endocrinology* 138: 1780-1786.

[31] Quesada I, Fuentes E, Viso-Leon MC, Soria B, Ripoll C, Nadal A. (2002) Low doses of the endocrine disruptor bisphenol A and the native hormone 17 beta-estradiol rapidly activate transcription factor CREB. *FASEB J.* 16:1671-1673.

[32] Zsarnovszky A, Le HH, Wang HS, Belcher SM. (2005) Ontogeny of rapid estrogen-mediated extracellular signal-regulated kinase signaling in the rat cerebellar cortex: Potent nongenomic agonist and endocrine disrupting activity of the xenoestrogen bisphenol A. *Endocrinology* 146:5388-5396.

[33] Takayanagi S, Tokunaga T, Liu X, Okada H, Matsushima A, Shimohigashi Y. (2006) Endocrine disruptor bisphenol A strongly binds to human estrogen-related receptor γ (ERRγ) with high constitutive activity. *Toxicol. Lett.* 167:95-105.

[34] Selevan SG, Kimmel CA, Mendola P. (2000) Identifying critical windows of exposure for children's health. *Environ. Health Perspect.* 108(suppl 3):451-455.

[35] Cooper JR, Bloom FE, Roth RH. (2003) Dopamine. In *The biochemical basis of neuropharmacology*, Oxford Univ. Press, NY. 225-270.

[36] Martinez S, Simeone A.(1999) Specification and patterning of the rostral neural tube. In *Development of dopaminergic neurons.* di Porzio, Pernas-Alonso R, and Perrone-Capano (eds) R.G. Landes Company, TX. 1999; 1-14.

[37] Anderson E, Tryggvason U, Deng Q, Friling, Alekseenko Z, Robert B, Perlmann T, Ericson J. (2006) Identification of intrinsic determinants of midbrain dopamine neurons. *Cell* 124: 393-405.

[38] Rice DC, Barone S. Jr. (2000) Critical periods of vulnerability for the developing nervous system: evidence from humans and animal models. *Environ. Health Perspect.* 108, (suppl. 3) 511-533.

[39] Borges CR, Geddes T, Watson JT, Kuhn DM. (2002) Dopamine biosynthesis is regulated by *S*-glutathionylation. *J. Biol. Chem.* 277: 48295-48302.

[40] Langston JW, Ballard P, Tetrud JW, Irwin I. (1983) Chronic Parkinsonism in humans due to a product of meperidine-analog synthesis. *Science* 219: 979-980.

[41] Betarbet R, Sherer TB, MacKenzie G., Garcia-Osuna M, Pabov AV, Greenamyre JT. (2000) Chronic systemic pesticide exposure reproduces features of Parkinson's disease. *Nat. Neurosci.* 3: 1301-1306.

[42] Thiruchelvam M, Richfield EK, Baggs RB, Tank AW, Cory-Slechta DA. (2000) The nigrostriatal dopaminergic system as a preferential target of repeated exposure to combined paraquat and maneb: Implications for Parkinson's disease. *J Neurosci.* 20: 9207-9214.

[43] Obata T, Kubota S. (2000) Formation of hydroxyl radicals by environmental estrogen-like chemicals in rat striatum. *Neurosci. Lett.* 296: 41-44.

[44] Obata T, Kinemuchi H, Aomine M. (2002) Protective effect of diltiazem, an L-type calcium channel antagonist, on bisphenol A-enhanced hydroxyl radical generation by 1-methyl-4-phenylpyridium ion in rat striatum. *Neurosci. Lett.* 334: 211-213.

[45] Xu M, Koeltzow TE, Santiago GT, Moraralla R, Cooper DC, Hu XT, White NM, Graybiel AM, White FJ, Tonegawa S. (1997) Dopamine D3 receptor mutant mice exhibit increased behavioral sensitivity to concurrent stimulation of D1 and D2 receptors. *Cell* 19: 837-848.

[46] Giros B, Jaber M, Jones SR, Wightman RM, Caron MG. (1996) Hyperlocomotion and indifference to cocaine and amphetamine in mice lacking the dopamine transporter. *Nature* 379: 606-612.

[47] Xu M, Hu XT, Cooper DC, Moratalla R, Graybiel AM, White FJ, Tonegawa S. (1994) Elimination of cocaine-induced hyperactivity and dopamine-mediated neurophysiological effects in dopamine D1 receptor mutant mice. *Cell* 79: 945-955.

[48] Baik J-H, Picetti R, Saiardi A, Thiriet G, Dierich A, Depaulis A, Meur ML, Borrelli E. (1995) Parkinsonian-like locomotor impairment in mice lacking dopamine D2 receptors. *Nature* 377: 424-428.

[49] Dulawa SC, Grandy DK, Low MJ, Paulus MP, Geyer MA. (1999) Dopamine D4 receptor-knock-out mice exhibit reduced exploration of novel stimuli. *J. Neurosci.* 19: 9550-9556.

[50] Viggiano D, Ruocco LA, Sadile AG.. (2003) Dopamine phenotype and behavior in animal models: in relation to attention deficit hyperactivity disorder. *Neurosci. Biobehav. Rev.* 27: 623-637.

[51] von Economo C. (1931) In: *Encephalitis Lethargica: Its Sequelae and Treatment.* Translated by K. O. Newman, K. O. Oxford University Press, London.

[52] Elia J, Ambrosini PJ, Rapoport J. (1999) Treatment of attention-deficit-hyperactivity disorder. *N. Eng. J. Med.* 340:780-788.

[53] LaHoste GJ, Swanson JM, Wigal SB, Galbe C, Wigal T, King N, Kennedy J. (1996) Dopamine D4 receptor gene polymorphism is associated with attention deficit hyperactivity disorder. *Mol. Psychiatry* 1:121-124.

In: Attention Deficit Hyperactivity Disorder (ADHD)
Editors: Stuart M. Gordon and Aileen E. Mitchell
ISBN 978-1-60741-581-7

Chapter 10

Chronic Methylphenidate Modulates the Circadian Activity Pattern of Adolescent SD Male Rats

Mohamed F. Algahim, Pamela B. Yang, Victor T. Wilcox, Keith M. Burau*, Alan C. Swann and Nachum Dafny†
Department of Neurobiology and Anatomy
The University of Texas Medical School at Houston
P.O. Box 20708, Houston, Texas 77225

ABSTRACT

The psychostimulant methylphenidate (MPD) is the drug most often used to treat Attention Deficit Hyperactivity Disorder (ADHD), a common behavioral disorder of children. Psychostimulant exposure to children at the time of neuronal development can cause behavioral and physiological changes enduring during adulthood. Most of the studies on psychostimulant investigate short term effects of the drug, 5 to 120 minutes post injection. The objective of this study was to investigate whether acute or chronic exposure to MPD will modulate the circadian activity pattern. Maintaining the circadian activity pattern is a physiological process that regulates the internal homeostasis. Dose response protocol was used to study the effect of acute and chronic MPD in four groups of rats, each N=8, as follows: saline (control) group, and 0.6, 2.5, or 10.0 mg/kg i.p. MPD groups respectively. The experiment was performed over 11 consecutive days of continuous recording. All rats received saline on day 1, followed by saline or the assigned MPD dose (0.6, 2.5, or 10.0 mg/kg) on experimental days 2 through 7. After three washout days, a re-challenge of saline or MPD was injected. Each animal (of the MPD groups) received the same dose of MPD for re-challenge injection as the dose of MPD given on experimental day 2. The data evaluation was divided into four phases: acute, induction, washout and expression phases. There was a dose-dependent increase in

* School of Public Health and Science Center of Houston
† Corresponding author: nachum.dafny@uth.tmc.edu, 713-500-5616 (office), 713-500-2515 (Fax).

the average locomotor activity. Analysis of the circadian rhythmic pattern of locomotion in the three dose groups demonstrated that only the 10.0 mg/kg MPD elicited significant changes in circadian pattern activity in the washout and the expression phase. In addition, this study showed that chronic MPD treatment elicits dose dependent withdrawal and behavioral sensitization in adolescent rats.

Keywords: adolescent, methylphenidate, stimulants, behavior, locomotor activity

INTRODUCTION

Methylphenidate (MPD), also known as Ritalin, is one of the most prescribed drug therapies in the treatment of adolescent and adult with Attention Deficit Hypertension Disorder (ADHD) (Accardo and Blondis, 2001; Clure et. al., 1999; Levin and Kleber, 1995; Zito et. al., 2000). The response to psychostimulants has been reported to vary with age (Adriani et. al., 1998;; Bowman and Kuhn, 1996; Brandon et. al., 2001; Byrnes et al., 1993; Collins and Isenwasser, 2002; Durmans et. al., 2004; Fujiwara et. al., 1987; Laviola et. al., 1995; Robinson, 1984; Segal and Kuczenski, 1997). During normal development, overproduction of synaptic onnections and receptors occurs and is followed by their pruning or competitive elimination. The marked overproduction and elimination of synapses and receptors during adolescence may serve as a permissive factor for a number of behavioral disorders including ADHD (Anderson and Teicher, 2000; Hammano et. al., 1996). Between 5 to 15 years of age in humans, synaptic density in the prefrontal cortex decreases by approximately 40% (Huttenlocher, 1979; Rakic, 1986). The time course and nature of ADHD parallel this pattern of overproduction and regressive synaptic elimination (Anderson and Teicher, 2000). There is concern that psychostimulant therapy given to adolescents and young adults may result in an increased risk of behavioral disorders (Anderson et. al., 2002; Grund et. al., 2006; Lambert and Hartsongh, 1998; Robinson and Berridge, 1993; Schenk and Isenwasser, 2002). However, other reports show that pyshcostimulant treatment may protect adolescents with ADHD from subsequent substance use disorders (Biederman et. al., 1994; Wilens et. al., 2003).

Most physiological and behavioral activity exhibits cyclical rhythmical cycles. Internal biological clocks regulate this activity and are thought to have a significant adaptive mechanism to response to internal and external conditions (Gillian et al, 2000; Moore, 2003). One of the main internal clocks, that integrates physiological and behavioral processes, is located in the suprachiasmatic nucleus (SCN), which responds to internal and external cues to regulate the timing of physiological and behavioral activities. These circadian functions are controlled genetically through a molecular mechanism maintained by the expression of clock genes that code for specific proteins which feed back on the nucleus to control their own production (Moore 2003).

Most, if not all, studies investigate the effect of MPD that occurs from 5 min to 2 h after injection. We know of no investigations of its longer term effects, such as those on the 24 hr rhythm of motor activity during repeated MPD treatment. The objective of this study is to investigate acute and chronic effects of MPD on the 24 hr circadian activity pattern of adolescent male SD rats during consecutive eleven days of continuous nonstop recording of locomotor activity, using measurements of infrared beam crossings in an open field (Algahim et. al., 2007; Amini et. al., 2003; Gaytan et. al., 1997; Yang et. al., 2003). The hypothesis of this study is that alteration of circadian activity pattern is an experimental indicator of long term MPD effects. The aim of this study is to find out whether MPD treatment modulates the circadian activity pattern of locomotor activity using the open field assay.

METHODS

Animals: Sprague-Dawley (SD) male adolescent rats post natal day 38 (P-38) were purchased and housed 4 in a cage in a sound proof control room. Temperature, humidity and light were kept constant at 21˚C, 37% to 42%, and 12:12 light/dark schedule (light on at 06:00) respectively for about 5 days for adaption prior to the recording sessions. On the last day of acclimatization, rats were weighed and randomly divided into 4 groups as follows: control (saline), 0.6 mg/kg MPD, 2.5 mg/kg MPD and 10.0 mg/kg MPD group (n=8 in each group) and placed in the open field cages located in the same room that became their home cages for additional 16 to 20 hrs for acclimation prior to the beginning of the consecutive 11 day recording session.

The open field Assay: Sixteen open field cages (40.5 x 4.5 x 31.5 cm each) equipped with two tears of 16 infrared beams each with their sensors at 6 cm and 12.5 cm above the floor (AccuScan Instruments, Inc. Columbus, Ohio) were used to record the locomotor activity (horizontal activity) 24 hrs/day continuously for 11 days (Table 1). Interruption of any beam above 100 Hz were counted as an activity score by Accusan Analyzer. Cumulative counts for each 10 min was compiled and downloaded every 10 minutes to PC using the Oasis software.

Experimental Protocol: The duration of the recording was 11 consecutive days as follows: Experimental day 1 was the same in all the 4 groups and consisted of the locomotor recording of 24 hrs post saline (0.9%) injection. Experimental days 2 to 7 were the recording post saline (the control group) or, 06, 2.5 or 10.0 mg/kg MPD injection. Experimental days 8 to 10 were washout days followed by additional treatment on experimental day 11 of either saline (to the control group) or 0.6, 2.5 or 10.0 mg/kg MPD injection as was given on experimental day 2. Locomotor activity recording started 1 hr into the light phase immediately post injection without interruption for consecutive 11 days except during cage cleaning and animal handling between 06:30 and 07:00 (Table I).

Drug: Methylphenidate (MPD) hydrochloride (Mallinkrot Hazelwood, MD) was dissolved in 0.9% saline to provide a volume of 0.8 ml per injection. Dosages were calculated as freebase. Each animal was injected intra-peritoneally (i.p). All injections were made between 06:30 to 07:00 in the same volume using a 26g needle. All efforts were made to minimize the animal suffering and to reduce the number of animals for the experiment. The study was conducted according to the declaration of Helsinki and approved by the local Animal Welfare Committee.

Data Analysis: The data analysis was divided to 4 phases: acute, induction, washout and expression phase to look for tolerance, withdrawal or behavioral sensitization.

Two forms of data analysis were used to analyze the dose response characteristics following saline and MPD administration. 1) Six 10 min counts of the locomotor activity were summed to produce hourly histograms for experimental days 1,2,7,8 and 11. Figure 1 shows the resulting histograms with means ± 2 standard errors (SE). The mean and 2±SE were used to compare and analyzing for significant shift between the hourly activity within each experimental phase. 2)The second evaluation used the 10 min count bins for statistical analysis using the Cosine Curve Statistical Analysis (CCSA) test (Bingham et al., 1982) to perform statistical comparison by parameterizing the 23-hour activity pattern curve. Such curves are typically parameterized by estimating the mesor (average activity representing by the curve); amplitude (distance from mesor to the highest point – the peak activity), and acrophase (time at which the maximum amplitude occurs). The estimates of these three parameters provide the ability to test for statistical significant change in locomotor activity patterns with respect to time and intensity within the 24 hrs of each day. It is therefore possible to determine whether a significant shift in locomotor activity circadian rhythm pattern occurred in the treatment phases (Bingham et al, 1982).

Table 1

		Experiment days			
		Day 1	**Days 2-7**	**Days 8 – 10**	**Day 11**
Groups	**One: Control**	Saline	Saline	Washout	Saline
	Two: 0.6 mg/kg MPD	Saline	0.6 mg/kg MPD	Washout	0.6 mg/kg MPD
	Three: 2.5 mg/kg MPD	Saline	2.5 mg/kg MPD	Washout	2.5 mg/kg MPD
	Four: 10.0 mg/kg MPD	Saline	10.0 mg/kg MPD	Washout	10.0 mg/kg MPD

Table 1 describes the 11 day experimental protocol for the four experimental groups. The baseline was recorded on experimental day 1 following saline injection for all groups. Then, the groups received six days of saline (control – group I) or 0.6 mg/kg MPD (group II), 2.5 mg/kg MPD (group III) or 10.0 mg/kg MPD (group IV) for six days. Experimental days 8 to 10 were washout days, where no injections were administered. On the last experimental day, the groups received either saline (to the control group) or 0.6, 2.5 or 10.0 mg/kg MPD injection as was given on experimental day 2

RESULTS: ADOLESCENT

CONTROL: (saline injection)

Locomotor activity of 8 adolescent male rats injected with saline, as described in Methods, served as the control group (Table 1). Analysis of the activity of the control group (Figure 1 left side) shows a consistent diurnal pattern of increased activity during the dark period followed by decreased activity during the light period, as expected from nocturnal animals. The right part of figure 1 summarizes (N=8) the 10 min count of locomotor activity over about 24 hrs. The observed histograms and CCSA test parameters i.e. the cosine curves, expressed consistency in the locomotor activity rhythm between all of the experimental days receiving saline. This consistency was considered the baseline of a typical locomotor activity rhythm for these rats; therefore any major deviations from this rhythmicity were attributed to the MPD treatment. Since the locomotor activity following saline injection in experimental day 1 was the same as the other experimental days following saline injection, in the MPD groups, experimental day 1 following saline injection was used as its own control within each rat group.

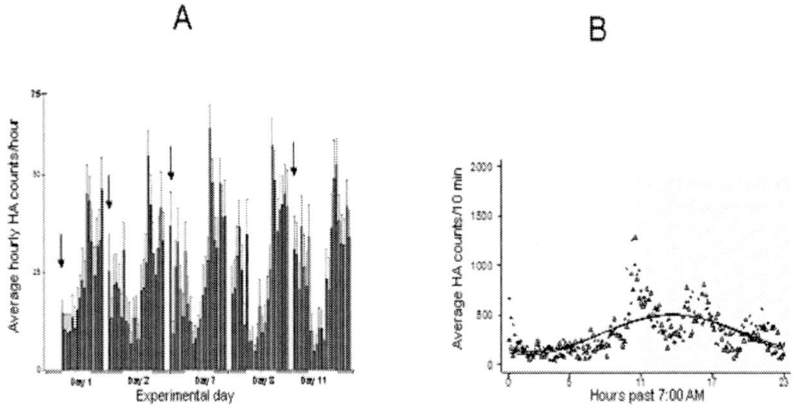

Figure 1: Control histogram reflecting the consistent rhythmic of the average horizontal activity counts per hour of experimental days, 1, 2, 7, 8, and 11. Arrows indicate time of injection (saline) and shaded areas indicate dark period of 23 h experimental period; experimental day 1 begins at 06:00 h whereas all other days thereafter begin at 00:00 h **B**: Twenty-four hour cosine curve of the horizontal activity circadian rhythm pattern in counts per 10 min, post-injection, of control days 2, 3, and 4. Time 0=07:00 h; shaded area indicates dark period of the 24 h experimental period.

MPD ACUTE PHASE: (experimental day 2 vs. experimental day 1)

Comparing activity in day 2 (first MPD injection) with effects of saline given on day 1 provided information about the acute effects of MPD. At 0.6 mg/kg, MPD did not elicit any significant changes in locomotor activity neither in the initial post-injection hours nor in the activity pattern over the 23 h post-injection (Figure 2A). MPD at 2.5 mg/kg elicited an increase in HA counts between 07:00 and 09:00 h (Figure 2A). Some differences in the circadian activity pattern over the 23 h post-injection between 09:00 h and 11:00 h as well as between 12:00 h and 14:00 h were observed compared to experimental day 1 (Figure 2A). This data was analyzed by the CCSA test and showed that these differences were statistically non-significant (Table 2). MPD at 10.0 mg/kg induced a robust increase in the locomotor activity, lasting about 3 h. (07:00 to 10:00 h) followed by a decrease in activity during the light period (10:00 h-12:00 h) (Figure 2A).Analysis of the CCSA test curves rendered this observation to be significant (Fig 2B 10.0 mg/kg MPD).

It became evident that the responses immediately post injection distorted the cosine curve (Figure 2B). Therefore, in order to accurately evaluate the locomotor activities throughout the entire experimental day, the initial 3 h post-injection was eliminated (Figure 2C). This adjustment was done to eliminate the acute MPD effect and to evaluate the rest of post injection time in all dose groups to obtain accurate comparison of the long term effects of MPD in the 3 dose groups. Therefore, unless otherwise indicated, the statistical analysis for each experimental day presented below is based on the cosine curves beginning 3 h after injection (Table 2). The CCSA test curves prior to the 3 h elimination are provided for comparison (Figure 2B). This adjustment shows that the acute MPD treatment did not alter the circadian pattern activity at any dose (Figure 2C and Table 2).

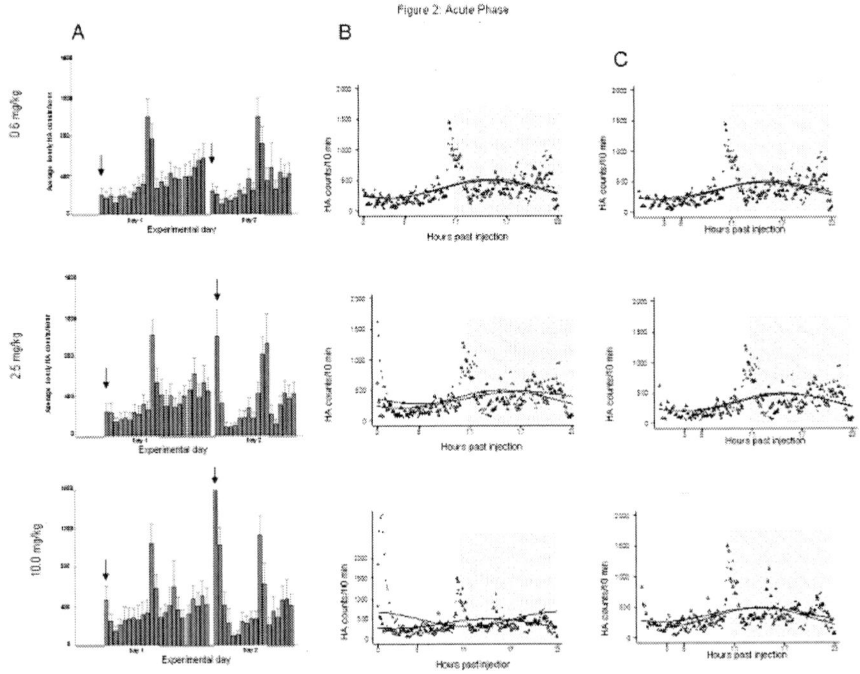

Figure 2: Acute phase effect in the 3 experimental dose groups: **A**) histogram representation of HA counts/h of experimental days 1 and 2. Arrows indicate time of injection (saline on experimental day 1 and MPD on experimental day 2); shaded areas indicate dark period of the 23 h experimental period. **B**) Cosine curve comparing experimental days 1 and 2 over a 23 h period post-drug injection; time 0=07:00 h, shaded area indicates dark period of the 23 h experimental period. **C**) Cosine curves corrected for the first 3 hours of high HA due to immediate effect of MPD injection.

Table 2

Dosage	Treatment day	N	MESOR	Amplitude	P-value (Ho: Amp. = 0)	Acrophase (hours)	R-Squared	Days compared	Ho: Equal Parameter	F-Statistic	(df)	P-value
---		278	505.78	163.72	<0.001	14.16	0.1905	(1,2)	Mesor	1.841	(1, 272)	0.176
	Day 1	139	486.44	123.81	<0.001	13.86	0.1242		Amplitude	3.835	(1, 272)	0.051
	Day 2	139	525.11	204.25	<0.001	14.35	0.2664		Acrophase	0.229	(1, 272)	0.633
	ACUTE PHASE (experimental day 2 vs experimental day 1)											
Dosage	**Treatment day**	**N**	**MESOR**	**Amplitude**	**P-value (Ho: Amp. = 0)**	**Acrophase (hours)**	**R-Squared**	**Days compared**	**Ho: Equal Parameter**	**F-Statistic**	**(df)**	**P-value**
0.6 mg/kg MPD		278	355.47	146.76	<0.001	15.04	0.1851	(1,2)	Mesor	0.42	(1, 272)	0.518
	Day 1	139	346.89	140.54	<0.001	14.94	0.1738		Amplitude	0.108	(1, 272)	0.743
	Day 2	139	364.05	153.07	<0.001	15.13	0.1971		Acrophase	0.039	(1, 272)	0.843
2.5 mg/kg MPD		278	363.36	116.61	<0.001	15.80	0.1016	(1,2)	Mesor	0.057	(1, 254)	0.812
	Day 1	139	348.79	144.39	<0.001	14.77	0.2073		Amplitude	0.041	(1, 254)	0.839
	Day 2	139	377.93	101.62	<0.013	17.28	0.0622		Acrophase	0.156	(1, 254)	0.693
10.0 mg/kg MPD		278	434.77	60.45	<0.230	20.77	0.0106	(1,2)	Mesor	3.243	(1, 254)	0.073
	Day 1	139	379.32	115.42	<0.001	14.16	0.1237		Amplitude	0.966	(1, 254)	0.327
	Day 2	139	490.22	179.92	<0.021	23.39	0.055		Acrophase	0.005	(1, 254)	0.943

Table 2. (Continued)

	INDUCTION PHASE (experimental day 7 vs experimental day 2)											
Dosage	**Treatment day**	**N**	**MESOR**	**Amplitude**	**P-value (Ho: Amp. = 0)**	**Acrophase (hours)**	**R-Squared**	**Days compared**	**Ho: Equal Parameter**	**F-Statistic**	**(df)**	**P-value**
0.6 mg/kg MPD		278	363.09	172.45	<0.001	15.27	0.1928	(2,7)	Mesor	0.117	(1, 236)	0.732
	Day 2	139	364.05	153.07	<0.001	15.13	0.1971		Amplitude	1.031	(1, 236)	0.311
	Day 7	139	362.13	192.01	<0.001	15.38	0.1945		Acrophase	0	(1, 236)	0.990
2.5 mg/kg MPD		278	381.57	132.59	<0.001	16.17	0.1197	(2,7)	Mesor	0.466	(1, 236)	0.495
	Day 2	139	377.93	101.62	<0.013	17.28	0.0622		Amplitude	2.029	(1, 236)	0.156
	Day 7	139	385.22	170.35	<0.001	15.51	0.228		Acrophase	0.141	(1, 236)	0.707
10.0 mg/kg MPD		278	510.70	107.61	<0.044	23.16	0.0225	(2,7)	Mesor	3.37	(1, 236)	0.068
	Day 2	139	490.22	179.92	<0.021	23.39	0.055		Amplitude	2.634	(1, 236)	0.106
	Day 7	139	531.19	37.25	<0.805	22.03	0.0032		Acrophase	1.037	(1, 236)	0.310
	WASHOUT PHASE (experimental day 8 vs. experimental 1)											
Dosage	**Treatment day**	**N**	**MESOR**	**Amplitude**	**P-value (Ho: Amp. = 0)**	**Acrophase (hours)**	**R-Squared**	**Days compared**	**Ho: Equal Parameter**	**F-Statistic**	**(df)**	**P-value**
0.6 mg/kg MPD		278	346.82	171.89	<0.001	15.09	0.2472	(1, 8)	Mesor	0.094	(1, 254)	0.759
	Day 1	139	346.89	140.54	<0.001	14.94	0.1738		Amplitude	2.924	(1, 254)	0.088
	Day 8	139	346.75	203.43	<0.001	15.20	0.3298		Acrophase	0.008	(1, 254)	0.928
2.5 mg/kg MPD		278	354.00	163.79	<0.001	15.01	0.2343	(1, 8)	Mesor	0.136	(1, 254)	0.712
	Day 1	139	348.79	144.39	<0.001	14.77	0.2073		Amplitude	2.827	(1, 254)	0.094
	Day 8	139	359.21	183.73	<0.001	15.20	0.2631		Acrophase	0.01	(1, 254)	0.919

Table 2. (Continued)

Dosage	WASHOUT PHASE (experimental day 8 vs. experimental 1)											
Dosage	**Treatment day**	**N**	**MESOR**	**Amplitude**	**P-value (Ho: Amp. = 0)**	**Acrophase (hours)**	**R-Squared**	**Days compared**	**Ho: Equal Parameter**	**F-Statistic**	**(df)**	**P-value**
10.0		278	476.55	120.08	<0.001	14.75	0.0954	(1, 8)	Mesor	29.22	(1, 254)	0.001
mg/kg	Day 1	139	379.32	115.42	<0.001	14.16	0.1237		Amplitude	2.394	(1, 254)	0.123
MPD	Day 8	139	573.77	127.31	<0.001	15.28	0.1033		Acrophase	0.03	(1, 254)	0.862
	EXRESSION PHASE (experimental day 11 vs. experimental 2)											
Dosage	**Treatment day**	**N**	**MESOR**	**Amplitude**	**P-value (Ho: Amp. = 0)**	**Acrophase (hours)**	**R-Squared**	**Days compared**	**Ho: Equal Parameter**	**F-Statistic**	**(df)**	**P-value**
0.6		278	362.52	169.28	<0.001	15.44	0.2169	(2,11)	Mesor	0	(1, 236)	0.991
mg/kg	Day 2	139	364.05	153.07	<0.001	15.13	0.1971		Amplitude	0.344	(1, 236)	0.558
MPD	Day 11	139	360.99	186.43	<0.001	15.70	0.239		Acrophase	0.37	(1, 236)	0.543
2.5		278	374.47	126.68	<0.001	16.66	0.108	(2,11)	Mesor	0.09	(1, 236)	0.765
mg/kg	Day 2	139	377.93	101.62	<0.013	17.28	0.0622		Amplitude	2.132	(1, 236)	0.146
MPD	Day 11	139	371.00	153.92	<0.001	16.26	0.1807		Acrophase	0.032	(1, 236)	0.859
		278	553.84	162.83	<0.004	22.66	0.0395	(2,11)	Mesor	22.02	(1, 236)	0.001
10.0	Day 2	139	490.22	179.92	<0.021	23.39	0.055		Amplitude	1.679	(1, 236)	0.196
mg/kg	Day 11	139	617.45	152.90	<0.120	21.80	0.032		Acrophase	0.009	(1, 236)	0.923
MPD												

INDUCTION PHASE: (experimental day 7 vs. experimental day 2)

Comparison of the locomotor activity obtained after the six MPD injection (experimental day 7) to that obtained after acute administration (experimental day 2) permitted evaluation of any effects induced by the 6 repetitive MPD treatments, such as behavioral sensitization or tolerance.

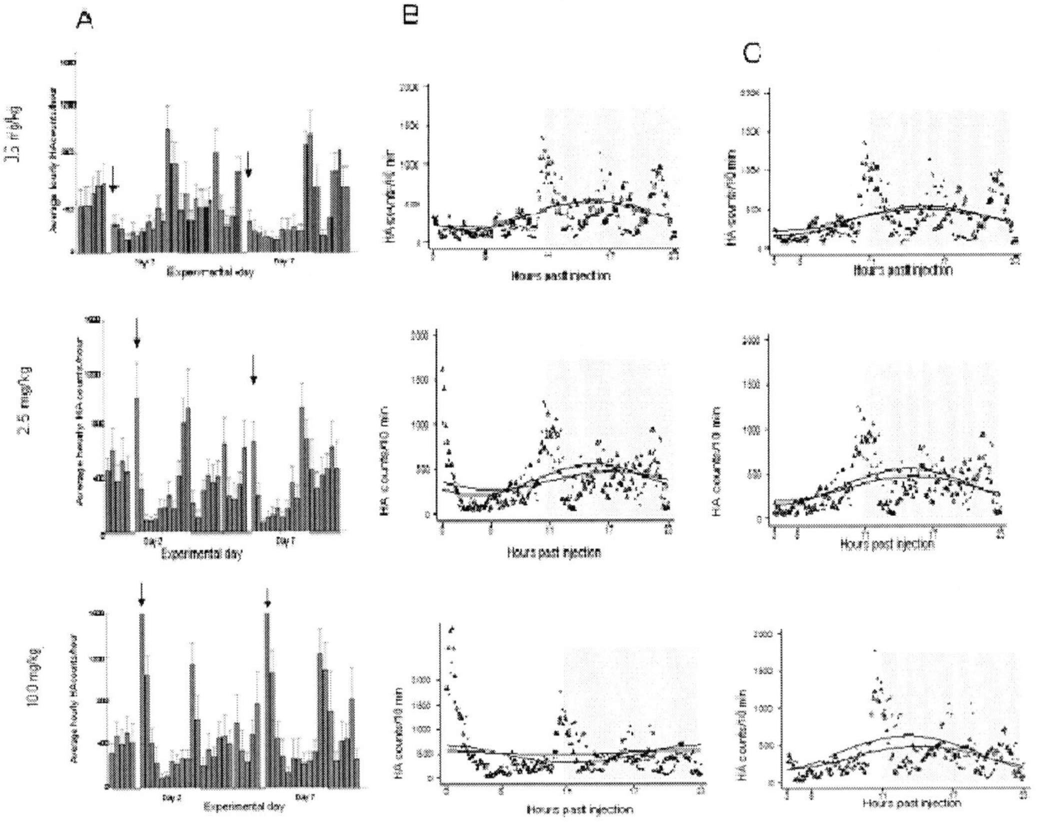

Figure 3: Induction phase effect in the 3 experimental dose groups: **A**) histogram representation of HA counts/h of experimental days 1 and 2. Arrows indicate time of injection (MPD); shaded areas indicate dark period of the 23 h experimental period. **B**) Cosine curve comparing experimental days 1 and 2 over a 23 h period post-drug injection; time 0=07:00 h, shaded area indicates dark period of the 23 h experimental period. **C**) Cosine curves corrected for the first 3 hours of high HA due to immediate effect of MPD injection.

Comparing the locomotor recordings of experimental day 7 to experimental day 2 of the group treated with 0.6 mg/kg MPD indicated a decrease in activity prior to injection, between 02:00 and 04:00 h, and again between 14:00 h and 17:00. On experimental day 7 there was an increase in activity between 21:00 and 23:00 h compared to experimental day 2 (Figure 3A). But the CCSA analysis test showed that these changes were not statistically significant (Fig 3C and Table 2). Chronic administration of 2.5 mg/kg MPD elicited an increase in locomotor activity similar to that observed in the acute phase immediately post injection. The histogram exhibited some decrease in locomotion between 01:00 h to 04:00 h and again between 12:00 h and 14:00 h, as well as an increase in activity between 18:00 h and 21:00 h, on experimental day 7 compared to experimental day 2 (Figure 3A). CCSA analysis showed that there were no significant changes in rhythmicity over the 6 days of injection (Figure 3C and Table 2). MPD at 10 mg/kg elicited a robust increase in locomotor activity during the initial hours post injection, similar to that observed in the acute phase. The histogram suggested increased activity between 10:00 h and 12:00 h and 17:00 h and 19:00 h as well (Figure 3A), but CCSA analysis showed that these deviations were statistically non-significant (Figure 3C, and Table 2).

These results showed that, while MPD elicited a dose-dependent increase in motor activity immediately after each injection, it had no effect on the circadian activity rhythm pattern of motor activity in juvenile rats.

WASHOUT PHASE: (experimental day 8 vs. experimental day 1)

Observation of motor activity during experimental days 8-10, when no MPD was given, made it possible to determine 1) whether there was an anticipation conditioned to obtain the drug in and the usual time of previous injection and/or 2) whether withdrawal from MPD will express by increase in locomotion or by changes in the circadian activity pattern compare to experimental day 1.

MPD at 0.6 mg/kg did not elicit any significant changes in locomotor activity in experimental day 8 compared to experimental day 1, although the histogram of experimental day 8 indicated a decrease in activity between 10:00 h and 12:00 h, relative to experimental day 1 (Figure 5A). Rats that had received 2.5 mg/kg MPD exhibited an increase in activity at 07:00, the time that in the previous 6 days the animals were injected with MPD. This increase in activity suggested an anticipation of MPD injection by the rats. In addition, the hourly histogram of the entire 23 h period between experimental day 8 and experimental day 1 indicated a decrease of activity between 08:00 h and 10:00 h followed by an increase in locomotion later on, between 21:00 h and 23:00 h, but these differences were statistically non-significant as indicated by CCSA analysis of both experimental days (Figure 4A, and -B, Table 2). The 10.0 mg/kg MPD group exhibited an increase in locomotion between 07:00 h and 10:00 h suggesting a greater anticipation of MPD administration effect compared to what was observed in the lower doses. Evaluation of this data using the CCSA test for both experimental days showed a significant change (p=0.001) in the average locomotion. Experimental day 8 expressed a mesor of 574 locomotor activity counts/10 min, a 66.0 % increase from that expressed on experimental day 1 (379 locomotor activity counts/10 min) (Figure 4A and –B, Table 2). Furthermore, there was a nonsignificant shift in peak activity of 48 minutes (table 2) when comparing experimental day 8 (15:28 hrs) and experimental day 1 (14:16).

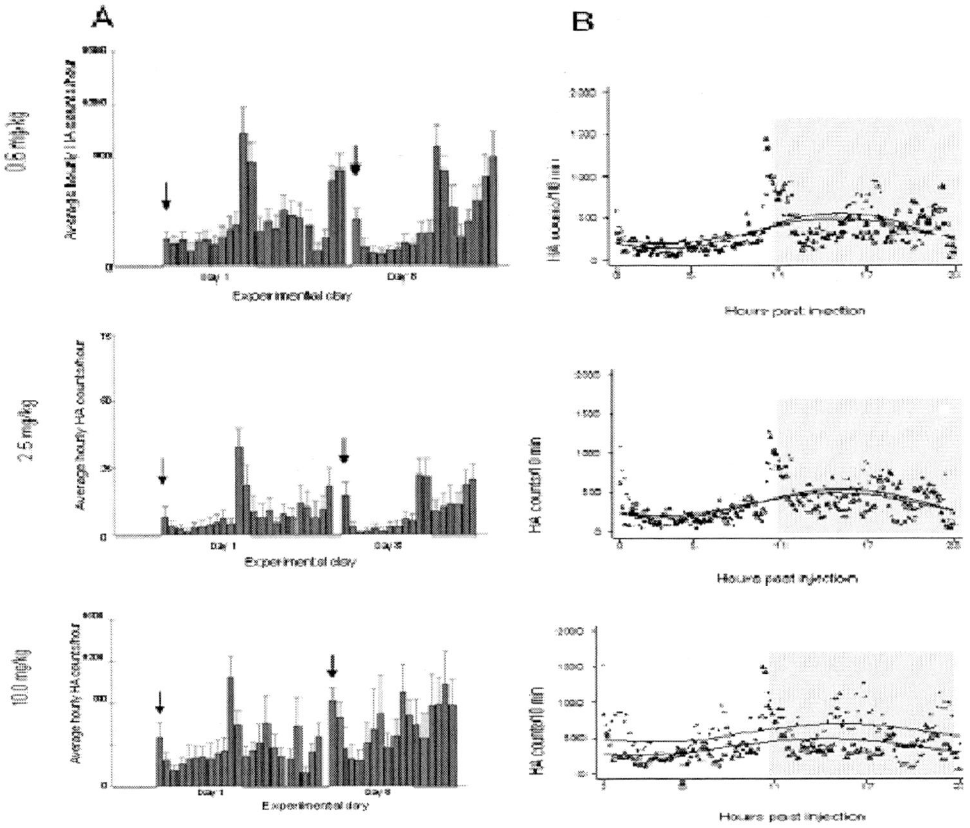

Figure 4: Washout phase effect in the 3 experimental dose groups: **A**) histogram representation of HA counts/h of experimental days 1 and 8. Arrows indicates time of injection (saline on experimental day 1); shaded areas indicate dark period of the 23 h experimental period. **B**) Cosine curve comparing experimental days 1 and 2 over a 23 h period beginning at 07:00 (time 0).

EXPRESSION PHASE: (experimental day 11 vs. experimental day 2)

To observe whether the induced changes caused by MPD in the previous phases (i.e. induction phase – comparing experimental day 7 to experimental day 2) were transient or prolonged, a re-challenge of MPD at each dose was given on experimental day 11. The effects of MPD post-re-challenge injection were then compared to the initial effects observed on experimental day 2.

The group treated with 0.6 mg/kg MPD exhibited a non-significant increase in activity in the first hour post injection on experimental day 11 compared to experimental 2 (Figure 5). Over the 23 h rhythmic period, a notable decrease in locomotor activity was observed between 02:00 h and 04:00 h followed by an increase in activity between 04:00 h and 06:00 h on experimental day 11 compared to experimental day 2 (Figure 5A). CCSA analysis showed that these differences were non-significant. The 2.5 mg/kg dose group exhibited a moderate increase in locomotor activity in the initial hour post injection on both experimental days 11 and 2 (Figure 5A). The hourly histograms showed a similar alteration in the 23 h locomotion activity pattern as observed in the 0.6 mg/kg MPD group between the two experimental days, i.e. a decrease in activity between 01:00 h and 04:00 h followed by an increase in activity between 04:00 h and 06:00 h, as well as an increase in activity between 20:00 h and 23:00 h (Figure 5A). The CCSA analysis comparing experimental days 11 and 2 demonstrated no significant differences (Figure 5B and –C). Re-challenge with 10.0 mg/kg MPD elicited a strong increase in locomotion post injection (07:00 h to 09:00 h) (Figure 4A). The re-challenge was associated with significant changes in the rhythmic pattern of the locomotor activity between experimental day 11 and experimental day 2. The average locomotor activity on experimental day 11 was significantly higher (p=001) than that observed on experimental day 2 (Figure 5 and Table 2). Also, experimental day 11 followed the trend seen on the same day for the lower doses of an increase in activity between 04:00 h and 06:00 h, but also increases in activity were seen between 11:00 h and 14:00 as well as between 18:00 and 21:00 h. CCSA analysis of motor activity over the 23 h period showed a significant (Table 2) difference between experimental days 11 and experimental day 2.

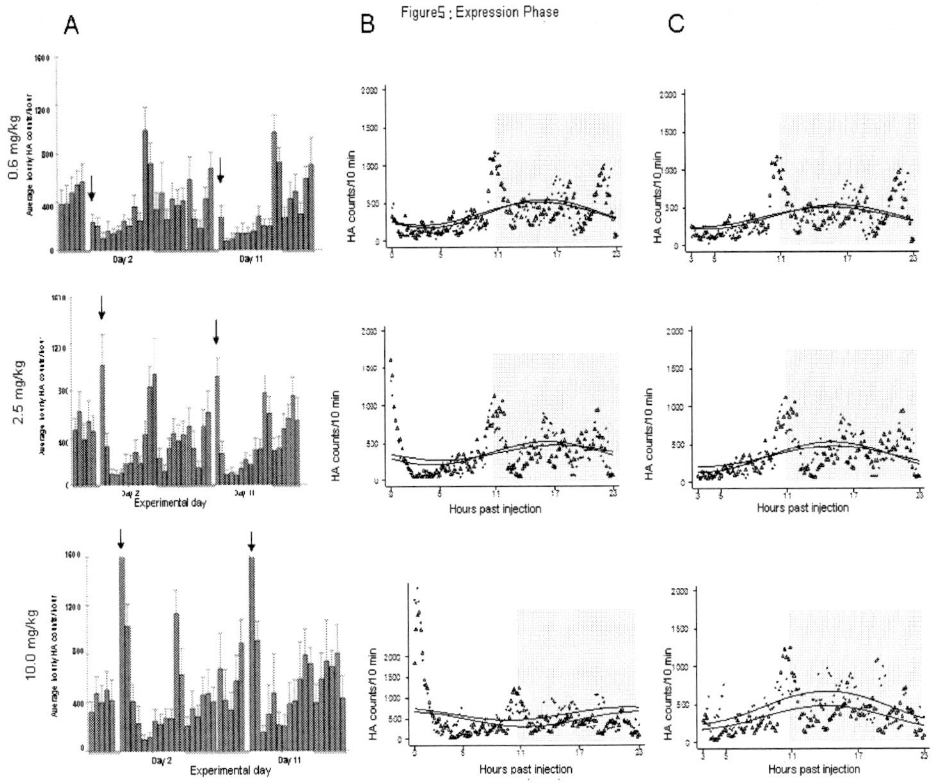

Figure 5: Expression phase effect in the 3 experimental dose groups: **A**) histogram representation of HA counts/h of experimental days 2 and 11. Arrows indicate time of injection (MPD); shaded areas indicate dark period of the 23 h experimental period. **B**) Cosine curve comparing experimental days 2 and 11 over a 23 h period post-drug injection; time 0=07:00 h, shaded area indicates dark period of the 23 h experimental period. **C**) Cosine curves corrected for the first 3 hours of high HA due to immediate effect of MPD injection.

DISCUSSION

Treatment with psychostimulants during the adolescent period of rats may cause transient or permanent changes in the central nervous system (CNS) (Yang et al, 2006). These changes may be reflected in the receptor binding and sensitivity of various neurotransmitter systems (Izenwasser and French, 2002). Rats exposed to MPD during the period of neurodevelopment experienced behavioral changes that endured into adulthood; suggesting prolonged MPD effect on neuronal maturation (Dafny and Yang, 2006).

In view of the wide use of MPD and the possibility of misdiagnosis of ADHD in children (Brandon et al., 2003; Dafny and Yang, 2006; Marshall, 2000), it is critical to understand the effects of this drug on the developing brain. The present study explores the effects of MPD on the circadian pattern of locomotor activity in the adolescent rat.

The effects of MPD on locomotor activity were evaluated for 1) the acute phase (experimental day 2 vs. experimental day 1). 2) Induction phase (experimental day 7 vs. experimental day 2), and 3) expression phase (experimental day 11 vs. experimental day 2) to verify whether any induced MPD effect was transient or prolonged. 4) The washout phase (experimental day 8 vs. experimental day 1) was used to determine whether six daily treatments elicited long term effect such as anticipation or withdrawal behavior.

MPD in the 0.6 mg/kg dose group exhibited non-significant changes in locomotor activity in the acute, induction and expression phases – unlike what was observed in the adult for this dose group, which demonstrated increased level of locomotor activity immediately after MPD injection (Algahim et. al., 2009). In the 11-day experimental period, analysis of the 23 h HA pattern in each of the challenge phases showed a consistent circadian rhythm activity pattern, with minor fluctuations suggesting that the low dose of MPD (0.6 mg/kg) did not alter the circadian activity pattern. However, during the washout phase, comparing the locomotor activity recording on experimental day 8 to experimental day 1, the circadian activity pattern exhibited significant increase in locomotion in the morning (the time of drug administration during the previous day). This increase in locomotion suggests that the rats anticipated the drug (0.6 mg/kg of MPD) or exhibited withdrawal behavior without modification in the total pattern of the 23 hr activity pattern.

Increasing the dose to 2.5 mg/kg MPD yielded significant increase in locomotion post injection and some variability in the hourly histogram of the locomotor activity pattern when compared to the 0.6 mg/kg MPD dose group. MPD treatment of 2.5 mg/kg dose induced a robust increase in activity in the rats during the initial hours post injection. The increase was drastic and distorted the cosine curve since the objective of this study was mainly to look for long term changes. This increase in activity 3hr post injection was deleted for statistical analysis of the circadian activity pattern. Once this increase was eliminated, the CCSA test showed that the 2.5 mg/kg MPD dose did not alter the circadian activity pattern. However, the initial robust activity on experimental days 7 and 11 compared to experimental day 2 indicates that behavioral sensitization was developed for this MPD dose.

In the 10.0 mg/kg MPD group, MPD treatment in the acute and induction phase, after elimination of the initial increase in activity, did not demonstrate any significant changes in locomotor activity rhythmicity pattern. However, in the washout and expression phase, the challenge with the 10 mg/kg MPD dose elicited significant modulation of circadian pattern using the CCSA test. The change in the washout phase suggests that the 6 consecutive MPD injections elicited an anticipation effect. Similar observations were seen in the adult (Algahim et al, 2009). This anticipation behavior can be interpreted as withdrawal behavior, a phenomenon that was not reported before following MPD treatment.

As opposed to the adult rats, which expressed the most significant change following the 2.5 mg/kg dose group, in the adolescent group, the 10.0 mg/kg dose group elicited the most significant changes of all the four experimental phases. This difference is reflected in the greater distortion of the CCSA test curves of the 10 mg/kg MPD challenge dose on experimental day 11 compared to experimental day 2 in the adolescent group. The adult rat group treated with 10 mg/kg on experimental day 11 exhibited tolerance to this dose compared to experimental day 2 and no significant change in the circadian activity pattern, while the adolescent 10 mg/kg MPD group exhibited behavioral sensitization and significant change in the circadian rhythm activity pattern.

It can be summarized that in the adolescent rat, there was a dose-dependent increase in the degree of locomotor activity to the acute MPD treatment and changes in the rhythmicity of locomotion activity pattern only to the higher MPD dose, contrary to what was observed in the adult group, which exhibited increase in locomotor activity following low to moderate MPD doses (0.6 and 2.5 mg/kg) and tolerance for the 10 mg/kg MPD.

The reduced behavioral responses to low doses of MPD in adolescent compared to adult rats may be related to lower density of dopamine receptors in the younger animals (Brandon et. al., 2003, Laviola et. al., 1995; Ujike et. al., 1995). The notably high anticipation behavior in the washout day at 10.0 mg/kg MPD suggests a new baseline of locomotor activity was established due to high levels of dopamine release. This effect was also demonstrated by Brandon and Steiner, (2003), who noted during early withdrawal from high doses of MPD, there were transient changes in midbrain dopamine neurons, particularly an increase in firing rate of dopaminergic neurons in the ventral tegmentum (VTA). In other words, in response to immediate abstention of MPD, the VTA is trying to sustain the new baseline level of extracellular dopamine that had been induced by chronic administration of 10.0 mg/kg MPD. Furthermore, the chronic administration of 10.0 mg/kg MPD on experimental day 11 elicits robust increase in locomotion suggesting that sensitization was developed, as well as alteration in the hourly histogram and the circadian rhythm of locomotor activity.

In the adult group, we suggested that MPD, like other psychostimulants, may possess the ability to impose molecular changes, possibly changing in the expression of the clock genes. Adolescent rats appeared less sensitive to the effects of MPD. Previous studies have reported that increased DA release caused by stimulants was associated with changes in gene expression in dopamine-receptive neurons (Berk and Hyman, 2000; Brandon and Steiner, 2003, Hymann and Nestler, 1996; Nestler, 2001; White and Kalivas, 1998). Furthermore, Brandon and Steiner (2003) demonstrated that, in adolescent rats, acute and repeated MPD treatment can produce molecular alterations. Therefore, it can be suggested that, although MPD has the ability to enforce molecular changes, its efficacy in altering the circadian clock genes in the adolescent rat may be lower than in the adult. This warrants further investigation.

Acknowledgments

This research was supported in part by the NIH-DA 14441 and 027222. We also wish to thank Molinckrodt, Inc. for their gift of methylphenidate; Dr. M. Smolinski for his constructive comments; Ms. Sheshali Wanchoo for manuscript preparation.

References

Accardo, P., and Blondis, T. A. What's all the fuss about Ritalin? J Pediatr 2001; 138: 6-9.

Adriani, W., Chiarotti, F., and Laviola, G. Elevated novelty seeking and typical d-amphetamine sensitization in periadolescent compared to adult mice. Behav Neurosci 1998; 112: 1152-1156.

Algahim, M.F., Yang, P.B., Wilcox, V.T., Burau, K.D., Swann, A.C. and Dafny, N. Prolonged methylphenidate treatment alters the behavioral diurnal activity pattern of adult male Sprague-Dawley rats. Pharmacology, biochemistry, and behavior 2009; 92(1): 93-9.

Amini, B, Yang, P.B., Swann, A.C. and Dafny, N., Differential locomotor responses in male rats from three strain to acute methylphenidate. Int. J. Neurosci., 2004, 114:1063-1084.

Andersen, S.L., Arvaniitaglannis, S.A., Pliakas, A.M., LeBlance, C., Carleron, W.A. Altered responsiveness to cocaine in rats exposed to methylphenidate during development. Nat Neurosci 2002; 51:13-14.

Andersen, S.L. and Teicher, M.H. Sex differences in dopamine receptors and their relevance to ADHD. Neurosci, Biobehav. Rev 2000; 24:137-141.

Berk, J.D. and Hyman, S.E. Addiction, dopamine, and the molecular mechanisms of memory. Neuron. 2000; 25: 515-532.

Biederman, J., Faraone, S.V., Spencer, T., Wilenes, T, Mich E. and Lapey, K.A. Gender differences in a sample of adult with attention deficit hyperactivity disorder. Psychiatry Rev., 1994, 53:13-29.

Bingham, C., Arbogas, A., and Guillaume, B. Influential statistical methods for estimating and comparing cosine parameters. Chronobiologia, 1982; 9:397-439.

Bowman, B. P. and Kuhn, C. M. Age-related differences in the chronic and acute response to cocaine in the rat. Dev Psychobiol 1996; 29: 597-611.

Brandon, C. L., Marinelli, M., Baker, L. K., and White, F. J. Enhanced reactivity and vulnerability to cocaine following methylphenidate treatment in adolescent rats. Neuropsychopharmacol, 2001; 25: 651-661.

Brandon C.L., Steiner H. Repeated methylphenidate treatment in adolescent rats alter gene regulation in the striatum. European Journal of Neuroscience, 2003; 18 (6):1584-1592.

Byrnes, J. J., Pritchard, G. A., Koff, J. M., and Miller, L. G. Prenatal cocaine exposure: Decreased sensitization to cocaine and decreased striatal dopamine transporter binding in offspring. Neuropharmacology 1993; 32: 721-723.

Clure, C., Brady, K. T., Saladin, M. E., Johnson, D., Waid, R., and Rittenbury, M. Attention deficit/hyperactivity disorder and substance use: symptoms patterns and drug choice. Am J Drug Alcohol Abuse 1999; 25: 441-448.

Collins, S.L., Izenwasser, S. Cocaine differentially alters behavioral and Neurochemistry in periadolescent versus adult rats. Developmental Brain Research. 2002; 138: 27-34.

Dafny, N. and Yang, P.B. The role of age, genotype, sex and route of acute and chronic administration of methylphenidate: A review of its locomotor effects. Brain Research Bull. 2006; 68: 393-405.

Durmans, T. L., Varlinskaya, E. I., and Spears, L.P. Age related differences in elevated plus maze behaviors between adolescent and adult rats. Ann NY Acad Sci 2004; 1021: 427-430.

Gaytan, O., al-Rahim, S., Swann, A.C. and Dafny, N. Sensitization to locomotor effects of methylphenidate in the rat. Life Sciences 1977; 61: 101-107.

Fujiwara, Y., Kazahaya, Y., Nakashima, M., Sato, M., and Otsuki, S. Behavioral sensitization to methamphetamine in the rat: an ontogenic study. Psychopharmacology 1987; 91: 316-319.

Gillian, T.C., Kandel, E.R., and Jessell, T.M., Gene and Behavior. In Principles of Neural Science. E.R. Kandel, E.R., J.H. Schwartz and T.M. Jessel Gds. McGraw-Hill Com. Inc., 4th Edition, 2000 pp.36-60.

Grund, T., Lehmann, K., Bock, N., Rothenberger, A., Teuchert-Nood, G. Influence of methylphenidate on brain development—an update of recent animal experiments. Behavioral Function. 2006; 2: 2.

Hammano, K., Iwasaki, N, Takeya, T. A quantitive analysis of rat central nervous system myelination using the immunochistochemical method for MBP. Developmental Brain research. 2006; 93: 18-22.

Huttenlocher, P. R. Synaptic density in human frontal cortex-developmental changes and effects of aging. Brain Res 1979; 163: 195-205.

Hyman, S.E. and Nestler, E.J. Initiation and adaptation: a paradigm for understanding psychotropic drug action. American Journal Psychiatry. 1996; 153: 151- 162.

Izenwasser, S. and French, D. Tolerance and sensitization to the locomotor – activating effects of cocaine are mediated via independent mechanisms. Pharmacol. Biochem and Behav. 2002, 73:877-882.

Lambert, N.M., and Hartsongh, C.S. Prospective study of tobacco smoking and substance dependencies among samples of ADHD and non ADHD participants. J Learn Disabil. 1998; 31: 533-544.

Laviola, G., Wood, R.D., Kuhn, C., Francis, R., Spear, L.P. Cocaine sensitization in periadolescent and adult rats. Journal of Pharmacol. Exp. Ther. 1995; 275: 345-357.

Levin, F.R. and Kleber, H.D. Attention-deficit hyperactivity disorder and substance abuse; relationships and implications for treatment. Havard Rev. Psychiatry 1995; 2: 246-258.

Marshall, E. Duke study faults overuse of stimulants for children. Science. 2000; 289:721.

Moore, R.Y. Circadian Timing In Fundamental Neuroscience. L.R, Squire, F.E., Bloom, S.K.,

McConnel, J.L. Roberts, Nic. Spitzer and M.J.Zigmond Eds., Academic Press, 2nd Edition, 2003; 1067-1084.

Nestler, E.J. Molecular basis of long-term plasticity underlying addiction. Nature Rev. Neurosci. 2001; 2: 119-128.

Rakie, P. Development of the primate cerebral cortex. In Lewis, M. ed. Child and adolescent psychiatry. Baltimore, Williams and Wilkins. 1986.

Robinson, T. E. Behavioral sensitization: characterization of enduring changes in rotational behavioral produced by intermittent injections of amphetamine in male and female rats. Psychopharmacology (Berl) 1984; 84: 466-475.

Robinson, T.E. and Berridge, K.C. The neural basis of drug craving; an incentive-sensitization theory of addiction. Brain Res. Rev. 1993; 18: 247-291.

Rosenberg, D.R., Lewis, D.A. Postnatal maturation in the dopaminergic innervation of monkey prefrontal and motor cortices: a tyrosine hydroxylase immunohistochemical analysis. J. Comp.Neurol, 1995; 358: 383-400.

Schenk, S., and Isenwasser, S. Pretreatment with methylphenidate sensitizes rats to the reinforcing effects of cocaine Pharacol. Biochem. Behave. 2002; 72: 651-657.

Segal, D. S., and Kuczenski, R. Repeated binge exposure to amphetamine and methamphetamine: Behavioral and neurochemical characterization. J Pharmacol Exp Ther 1997; 282: 561-573.

Teicher, M.H., Andersen, S.L., Hostetter Jr., J.C. Evidence for dopamine receptor pruning between adolescence and adulthood in striatum but not nucleus accumbens. Developmental Brain Research. 1995; 89: 167-72.

Ujike, H., Tuschida, K., Akiyama, K., Fujiwara, Y., Kuroda, S. Ontogeny of behavioral sensitization to cocaine. Pharmacol. Biochem Behav. 1995; 50: 613-617.

Wilens, T.E., Faraone, S.V., Biederman, J., and Gunawardoene, S. Does stimulant therapy of attention deficit/hyperactive disorder beget later substance abuse, A meta-analytic review of the literature. Pediatrics, 2003; 111: 179-185.

Yang, P.B., Swann, A.C, Dafny, N. Acute and Chronic Methylphenidate dose-response assessment on three adolescent rat strains. Brain Res. Bull. 2006; 71: 301-310.

Yang, P.B., Behrang, A., Swann, A.C., and Dafny, N. Strain differences in the behavioral responses of male rat to chronically administered methylphenidate. Brain Res., 2003, 971: 139-152.

Zito, J. M., Safer, D. J., dosReis, S., Gardner, J. F., Boles, M., and Lynch, F. Trends in the prescribing of psychotropic medications to preschoolers. Amer Med Assoc 2000; 283: 1025-1030.

In: Attention Deficit Hyperactivity Disorder (ADHD) ISBN 978-1-60741-581-7
Editors: Stuart M. Gordon and Aileen E. Mitchell

Chapter 11

Psychopharmacology in Children, Adolescents and Adults with Attention Deficit Hyperactivity Disorder (ADHD)

Donald E Greydanus1 **and Joav Merrick**2,3*

[1]Michigan State University College of Human Medicine, Pediatrics Program, Michigan State University/Kalamazoo Center for Medical Studies, Kalamazoo, Michigan, United States,

[2]National Institute of Child Health and Human Development, Office of the Medical Director, Division for Mental Retardation, Ministry of Social Affairs, Jerusalem, Israel

[3]Kentucky Children's Hospital, University of Kentucky, Lexington, United States

Abstract

Attention deficit hyperactivity disorder (ADHD) is a neurobehavioral developmental disorder affecting several percent of the population, which usually presents itself during childhood, but can persist into adulthood or be diagnosed in adulthood also. Treatment of the male or female child, adolescent, young adult, or older adult with ADHD begins with a careful assessment to establish a correct diagnosis and what potential co-morbid conditions may also complicate the clinical picture. If a psychopharmacologic approach is chosen as part of the management strategy for this common conundrum, the clinician should understand that the medications noted by research to help many patients improve their attention dysfunction are stimulants, norepinephrine reuptake inhibitors, and antidepressants; alpha-2 agonists may improve the classic insomniac effect of stimulants. The most popular drugs and the ones with the most underlying research support are the

* Correspondence: Donald E Greydanus, MD, Professor, Pediatrics and Human Development, Michigan State University College of Human Medicine, Pediatrics Program Director, Michigan State University/Kalamazoo Center for Medical Studies, 1000 Oakland Drive, Kalamazoo, MI 49008-1284 United States. E-mail: Greydanus@kcms.msu.edu and Professor Joav Merrick, MD, MMedSci, DMSc, Medical Director, Division for Mental Retardation, Ministry of Social Affairs, POBox 1260, IL-91012 Jerusalem, Israel. E-mail: jmerrick@zahav.net.il.

stimulants, *methylphenidate* (available since 1957) and *amphetamine* (with observational data on its effectiveness starting in 1937). A number of newer, long-acting stimulants have been introduced in the past decade.

Introduction

Attention deficit hyperactivity disorder (ADHD) is a neurobehavioral developmental disorder affecting several percent of the population, which usually present itself during childhood by a persistent pattern of inattention and/or hyperactivity, but also forgetfulness, poor impulse control or impulsivity and distractibility. It is considered a chronic condition, usually diagnosed in children with a generally continuation into adulthood, but over the past decade also diagnosed in adults.

Heinrich Hoffman (1809-1894) was a German physician and medical writer/illustrator who in 1844 wrote about a young child, *Fidgety Phillip (Struwwelpeter)*, who had traits of what was later called attention deficit hyperactivity disorder (ADHD) or attention deficit disorder (ADD) [1]. In this chapter, the terms ADD and ADHD are used interchangeably. Epidemiologic data today suggest that ADHD affects 3%-10% of the population at all ages, including children, adolescents, and adults [2-5]. Some clinicians have considered ADHD to be a "pediatric" disorder and a condition not found in adolescents or adults. However, the "older" student (i.e., high school, college, or graduate student) and the "mature" adult may also have ADHD and such a diagnosis should be suspected, if the clinician sees a patient of any age, who presents with marked problems in concentration. For example, such students may be seen in the college health service complaining of limited academic success and secondary anxiety as well as concern over problems adjusting to the educational demands of college/university life [6]. The adult may present to the primary care clinician's office complaining of problems with his or her job, because of concentration dysfunction with some unable to keep a job, because of such attentional problems.

A careful evaluation is necessary to identify if ADHD is present in such a situation [7-9]. Management of ADHD in the child, adolescent, or adult includes a variety of modalities, including helping the patient of any age accept this diagnosis (if present), placing the individual in the correct academic or work environment, considering the role of psychosocial or psychological guidance or therapy, and assessing the potential role of psychopharmacology. This chapter reviews medications that research has shown improves the attentional dysfunction of many individuals with ADHD, including children, adolescents, and adults.

Psychopharmacology of ADD/ADHD

Over a half century of research has identified a number of medications that can benefit the concentration ability of a child, adolescent, or adult with ADHD (see table 1): stimulants, norepinephrine reuptake inhibitors, antidepressants and alpha-2 agonists [6,10-14].

Stimulant Medications

Hundreds of randomized, controlled, research studies have revealed that stimulant medications can improve the concentration ability of 75% to 95% of children, adolescents and adults with ADD/ADHD [10-15]. Surveys suggested that approximately 6% of those between 5 and 15 years of age in the United States take stimulant medication [16]. It is unknown how many adults with ADHD are on such medication, but the number is much smaller, since there are fewer clinicians recognizing this disorder in adults and fewer who are willing to place their adult patients on anti-ADHD medications

Table 1. Medications with research support for use in attention disorders. Modified with permission from Greydanus DE, Sloane M, Rappley M. Psychopharmacology of ADHD in adolescents. Adolesc Med 2002;13:600

Medication	Daily dose (mg/kg) schedule	Common untoward effects
Stimulants		
Methylphenidate	0.3-2.0 (10-80 mg/day) in 2-4 divided doses	Insomnia, decreased appetite, abdominal pain, headache, depression, loss of weight, rebound symptoms, decreased velocity versus growth delay; See text
Magnesium pemoline	0.5-3.0 (37.5 to 131.25 mg/day) In 1-2 divided doses	Same as methylphenidate + possible liver toxicity (new FDA "black box" warning)
Dextroamphetamine	0.1-1.5 (5-80 mg/day) in 2-4 divided doses	Same as methylphenidate but more depression
Antidepressants		
Tricyclic Antidepressants		Anticholinergic effects, others. See text
imipramine	1-5	
desipramine	1-5	
nortriptyline	0.5 to 3	
Bupropion	3-6 (50-300 mg/day) in 2-3 divided doses	Insomnia, irritability, drug induced seizures (with doses >6 mg/kg) : contraindicated in bulimic patients
a$_2$ –agonists		
Clonidine	3-10 ug/kg (.05-.4 mg/day) in 2-4 divided doses	Sedation (very frequent), depression, dry mouth, rebound hypertension, hypotension (rare), confusion (with high doses), localized irritation with transdermal preparation
Guanfacine	15-43 ug/kg (0.5-4.0 mg/day) in 1-2 divided doses	Same as clonidine but much less sedation, less hypotension
Norepinephrine Reuptake Inhibitors		
Atomoxetine	0.5-1.4 mg/kg/day in 1-2 divided doses	Decreased appetite, dyspepsia, dizziness, fatigue, sedation, nausea emesis, mood swings, growth delay

Methylphenidate

Methylphenidate (MPH), a schedule II medication first introduced in 1957, remains the most widely prescribed psychostimulant [6,10-14]. Until recently, the most common form of MPH has been Ritalin®, though other longer-acting formulations are now available (see table 2). An advantageous effect on attention dysfunction is related to an increase in extracellular dopamine in the central nervous system (CNS) because of selective binding of the presynaptic dopamine transporter in the striatal and prefrontal areas of the CNS; there is also a blockade of the norepinephrine transporter in the CNS [13,15].

MPH, as Ritalin® or its generic equvalent, is taken by mouth and becomes pharmacologically active in 30 to 45 minutes; it peaks in 1-2 hours and fades over 3 to 5 hours. It (or its generic equivalent) is given one to three times a day, depending on when the stimulant effects are necessary or desired. Guidelines are how to prescribe short-acting MPH is widely-available [10-14]. The patient must be individually titrated to the dose and schedule best suited for his or her schedule and needs. A single dose of over 20 mg or a total daily dose of over 60-80 mg is not recommended.

Table 2. Available methylphenidate medications. Modified with permission from: Greydanus DE, Pratt HD, Sloane M, Rappley M. Attention-deficit/hyperactivity disorder in children and adolescents: interventions for a complex costly clinical condundrum. Pediatr Clin N Am 2003;50:1063

Available Methylphenidate Medications
Ritalin® (methylphenidate-immediate-release; 5 mg, 10mg, 20 mg tablets) (Novartis)
Ritalin SR® (20 mg methylphenidate tablet, sustained-release) (Novartis)
Generic MPH (both immediate-release and sustained-release; tablet options same as Ritalin®) (Geneva)
Ritalin® LA (Ritalin® developed for 8 to 9 hours duration; 20 mg, 30 mg, 40 mg capsules) (Novartis)
Metadate™ ER (sustained-release [8 hours] MPH; 20 mg tablets) (Celltech)
Methylin® ER (sustained-release [8 hours] MPH; 10 mg, 20 mg tablets) (Mallinckrodt)
Concerta ™ (MPH HCL: extended release tablets: 18mg, 36 mg, 54 mg; up to 12 hours MPH duration) (Alza-McNeil)
Metadate® CD (MPH HCL: extended-release 20 mg capsules; 8-9 hours of MPH duration) (Celltech)
Focalin™ (dexmethylphenidate [purifed d-methylphenidate] to last 4-6 hours at half the usual dose; 2.5 mg, 5 mg, 10 mg tablets) (Novartis)
Daytrana® (once a day MPH patch) (Noven)

Stimulant Side Effects

Table 3 provides known side effects of stimulant medication, whether MPH or amphetamines (see next section) [6,10-14]. Adverse effects (see table 3) are noted with both short-acting and sustained-release stimulants. Starting at a low dose and carefully increasing the stimulant dose may ameliorate many of these adverse events. Contraindications to stimulant use are listed in table 4. A limited number of case reports of death have occurred in children or adolescents on both MPH and a tricyclic antidepressant [17,18]. Caution should be used in placed patients with heart problems on stimulant medications and sudden deaths have been reported on rare occasions. Some have suggested that an EKG be given to patients prior to stimulant prescription, though this remains controversial [19]. Also, MPH can interact with some anticonvulsants, such as ethosuximide, phenytoin, and phenobarbital.

Approximately 50% to 75% of those with Tourette Syndrome also have ADHD and the presence of tics is a relative, not absolute contraindication to stimulant use [20]. If the stimulant is helping the ADHD symptoms, but worsening or inducing tics, anti-tic medication may be added or adjusted, such as pimozide, haloperidol or risperidone. Other anti-ADHD medications can be used that do not induce tics, such as tricyclic antidepressants, α_2 agonists (as clonidine or guanfacine), and atomoxetine. Stimulants may induce mania in a student with latent bipolar disorder or psychosis in one with latent schizophrenia.

There is no clear evidence that prescription of stimulant medication for those with ADHD increases the risk of substance abuse in these ADHD patients. However, clinicians must understand that some stimulant abuse or the non-medical use of prescription stimulants does occur in our current society that is characterized by widespread substance abuse in general; thus, *close* observation of prescription patterns is important and mandatory if stimulants are medically prescribed [21-24].

Table 3. Potential side effects of methylphenidate. Modified with permission from: Greydanus DE, Sloane M, Rappley M. Psychopharmacology of ADHD in adolescents. Adolesc Med 2002;13:607. *Common side effects

Potential side effects of Methylphenidate**
Headache*
Abdominal pain*
Jitteriness*
Dizziness
Anorexia *
Insomnia (delayed onset of sleep)*
Social withdrawal*
Weight loss (due to decreased appetite)*
Moodiness (irritability)
Nausea
Dry mouth
Constipation
Increase in heart rate, blood pressure and palpitations
"Unmasking" of Tourette's syndrome
Appearance of being "dazed or drugged"; perseveration and withdrawal

Table 3. (Continued)

Potential side effects of Methylphenidate**
Rebound phenomenon
Increased hyperactivity
Appearance of psychosis or psychotic features
Personality change
Tolerance
Skin rash (rare)

Tolerance has been observed in some patients taking high doses of stimulants, so trying another stimulant or using a lower dose of the same stimulant may help this problem. Rebound refers to the development of a worsening ADHD state as the stimulant is lowered in dose or blood levels become reduced from the last dose. Changing the combination of short-acting and/or long-acting stimulant doses may help. Early evening rebound may be difficult to improve and sleep dysfunction may arise, if stimulant effect is still present in the evening, when sleep is needed or desired. Stimulant-induced sleep disturbances may be helped with other anti-ADHD medications (as tricyclic antidepressants, bupropion, or an alpha-2-agonist). Medications that have been added to the stimulant regimen to induce sleep include melatonin (3-6 mg before bedtime), trazodone (25-50 mg before sleep) or mirtazepine (Remeron®, 7.5 mg-15 mg before sleep).

Table 4. Contradictions to stimulant use

Contraindications to stimulant use
Overt sensitivity to these medications
Psychosis
Hyperthyroidism
Drug dependence
Uncontrolled hypertension
Symptomatic cardiovascular disease
Glaucoma;
Concomitant use with monoamine oxidase inhibitors,

MPH Preparations

Ritalin® and Ritalin-SR® have been the most popular MPH brands until recently. Many patients do not like to take short acting MPH several times a day. Ritalin-SR ® is a 20 mg sustained release (SR) MPH tablet that allows release of 7 mg of short-acting MPH over several hours. Because Ritalin-SR is only made as a 20 mg tablet and has unpredictable absorption in half or more of users, an intense search has been conducted by pharmaceutical companies over the past 15 years for more reliable, long-acting stimulant medication. Table 2 lists these products and table 5 identifies the basic duration of action of these and other long-acting amphetamine products [6,10-14].

Newer MPH Formulations

Concerta™ has a tri-layer core covered by a semi-permeable membrane with a laser-drilled hole on one end that results in gradual release of MPH [6,10-14]. This OROS mechanism (osmotic time-release process) allows immediate release of 22% of MPH in the overcoat leading to a plasma MPH peak in 1-2 hours. Then, this extended-release capsule leads to further MPH release over 10 to 16 hours with an ascending MPH profile. The capsule is difficult to alter and use as a drug of abuse. It comes as 18 mg, 36 mg, and 54 mg capsules that are taken once a day.

Ritalin® LA is made as a 20 mg, 30 mg, or 40 mg MPH capsule that has similar amounts of immediate release (IR) and sustained release (SR) beads; this allows MPH release for up to 8 hours, based on the release of two doses four hours apart. Start with a 20 mg capsule and do not exceed 60 mg per day. Methylin® is available as 5, 10, and 20 mg tablets with short-acting MPH. Methylin® ER is an extended-release 10 mg and 20 mg MPH tablets for up to 8 hours of MPH effect. Metadate® CD is a long-acting 20 mg MPH capsule with coated beads; 30% of the MPH is released immediately and the remaining MPH is released over the next 6 to 10 hours. The patient starts with the 20 mg capsule and can gradually increase, if necessary, up to 60 mg a day. Focalin™ (dexmethylphenidate HCL) is the d-threo-enantiomer of racemic MPH; this MPH formulation may be more pharmacologically active than the l-threo-enantiomer and perhaps with fewer adverse effects. It comes as 2.5 mg, 5 mg, and 10 mg tablets (half the regular dose of MPH) that may last 4 to 6 hours.

Some data suggests that medication compliance for some patients with ADHD is better with extended-release MPH formulations versus immediate-release types [25]. However, there are no current valid scientific studies comparing the long-acting stimulant products to each other, to determine which one is the best to use. This is important for clinicians and consumers to understand, especially in the light of aggressive company advertisements or potentially biased opinions of some speakers who are paid by companies for research and/or lectures. A trial and error method is necessary to determine which product (IR or SR) is the best for an individual patient. The cost of these various products must also be carefully considered

Table 5. Stimulants: Duration of action. Modified with permission from Greydanus DE, Pratt HD, Sloane M, Rappley M. Attention-deficit/hyperactivity disorder in children and adolescents: interventions for a complex costly clinical condundrum. Pediatr Clin N Am 2003;50:1065

A. Short-acting (3-6 hours)
1 Ritalin®
2 Methylin®

Table 5. (Continued)

3 Dexadrine®
4 Dextrostat®
5 Focalin™
B. Intermediate-acting (6-8 hours)
1 Ritalin-SR®
2 Methylin® ER
3 Adderall®
4 Metadate™ ER
C. Once-Daily (8+ hours)
1 Dexedrine Spansules®
2 Concerta™
3 Adderall XR™
4 Metadate® CD
5 Ritalin® LA
6 Methylphenidate patch (Daytrana®)

Amphetamine Products

Medicinal applications of amphetamines have been recorded since the late 1800s, though observation of their effect on behavioral issues dates back to the classic paper of Bradley in 1937 on Benzedrine [6,26]. Dextroamphetamine (Dexedrine®; Dextrostat®) is an MPH alternative and is used for those who are not helped with MPH products or who cannot tolerate the MPH side effects; its stimulant effect is 3 to 6 hours (average of 5 hours). Amphetamine use leads to inhibition of norepinephrine reuptake and dopamine transporter binding with increase release of dopamine; serotonin effects are also noted, though they are not robust [10-15]. In general, MPH and amphetamine side effects are similar, though amphetamines may lead to more depression and have a well-known addiction potential. Available amphetamine products are listed in table 6.

Dextroamphetamine is taken one to three times daily and is produced as 5 mg (Dexedrine®; Dextrostat®)and 10 mg scored tablets (Dextrostat®); a generic version is also available. Careful titration is suggested and the upper daily limit is 40 to 50 mg. Dexedrine Spansule® is available as 5 mg, 10 mg, and 15 mg capsules; it is taken once daily and stimulant effects may least 8 to 10 hours. These short-acting and long acting amphetamines may be combined if necessary. Vyvanse® (lisdexamfetamine) is a long-acting formuation of dextroamphetamine that has been available since 2007 and lasts ≥ 12 hours; it is difficult to alter to use as a drug of abuse.

Table 6. Available amphetamine stimulant medications. Modified with permission from Greydanus DE, Pratt HD, Sloane M, Rappley M. Attention-deficit/hyperactivity disorder in children and adolescents: interventions for a complex costly clinical condundrum. Pediatr Clin N Am 2003;50:1075

Available amphetamine stimulant medications
Dexedrine® (dextroamphetamine tablets; short-acting) (GlaxoSmithKline)
Dexedrine Spansule® (long-acting dextroamphetamine) (GlaxoSmithKline)
Dextroamphetamine generic (Barr)
Dextrostat® (dextroamphetamine) (Shire US)
Adderall ® (mixed-salts amphetamine with extended-release) (Shire US)
Adderall XR ™ (mixed-salts amphetamine with extended-release) (Shire US)
Desoxyn® (methamphetamine) (Abbott)
Vyvanse® (lisdexamfetamine) (Shire US)

Methamphetamine (Desoxyn® [5 mg tablets]) is a potent stimulant with effects lasting four hours; it has the highest addiction potential of the stimulants and is difficult to legally obtain in many parts of the United States. Adderall® is a mixed-salts amphetamine (75% of the d-isomer and 25% of the l-isomer) with an dextroamphetamine-like adverse effect profile. It is produced in scored tablets (5 mg, 7.5 mg, 10 mg, 12.5 mg, 15 mg, 20 mg and 30 mg) that have stimulant effects for up to 8 to 10 hours. Adderall XR™ is produced as 5 mg, 10 mg, 15 mg, 20 mg, 25 mg and 30 mg capsules; it produces a pulsed amphetamine salts release that leads to stimulant effects for up to 12 hours.

Pemoline

Pemoline (Cylert®) is a schedule III stimulant provided as magnesium pemoline that has been available in 18.75 mg, 37.5 mg (chewable form also) and 75 mg tablets. It is taken once daily up to maximum of 112.5 mg to 131.25 mg a day [11,12]. It is used sparingly today because of the rare, but well-known occurrence of irreversible liver failure associated with its use. Informed, written consent is necessary acknowledging the potential risk of liver failure and death for anyone on pemoline. Pemoline is no longer actively produced in the United States.

Atomoxetine

Atomoxetine (Strattera®) is a non-stimulant medication that is a norepinephrine reuptake inhibitor without primary affects on dopamine levels [6,27]. It was released in January of 2003 and is available as 10-,18-, 25-, 40-, and 60-mg capsules. Atomoxetine is FDA-approved for children (6 years and up), adolescents, and adults. However, it is currently recommended by some experts only in situations where stimulants are not effective, tolerated, or desired [6,28]. Table 7 lists known side effects of atomoxetine and it is given up to 100 mg a day in either a once a day or twice a day regimen [13,29,30]. In 2005, the FDA issued a black box warning for atomoxetine regarding an increased risk for suicidal thinking in children and adolescents and asked that a Patient Medication Guide (MediGuide) be provided to patients prescribed this medication to alert consumers to this potential risk [31]. Children and adolescents placed on this medication should be carefully observed for such features as agitation, irritability, suicidal thinking or behaviors, and unusual changes in behavior especially during the initial few months of starting the drug or at times of dosage change (increase or decrease) [31].

Table 7. Atomoxetine side effects

Atomoxetine side effects
Anorexia
Constipation
Dizziness
Dry mouth
Dyspepsia
Emesis
Fatigue
Heightened pulse and blood pressure
Mood swings (FDA Black Box warning on increased suicidal thinking in children and adolescents)
Nausea up to several weeks
Sedation or insomnia
Sexual dysfunction
Voiding difficulty

Alpha-2 Agonists

Clonidine

Clonidine (Catapres®) is an alpha$_2$-adrenergic agonist that is produced as a pill and as a patch in 0.1 mg, 0.2 mg and 0.3 mg dosages [6,10-14]. It may help some ADHD patients, because of its sedative effects, ameliorating the insomniac effects of MPH. However, patients who only have attentional dysfunction should not take clonidine, since it may lead to impaired neuropsychological functioning on this medication. Clonidine is prescibed two to four times a day or at bedtime; start at 0.1 mg once or twice a day and the daily dosage range is .05 to 0.4 mg a day. It is important to titrate slowly to reduce the potential side effects (see table 8). If clonidine is not reduced slowly when seeking to stop the medication, rebound hypertension may result. The patch is effective for 3 to 7 days.

Take a baseline blood pressure, pulse, and blood glucose; repeated these parameters periodically, particularly when changing doses. Also, obtain a baseline EKG and repeat every 6 months the patient remains on clonidine. There have been a few deaths of pediatric patients on both MPH and clonidine. The patch may improve or prevent sedative side effects and rebound blood pressure problems associated with oral clonidine.

Guanfacine

Guanfacine (Tenex®) is an $alpha_{2A}$-adrenergic agonist related to clonidine, and also without proven benefit for concentration deficits of ADHD [11-14]. In contrast to clonidine, guanfacine may induce less sedation and less hypotension; adverse effects are otherwise similar to clonidine, though more agitation and headaches can occur. Guanfacine is produced as 1 mg and 2 mg tablets and daily dosages range from 0.5 mg to 4.0 mg. A long-acting formulation will soon be available.

Table 8. Side effects of clonidine. Modified with permission from Greydanus DE, Sloane M, Rappley M. Psychopharmacology of ADHD in adolescents. Adolesc Med 2002;13:615

Side effects of clonidine
Sedation (50%)
Dry mouth
Headache
Attention impairment
Decreased glucose tolerance
Depression
Dermatitis (from the patch)
Dizziness
Dysphoria
Fatigue
Inconsistent effects
Irritability
Itchy eyes
Postural hypotension
Potentiation of neuroleptic anticholinergic side effects
Rebound Phenomenon
Tolerance
Weight gain
Withdrawal effects (rebound tachycardia and severe hypertension from sudden clonidine cessation)
Worsening of pre-existing cardiac arrhythmias

Antidepressants

Tricyclic Antidepressants (TCA)

Research has noted that tricyclic antidepressants (TCA) can benefit ADHD and some clinicians use TCA (see table 9) as alternatives to stimulant medication [6,10-14]. Table 10 lists some of the TCA side effects. Careful monitoring of the patient taking a TCA is important, such as monitoring of the vital signs, complete blood count, serum TCA levels, and electrocardiogram (ECG); management protocols are published [17,18,32].

Table 9. Tricyclic antidepressants

Tricyclic antidepressants Dosage Range
Imipramine (Tofranil®, others) 50-200 mg/day
Desipramine (Norpramin®, Desipramine®) 50-200 mg/day
Amitriptyline (Elavil®) 50-200 mg/day
Nortriptyline (Pamelor®) 20-100 mg/day

Table 10. Tricyclic antidepressant side effects. Modified with permission from Greydanus DE, Pratt HD, Sloane M, Rappley M. Attention-deficit/hyperactivity disorder in children and adolescents: interventions for a complex costly clinical condundrum. Pediatr Clin N Am 2003;50:1079

Tricyclic antidepressant side effects
Blood dyscrasias
Blurred vision (including cycloplegia and mydriasis)
Cholestatic jaundice
Confusion
Constipation
Delirium (in high doses)
Dizziness
Drowsiness and sedation
Drug interactions (as with SSRIs)
Dry mouth (with decreased salivary flow and increased tooth decay)
EKG changes (sinus tachycardia, AV blocks, increased QRS interval, increased QTc interval)
Exercise-induced tachycardia
Hypotension
Increase in heart rate (10-15 BPM) and blood pressure (up to 8 to 10 mm Hg)
Lowered seizure threshold
Peripheral neuropathy
Priapism
Respiratory failure and death from an overdose
Skin rash
Sudden death

Tachycardia
Tremor
Urinary retention
Weight gain

Bupropion

Bupropion (Wellbutrin®) (see table 1) is an antidepressant medication that may improve attention span [33], it is FDA-approved for use in adults with depression. Zyban® is an alternate formulation to Wellbutrin® used to help manage tobacco addiction [22]. Bupropion is available as 75 mg and 100 mg tablets; the daily dosage range is 50 to 300 mg. Wellbutrin SR® is a sustained-release form (100 mg and 150 mg) given twice a day, while Wellbutrin® XL is a once-a-day bupropion formulation. Bupropion side effects are listed in table 11.

Bupropion side effects are listed in table 11 and include seizures, 0.1% under 300 mg per day and 0.4% with doses over 300 mg a day. Seizure thresholds are reduced and bupropion is contraindicated in patients with seizure disorders and with eating disorders, such as bulimia nervosa. The risks for a seizure can also be reduced by not taking doses less than 8 hours apart, slow titration of the drug, using the SR formulation, and not using high doses of the regular formulation. Bupropion does not induce cardiac conduction delays and drug-to-drug interactions are minimal.

Table 11. Bupropion side effects

Bupropion side effects
Anorexia
Agitation
Nausea
Restlessness
Drowsiness
Headache
Tics (exacerbation)
Seizures (0.1% under 300 mg a day and 0.4% over 300 mg a day)

Conclusions

The attention dysfunction of ADD/ADHD appears to be a lifelong condition and does not disappear as Fidgety Phillip (Struwwelpeter) leaves childhood, when puberty occurs or as he becomes an adult [34]. Treatment of the male or female child, adolescent, young adult, or older adult with ADHD begins with a careful assessment to establish a correct diagnosis and what potential co-morbid conditions may also complicate the clinical picture. If a psychopharmacologic approach is chosen as part of the management strategy for this common conundrum, the clinician should understand that the medications noted by research to help many patients improve their attention dysfunction are stimulants, norepinephrine reuptake inhibitors, and antidepressants; alpha-2 agonists may improve the classic insomniac effect of stimulants.

The most popular drugs and the ones with the most underlying research support are the stimulants, *methylphenidate* (available since 1957) and *amphetamine* (with observational data on its effectiveness starting in 1937). A number of newer, long-acting stimulants have been introduced in the past decade. Despite intense pressure from various pharmaceutical companies to use a specific brand, there is limited neutral research to-date to inform the unbiased clinician and the consumer which one is the best; thus, a *trial and error* method (with the cost of these medications kept in mind) is necessary to find the best stimulant (short-acting or long-acting) for a specific patient. The issue of non-prescription use of stimulants in a society permeated with drug abuse must also be appreciated [22-24,35]. Finally, other anti-ADHD drugs (*pemoline, atomoxetine, antidepressants, alpha-2 agonists*) are considered in this chapter. Other recent products for treatment of ADHD include an MPH patch (Methylpatch), Guanfacine XR, Adderall XR^2 , and a form of modafinil. The latter is now available as Provigil and is used to treat narcolepsy; recent research suggests potential beneficial effects for this non-stimulant medication on ADHD, though it is not approved by the FDA for use in children or adolescents because of concerns over safety in children [36].

References

[1] Lin-Dyken DC, Wolraich ML. Attention deficit hyperactivity disorder. In: Greydanus DE, Wolraich ML, eds. Behavioral pediatrics.New York: *Springer,* 1992:167-93.

[2] Greydanus DE, Pratt HD, Patel DR.: Attention deficit hyperactivity disorder across the lifespan. Dis D Month 2007;53(2):65-132.

[3] Barkley RA. Attention-deficit/hyperactivity disorder. *Sci. Amer*. 1998; 66-71.

[4] Soileau EJ. Medications with adolescents with attention-deficit/hyperactivity disorder.*Adolesc. Med*. 2008;19:254-67.

[5] Wolraich ML, Wibbelsman CJ, Brown TE et al. Attention deficit/hyperactivity disorder among adolescents. *Pediatrics* 2005;115:1734.

[6] Staufer WB, Greydanus DE. Attention-deficit/hyperactivity disorder: Psychopharmacology for college students. *Pediatric. Clin. North Am.* 2005;52:71-84.

[7] Reiff MI, Stein MT. ADHD evaluation and diagnosis: A practical approach to office practice. *Pediatric. Clin .North Amer.* 2003;50:300.

[8] Robin A, Schubiner H, Coleman WL, eds. ADHD/learning disorders. *Adolesc. Med.* 2008;19(2):209-356..

[9] Epstein JN, Langberg JM, Lichtenstein PK, et al.Community-wide intervention to improve the attention-deficit/hyperactivity disorder assessment and treatment practices of community physicians. *Pediatrics* 2008;122:19-27.

[10] Greydanus DE, Sloane MA, Rappley MD. Psychopharmacology of ADHD in adolescents. *Adol. Med*. 2002;13:599-624.

[11] Greydanus DE, Pratt HD, Sloane MA et al. Attention-deficit/hyperactivity disorder in children and adolescents: Interventions for a complex costly clinical conundrum. *Pediatr. Clin. North Am.* 2003;50:1049-92.

[12] Greydanus DE. Psychopharmacology of ADHD in adolescents: Quo vadis? *Psychiatric Times* 2003;20:5-9.
[13] Greydanus DE. Pharmacologic treatment of Attention-deficit/hyperactivity disorder. *Indian J. Pediatrics* 2005;72:27-34.
[14] Greydanus DE, Pratt HD. ADHD in children and adolescents. In: Greydanus DE, Patel DR, Pratt HD, eds. Behavioral pediatrics, 2nd ed. New York: iUniverse Publishers, 2006.
[15] Solanto MV, Arnsten AFT, Castellanos FX. The Neuroscience of stimulant drug action in ADHD. In: Solanto MV, Arnsten AFT, Castellanos FX, eds. Stimulant drugs and ADHD. London: Oxford Univ Press, 2001:355-79.
[16] Zito JM, Safer DJ, dosReis S, et al. Psychotropic practice patterns for youth. A 10-year perspective. *Arch. Pediatr. Adolesc. Med.* 2003;157:17-25.
[17] Varley C. Sudden death of a child treated with imipramine. *J. Child Adolesc. Psychopharmacol.* 2000;10:321-25.
[18] Varley CK. Sudden death related to selected tricyclic antidepressants in children: Epidemiology, mechanisms and clinical implications. *Paediatr. Drugs* 2001;3:613-27.
[19] Perrin JM, Friedman RA, Knilans TD. The Black Box Working Group, and the Section on Cardiology and Cardiac Surgery. *Pediatrics* 2008;122:451-3.
[20] Jankovic J. Tourette's syndrome. *N. Engl. J. Med.* 2001;345:1184-92.
[21] Wilens TE, Faraone SV, Biederman J, et al. Does stimulant therapy of attention-deficit/hyperactivity disorder beget later substance abuse? A meta-analytic review of the literature. *Pediatrics* 2003;111:179-85.
[22] Greydanus DE, Patel DR. The adolescent and substance abuse: Current concepts. *Curr. Probl. Pediatr .Adolesc. Health Care* 2005;35(3):78-98.
[23] McCabe SE, Knight JR, Teter CJ, et al. Non-medical use of prescription stimulants among US college students: prevalence and correlates from a national survey. *Addiction* 2005;99:96-106.
[24] Fone KCF, Nutt DJ. Stimulants: use and abuse in the treatment of attention deficit hyperactivity disorder. *Curr. Opin. Pharmacol.* 2005;5:87-93.
[25] Marcus SC, Wan GJ, Kenmner JE, et al. Continuity of methylphenidate treatment for attention-deficit/hyperactivity disorder. *Arch. Pediatr. Adolesc. Med.* 2005;159:572-8.
[26] Bradley C. The behavior of children receiving Benzedrine. *Am. J. Psychiatry* 1937;577-85.
[27] Allen AJ, Spencer TJ, Heiligenstein JH, et al. Safety and efficacy of atomoxetine for AHDH in two double-blind, placebo-controlled trials. Biol Psychiatry 2001;49(Suppl 8): 32S-33S.
[28] Atomoxetine (Strattera) for ADHD. *Med. Lett* 2003;45:11-12.
[29] Michelson D, Allen AJ, Busner J, et al. Once-daily atomoxetine treatment for children and adolescents with ADHD: A randomized, placebo-controlled study. *Am. J. Psychiatry* 2002;159:1896-1901.
[30] Spencer T, Biederman J, Wilens T, et al. Effectiveness and tolerability of atomoxetine in adults with attention-deficit hyperactivity disorder. *Am. J. Psychiatry* 1998; 155:693-5.
[31] http:www.fda.gov/medwatch/safety/2005/safety05.htm#Strattera.

[32] Pliszka SR, Greenhill LL, Crismon ML, et al. The Texas Children's Medication Algorithm Project: Report of the Texas Consensus Conference Panel on medication treatment of childhood attention-deficit/hyperactivity disorder. Part I. *J. Am. Acad. Child Adolesc. Psychiatry* 2001;39:908-19.

[33] Daviss WB. Buproprion for adolescents with attention-deficit/hyperactivity disorder. *J. Am. Acad .Child Adolesc. Psychiatry* 2001;40:307-14.

[34] Conant-Norville DO, Tofler IR. Attention-deficit/hyperactivity disorder and psychopharmacologic treatments in the athlete. Clin Sports Med 2005;24:829-43.

[35] Greydanus DE, Patel DR. Substance abuse in adolescents: Current concepts. *Curr. Probl .Peds .Adolesc. Health* 2005;25:78-98.

[36] Turner DC, Clark L, Dowson J, et al. Modafinil improves cognition and response inhibition in adult attention-deficit/hyperactivity disorder. *Biol. Psychiatry* 2004;55:1031-40.

In: Attention Deficit Hyperactivity Disorder (ADHD)
Editors: Stuart M. Gordon and Aileen E. Mitchell
ISBN 978-1-60741-581-7

Chapter 12

The Genetics of ADHD

Mohd Shamsi, Aliya Shamsi, Sunanda Muralee and Rajesh R. Tampi
Yale University, New Haven, CT, USA

Abstract

Introduction: Attention Deficit Hyperactivity Disorder (ADHD) is shown to be a disorder that is both familial as well as heritable. Over the last decade, and since the advent of advanced genotyping techniques, a lot of research has been done to uncover the genetic basis of ADHD. Trying to understand the genetics of ADHD helps us get a better understanding of its pathophysiology, its heritability and gives clues to any genetic subtypes that might exist. By realizing that diverse genetic variations might still produce the same clinical syndrome, we get a better understanding as to how individuals respond differently to the same medication.

Methods: The aim of this chapter is to educate those readers who have a basic understanding of the principles of genetics, by virtue of having a clinical background, but still need to be made familiar with recent advances in the genetics of ADHD, current trends and future directions. The chapter will begin with a brief introduction of genetic principles in psychiatric disorders and will involve discussion of basic physiology of the genetic targets where relevant. A glossary of relevant terms will be included. Discussion will include the challenges to conducting genetic research in psychiatric disorders. Only the most commonly researched genetic targets with the most compelling evidence to date will be discussed. The chapter will also include a section on pharmacogenetics – the genetic explanation of how individuals respond differently to the same medication. The chapter will explain how research in genetics is providing new insights into the disorder and what needs to be done to improve the quality of research.

Conclusion: Recent advances in bio-computational techniques and cheaper genotyping methods have led to a plethora of studies and a huge amount of information. Some of this information is changing the way we understand psychiatric disorders. However, clinicians find it difficult to keep pace with rapid advances and run the risk of not being able to understand what the new information means. This chapter aims to help clinicians who have an interest in ADHD get a better grip of this informational avalanche in the field of genetics.

Glossary of Terms

(From the Human Genome Project Website)

Allele

Alternative form of a genetic locus; a single allele for each locus is inherited from each parent (e.g., at a locus for eye color the allele might result in blue or brown eyes).

Candidate gene

A gene located in a chromosome region suspected of being involved in a disease.

Chromosome

The self-replicating genetic structure of cells containing the cellular DNA that bears in its nucleotide sequence the linear array of genes. In prokaryotes, chromosomal DNA is circular, and the entire genome is carried on one chromosome. Eukaryotic genomes consist of a number of chromosomes whose DNA is associated with different kinds of proteins.

Deletion

A loss of part of the DNA from a chromosome; can lead to a disease or abnormality.

DNA (deoxyribonucleic acid)

The molecule that encodes genetic information. DNA is a double-stranded molecule held together by weak bonds between base pairs of nucleotides. The four nucleotides in DNA contain the bases adenine (A), guanine (G), cytosine (C), and thymine (T). In nature, base pairs form only between A and T and between G and C; thus the base sequence of each single strand can be deduced from that of its partner.

DNA sequence

The relative order of base pairs, whether in a DNA fragment, gene, chromosome, or an entire genome.

Dominant

An allele that is almost always expressed, even if only one copy is present.

Exon

The protein-coding DNA sequence of a gene.

Gene

The fundamental physical and functional unit of heredity. A gene is an ordered sequence of nucleotides located in a particular position on a particular chromosome that encodes a specific functional product (i.e., a protein or RNA molecule).

Genome

All the genetic material in the chromosomes of a particular organism; its size is generally given as its total number of base pairs.

Genotype

The genetic constitution of an organism, as distinguished from its physical appearance (its phenotype).

Intron

DNA sequence that interrupts the protein-coding sequence of a gene; an intron is transcribed into RNA but is cut out of the message before it is translated into protein.

Nucleotide

A subunit of DNA or RNA consisting of a nitrogenous base (adenine, guanine, thymine, or cytosine in DNA; adenine, guanine, uracil, or cytosine in RNA), a phosphate molecule, and a sugar molecule (deoxyribose in DNA and ribose in RNA). Thousands of nucleotides are linked to form a DNA or RNA molecule.

Pharmacogenomics

The study of the interaction of an individual's genetic makeup and response to a drug.

Phenotype

The physical characteristics of an organism or the presence of a disease that may or may not be genetic.

Polymorphism

Difference in DNA sequence among individuals that may underlie differences in health. Genetic variations occurring in more than 1% of a population would be considered useful polymorphisms for genetic linkage analysis.

Promoter

A DNA site to which RNA polymerase will bind and initiate transcription.

Single nucleotide polymorphism (SNP)

DNA sequence variations that occur when a single nucleotide (A, T, C, or G) in the genome sequence is altered.

Variable Number Tandem Repeat (VNTR) sequences

Multiple copies of the same base sequence on a chromosome; used as markers in physical mapping.

The Genetics of ADHD

Introduction

There have been a number of genetic association studies as well as genome wide scanning studies for ADHD which have reported varying results. A number of possible disease foci have been investigated but very few have been replicated. The scope of this chapter does not permit the discussion of all the targets and all the studies that have been conducted on the genetics of ADHD. We shall discuss those gene targets that have been extensively investigated, have shown strong statistical evidence, have generated interest or have been subjected to systematic reviews or meta-analysis. Although most of the research in the genetics of ADHD is focused on the dopamine neurotransmitter system, other neurotransmitter systems have also been researched. The dopamine transporter has been extensively researched as has been the dopamine receptor. Researchers have also investigated the genetic polymorphisms in the serotonergic system and have done whole genome scans which we shall talk about. We have also included a glossary of terms for those unfamiliar with the genetic terminology

The Genetic Component of ADHD

As is the case with most psychiatric disorders, ADHD is a disorder emerging out of a complex interplay of genetics and the environment. The evidence of the genetic nature of ADHD comes from its heritable and familial nature. A disease is considered familial if it is shown to run in families. Of course, families also share the same environment and one can then argue that the disease develops solely from exposure to the same environment. On the other hand, a disease is considered heritable if twin and adoption studies are able to prove that a substantial risk for the development of the disease comes from transmission to a child from the parent. A number of twin and adoption studies have shown enough evidence strongly indicating that ADHD has a definite genetic component. Recent studies on twin subjects have concluded that the genetic component of ADHD is as high as 80% [1]. Adoption studies, which control for environmental influences, have shown a higher rate of ADHD, as much a three times higher, in the biological parents of adopted subjects, as compared to the adoptive parents [2-5]. While there is strong evidence to prove that ADHD has a strong component of being transmitted genetically, the mode of that transmission is still unclear. Most of the data that does exist from segregation studies, points towards a possible Mendelian mode of inheritance [6, 7]. While ADHD is more common in boys, there is little evidence to conclude an exclusive X chromosome linked transmission, as shown by genome wide scans [8-10].

Genetic Research In Psychiatric Disorders

Gene mutations, by definition, are rare events. On the other hand, psychiatric disorders are complex symptom syndromes lacking biological markers. Therefore, when one tries to conduct research in gene polymorphisms and psychiatric disorders, one comes across a number of study design issues, some of which are peculiar to genetic research and some of which are peculiar to psychiatric conditions. Together, genetic research in psychiatric disorders becomes quite a formidable task.

Gene mutations being rare events, studies involving genetic mutations require large sample sizes in order to have a statistically relevant sample. However, designing and funding large studies is not easily accomplished. Most centers are not able to fund large subject numbers. We therefore see a plethora of studies that get published but lack statistical significance. While the cost of genotyping has fallen considerable over the last many years, the issue of funding large studies has mainly been unresolved. Researchers have tried to circumvent the problem by resorting to meta-analyses of smaller association studies but that raises its own set of questions. It is difficult to combine studies, even when tackling the same diseases and genes, as they vary widely in their approach in study design, diagnostic criteria, rating scales, genotyping techniques and last but not the least, they look at different populations that differ in race and ancestry.

Unlike other medical conditions, the diagnostic criteria for psychiatric disorders are mostly descriptive and most symptoms overlap across diagnostic categories. The challenge with psychiatric syndromes lies in defining the phenotype i.e. the clinical presentation of the underlying genetic defect. The lack of biological markers makes an objective assessment of most psychiatric conditions very difficult. There might be different pathological processes that might lead to the same symptom presentation. For example ADHD could, as much be a result of dysfunction in the norepinephrine system, as it might be due to dysfunction in the dopamine system. A study looking at the dopamine genes in the development of ADHD could be recruiting subjects with a clinical presentation of ADHD but have an underlying defect in the norepinephrine system. Although dopamine could have a definite role in the development of ADHD but such a study would show up a weak association with dopamine genes. Modify such a study to also include exploring for gene mutations in the norepinephrine system and suddenly the sample size would have to be increased and the budget would sky rocket. Most research studies, therefore, in psychiatric disorders, are association studies that have small sample sizes.

Dopamine

The catecholamine neurotransmitter system is considered central to the pathophysiology of Attention Deficit Hyperactive Disorder (ADHD). Within the catecholamine neurotransmitter system, it is Dopamine that is considered to be the key neurotransmitter involved in the regulation of attention and motor control. Proof of the central role of Dopamine comes from the therapeutic effect of Methylphenidate on the symptoms of ADHD. Methylphenidate, which has a high response rate for the treatment of ADHD, blocks the reuptake of dopamine resulting in an increase of levels of dopamine in the synapse, thereby exerting its therapeutic effect[11]. The dopaminergic system originates in the ventral tegmental area and the substantia nigra in the brainstem and projects to the prefrontal cortex, striatum, nucleus accumbens and other areas of the brain. The symptoms of ADHD are thought to arise from abnormalities in the Dorsolateral Prefrontal Cortex (DLPC) and the Anterior Cingulate Cortex (ACC). These are the parts of the brain involved in impulse control, problem solving and attention regulation.

The Dopamine Transporter

The dopamine transporter (DAT or DAT1) is a presynaptic reuptake pump which terminates the action of dopamine by removing it from the synapse back into the presynaptic nerve terminal. The DAT is allosterically inhibited by the anti ADHD drug, methylphenidate, thereby increasing the level of dopamine in the synapse. The gene for DAT is located on Chromosome 5 and consists of 15 coding exons. As the DAT is a Na/Cl coupled transporter, it belongs to the solute carrier gene family and is also known as SLC6A3 (Solute Carrier Family 6 Member 3). The DAT is a natural target of research as it directly influences the level of dopamine in the synapse and any functional alteration can have an effect on the dopaminergic tone in the prefrontal cortex. The polymorphisms of interest in the DAT are of a Variable Number Tandem Repeat (VNTR) type as well as of a Single Nucleotide Polymorphism (SNP) type. The VNTR is a short nucleotide sequence that is organized into clusters of tandem repeats. The number of these repeats varies and each variant is considered an allele. The VNTR polymorphisms of interest are the VNTR 9-repeat and the VNTR 10-repeat and have been subjected to a number of studies and meta-analyses [12-14]. Of the two, the VNTR 10-repeat form is shown to have a stronger association with ADHD as shown by a large, albeit heterogeneous, meta-analysis of 18 studies [15]. It is also suggested that the 10-repeat VNTR polymorphism might actually be in linkage disequilibrium with another locus which might be the actual functional site[16]. Some researchers have also reported a positive association between some Single Nucleotide Polymorphisms (SNPs) within the DAT gene and ADHD. The SNPs implicated are rs463379, rs6350, rs403636, rs463379 and rs27072 [17, 18].

The Dopamine Receptor

Among the various subtypes of the dopamine receptors, it is the D4 receptor subtype [19, 20] along with the D5, that have been the most investigated receptor subtypes and we shall focus our discussion on these subtypes. The D4 receptor is a postsynaptic G protein coupled transmembrane receptor and is expressed most highly in the prefrontal cortex [21]. The D4 receptor belongs to the D2 class of receptors and is, therefore, considered part of the inhibitory family. The gene coding for the D4 receptor is known as DRD4 and is present on chromosome 11. There is a VNTR polymorphism on exon 3 of DRD4 and is the subject of numerous association studies on ADHD. Of particular interest is the 7-repeat allele, which has reduced gene expression[22], has been shown to have a significant association with ADHD as shown by a number of meta-analyses [12, 14, 20].

Research on the dopamine D5 receptor has also shown interesting results. Like D4, the dopamine D5 receptor is also post synaptic. Unlike the D4 receptor, the D5 receptor belongs to the D1 family and is considered excitatory. The dopamine D5 receptor gene, known as DRD5, is located on chromosome 4. There is a 148-bp allele in the microsatellite polymorphic region towards the 5'end of the gene. This allele became the center of intense research. A large multicenter joint analysis of 14 independent samples combined into one, totaling 1980 children and 3072 parents, showed a significant association of the DRD5 148-

bp allele with ADHD but confined to the predominantly inattentive and combined clinical subtypes [23]. Interestingly, this allele remains non functional and the authors of the study concluded that the strong association of this allele with a subtype of ADHD is probably because this allele is in linkage disequilibrium with another active site.

Catechol-O-Methyltransferase (Comt) Enzyme

It is important to discuss the COMT enzyme polymorphisms and ADHD as it illustrates an important phenomenon seen in genetic research of mental illness. Many times smaller studies showed a positive association but larger meta-analysis failed to replicate the findings. The COMT enzyme is present in the post synaptic terminal and inactivates dopamine by catalyzing its methylation. The gene for this enzyme is known as COMT and is present on chromosome 22. The functional SNP, Val158/108Met, in the gene, increases the activity of the enzyme. The increased activity in turn causes a higher turnover of dopamine. As the Val/Met SNP directly results in a change in enzyme activity and, by extension, a change in the level of synaptic dopamine, researchers actively investigated the association of this polymorphism with ADHD. Except for one study [24] most studies did not report an association of the high activity Val allele with ADHD. Subsequent meta-analysis of thirteen studies failed to report an association [25]. The case illustrates how a functional polymorphism directly related to the presumed pathophysiology of a psychiatric disorder attracts research interest and a plethora of small association studies follow. Ultimately, a meta-analysis then tries to answer the question.

Serotonin

Polymorphisms in the serotonin system have been extensively investigated in almost all psychiatric disorders. It is therefore, important to discuss the results of the outcome of research done in the genetics of the serotonin system in patients with ADHD. Serotonin is widely present in the human body, both in the brain and the gastrointestinal tract. Interesting, as much as 98% of serotonin is actually present in the gut and the remaining elsewhere in the body, including the serotoninergic nuclei in the brain. The serotonin producing neurons are present in the midline raphe nuclei of the midbrain, pons and medulla. Projections from these nuclei ascend upwards to the cortex, thalamus, hypothalamus and the limbic system. Fibers from these nuclei also descend downwards to the spinal cord and are thought to modulate painful stimuli. The serotonin transporter, also known as SERT or 5HTTR, is a plasma membrane protein that takes up extracellular serotonin and transports it back into the cell. It therefore helps terminate the action of serotonin at the synapse and also helps in recycling serotonin. SERT is the site of action of a variety of antidepressants and is the target of the SSRI class of antidepressants. By inhibiting SERT activity, these drugs prolong serotoninergic signaling, the intended pharmacodynamic action. Drugs of abuse such as, cocaine and amphetamines also target SERT.

Polymorphisms in the Serotonin Transporter

A gene located on the long arm of the 17th chromosome synthesizes the SERT. This gene is called the SLC6A4 gene. SLC stands for the designation that the gene belongs to the solute carrier of proteins. This gene is 31 kilobases in size and is made up of 14 exons. A polymorphism in the SERT gene arises out of a deletion in the promoter region of the gene. The promoter region is located upstream to the gene and modulates gene transcription. It must be remembered that the promoter region is not part of the actual gene sequence but, nevertheless, plays a pivotal role in gene expression. Some individuals can have a deletion of 44 bases within this promoter region. This gives rise to the so called "deletion polymorphism". When the SLC6A4 gene has 44 bases missing, it is classified as a "short" or "s" allele. When the gene has no deletion, it is classified as the "long" or "l" allele. The homozygous long form of the gene is considered to have a greater expression of the SERT and more efficient reuptake of the serotonin molecule.

Research done on the association of the deletion polymorphism with ADHD has shown mixed results. A number of studies have indicated a positive outcome of the association of the long variant with ADHD [26-28]. Some studies, instead of showing a higher association of the long variant with ADHD, were able to show a lower association of the short variant with ADHD [29, 30]. Other studies were not able to show association of ADHD with either polymorphism [31, 32]. The issue therefore, of association of the SERT deletion polymorphisms with ADHD is at best, unresolved.

Genome Scans

In contrast to the candidate gene approach, researchers have also done genome wide linkage analysis on "candidate" chromosomes. The results of the genome scans have shown peak LOD (Logarithm of the Odds) scores on chromosomes 5, 7, 15, 16 and 17 [9, 10, 33-35]. Of interest is the site of the high LOD score on chromosome 5 which is close to the DAT gene for the dopamine transporter. While these peaks could be a reflection of the complex phenotype that ADHD is, the exact association of these peaks with the pathophysiology of ADHD needs to be explored.

Pharmacogenetics of ADHD

Pharmacogenetics, the way the term is mostly used, can best be described as the genetics of pharmacodynamics. In other words, it is the study of the effect of the drug on the human body, therapeutic as well as adverse, as determined by the genetic makeup of the individual, everything else remaining more or less constant. Over the years, most of the studies that have come out on the pharmacogenetics of ADHD have looked at the dopaminergic system. Other neurotransmitter systems, including the serotonergic system, have also been investigated. Clinical response to methylphenidate has been investigated with mixed outcome. Of the studies that have investigated the association of the polymorphisms in the dopamine transporter gene, most have reported a poor outcome [36, 37]with the VNTR 10-repeat polymorphism but some reported a favorable [38] outcome or no effect[39].

Clinical application of pharmacogenetics lies in not only identifying responder and non-responders to the drug but also identifying patients at risk for side effects. Considering that an overwhelming number of patients with ADHD are children and teens who are likely to use ADHD medications for a long time, possibly into adulthood, these are worthwhile goals. Challenges in the field of pharmacogenetics of ADHD arise from a multitude of issues. Defining the phenotype remains the central issue in any research involving genetics. In pharmacogenetics studies, the phenotype is not limited just to the description of the disease but also involves an objective assessment of response to the drug in question as well. Population stratification becomes a confounder as is variation in allele frequencies in different populations. Studies focusing on candidate gene polymorphisms also need to take into account polymorphisms in the metabolizing enzymes. The Pharmacogenetics Working Group of the ADHD Molecular Genetics Network proposed several principles to guide future research in the pharmacogenetics of ADHD. The proposals include, among others, use of large samples to look for gene environment interactions, random distribution of participants in placebo and control groups, analysis of multiple genes and use of quality control mechanisms in genotyping [40].

Conclusion

Although a large number of research studies have tried to investigate the genetics of ADHD, and some have identified loci with strong association with ADHD, specific causes directly related to and explaining the presumed pathophysiology of the illness remain elusive. Like ADHD, other medical conditions like hypertension and diabetes also have a complex interplay of genes and the environment. However, unlike psychiatric disorders, research in most other medical conditions is not hampered by the lack of an objective assessment of the disease. Diseases like diabetes and hypertension are easily identifiable using biological techniques, with very little ambiguity with regards to diagnosis, and are very easily quantified into objective measurable entities. Research in the genetics of ADHD has to confront not only the complex interplay of genes and the environment but also has to tackle issues raised by the absence of biological markers and the need of ensuring inter rater reliability, both within studies as well as across studies. For genetic research in ADHD to progress, it is absolutely imperative that future designs should have large subject numbers. Cluster analysis and latent class analysis should help identify subtypes of ADHD which might have a higher genetic correlation. Longitudinal studies need to be designed that would investigate the role of environmental stress on the development of mental illness, ADHD or otherwise. Such studies would also help in better understanding the effect of the environment on, not just the physiological disease process per se, but also the effect of the environment on gene switching. All clinical drug trials should involve a process of collecting genetic information of the research subjects in order to facilitate the development of research of the pharmacogenetics of ADHD.

Refernces

[1] Faraone, S.V. and J. Biederman, *Neurobiology of attention-deficit hyperactivity disorder.* Biol Psychiatry, 1998. 44(10): p. 951-8.

[2] Thapar, A., et al., *Genetic basis of attention deficit and hyperactivity.* Br J Psychiatry, 1999. 174: p. 105-11.

[3] Alberts-Corush, J., P. Firestone, and J.T. Goodman, *Attention and impulsivity characteristics of the biological and adoptive parents of hyperactive and normal control children.* Am J Orthopsychiatry, 1986. 56(3): p. 413-23.

[4] Cadoret, R.J. and M.A. Stewart, *An adoption study of attention deficit/hyperactivity/aggression and their relationship to adult antisocial personality.* Compr Psychiatry, 1991. 32(1): p. 73-82.

[5] Sprich, S., et al., *Adoptive and biological families of children and adolescents with ADHD.* J Am Acad Child Adolesc Psychiatry, 2000. 39(11): p. 1432-7.

[6] Maher, B.S., et al., *Segregation analysis of attention deficit hyperactivity disorder.* Am J Med Genet, 1999. 88(1): p. 71-8.

[7] Arcos-Burgos, M., et al., *Attention-deficit/hyperactivity disorder (ADHD): feasibility of linkage analysis in a genetic isolate using extended and multigenerational pedigrees.* Clin Genet, 2002. 61(5): p. 335-43.

[8] Ogdie, M.N., et al., *A genomewide scan for attention-deficit/hyperactivity disorder in an extended sample: suggestive linkage on 17p11.* Am J Hum Genet, 2003. 72(5): p. 1268-79.

[9] Bakker, S.C., et al., *A whole-genome scan in 164 Dutch sib pairs with attention-deficit/hyperactivity disorder: suggestive evidence for linkage on chromosomes 7p and 15q.* Am J Hum Genet, 2003. 72(5): p. 1251-60.

[10] Arcos-Burgos, M., et al., *Attention-deficit/hyperactivity disorder in a population isolate: linkage to loci at 4q13.2, 5q33.3, 11q22, and 17p11.* Am J Hum Genet, 2004. 75(6): p. 998-1014.

[11] Elia, J., P.J. Ambrosini, and J.L. Rapoport, *Treatment of attention-deficit-hyperactivity disorder.* N Engl J Med, 1999. 340(10): p. 780-8.

[12] Maher, B.S., et al., *Dopamine system genes and attention deficit hyperactivity disorder: a meta-analysis.* Psychiatr Genet, 2002. 12(4): p. 207-15.

[13] Purper-Ouakil, D., et al., *Meta-analysis of family-based association studies between the dopamine transporter gene and attention deficit hyperactivity disorder.* Psychiatr Genet, 2005. 15(1): p. 53-9.

[14] Li, D., et al., *Meta-analysis shows significant association between dopamine system genes and attention deficit hyperactivity disorder (ADHD).* Hum Mol Genet, 2006. 15(14): p. 2276-84.

[15] Yang, B., et al., *A meta-analysis of association studies between the 10-repeat allele of a VNTR polymorphism in the 3'-UTR of dopamine transporter gene and attention deficit hyperactivity disorder.* Am J Med Genet B Neuropsychiatr Genet, 2007. 144B(4): p. 541-50.

[16] Galili-Weisstub, E., et al., *Dopamine transporter haplotype and attention-deficit hyperactivity disorder.* Mol Psychiatry, 2005. 10(7): p. 617-8.

[17] Ouellet-Morin, I., et al., *Association of the dopamine transporter gene and ADHD symptoms in a Canadian population-based sample of same-age twins.* Am J Med Genet B Neuropsychiatr Genet, 2008. 147B(8): p. 1442-9.

[18] Friedel, S., et al., *Association and linkage of allelic variants of the dopamine transporter gene in ADHD.* Mol Psychiatry, 2007. 12(10): p. 923-33.

[19] Gornick, M.C., et al., *Association of the dopamine receptor D4 (DRD4) gene 7-repeat allele with children with attention-deficit/hyperactivity disorder (ADHD): an update.* Am J Med Genet B Neuropsychiatr Genet, 2007. 144B(3): p. 379-82.

[20] Faraone, S.V., et al., *Meta-analysis of the association between the 7-repeat allele of the dopamine D(4) receptor gene and attention deficit hyperactivity disorder.* Am J Psychiatry, 2001. 158(7): p. 1052-7.

[21] Falzone, T.L., et al., *Absence of dopamine D4 receptors results in enhanced reactivity to unconditioned, but not conditioned, fear.* Eur J Neurosci, 2002. 15(1): p. 158-64.

[22] Schoots, O. and H.H. Van Tol, *The human dopamine D4 receptor repeat sequences modulate expression.* Pharmacogenomics J, 2003. 3(6): p. 343-8.

[23] Lowe, N., et al., *Joint analysis of the DRD5 marker concludes association with attention-deficit/hyperactivity disorder confined to the predominantly inattentive and combined subtypes.* Am J Hum Genet, 2004. 74(2): p. 348-56.

[24] Eisenberg, J., et al., *Haplotype relative risk study of catechol-O-methyltransferase (COMT) and attention deficit hyperactivity disorder (ADHD): association of the high-enzyme activity Val allele with ADHD impulsive-hyperactive phenotype.* Am J Med Genet, 1999. 88(5): p. 497-502.

[25] Cheuk, D.K. and V. Wong, *Meta-analysis of association between a catechol-O-methyltransferase gene polymorphism and attention deficit hyperactivity disorder.* Behav Genet, 2006. 36(5): p. 651-9.

[26] Seeger, G., P. Schloss, and M.H. Schmidt, *Functional polymorphism within the promotor of the serotonin transporter gene is associated with severe hyperkinetic disorders.* Mol Psychiatry, 2001. 6(2): p. 235-8.

[27] Curran, S., et al., *The serotonin transporter gene as a QTL for ADHD.* Am J Med Genet B Neuropsychiatr Genet, 2005. 134B(1): p. 42-7.

[28] Kent, L., et al., *Evidence that variation at the serotonin transporter gene influences susceptibility to attention deficit hyperactivity disorder (ADHD): analysis and pooled analysis.* Mol Psychiatry, 2002. 7(8): p. 908-12.

[29] Manor, I., et al., *Family-based association study of the serotonin transporter promoter region polymorphism (5-HTTLPR) in attention deficit hyperactivity disorder.* Am J Med Genet, 2001. 105(1): p. 91-5.

[30] Zoroglu, S.S., et al., *Significance of serotonin transporter gene 5-HTTLPR and variable number of tandem repeat polymorphism in attention deficit hyperactivity disorder.* Neuropsychobiology, 2002. 45(4): p. 176-81.

[31] Heiser, P., et al., *Family-based association study of serotonergic candidate genes and attention-deficit/hyperactivity disorder in a German sample.* J Neural Transm, 2007. 114(4): p. 513-21.

[32] Langley, K., et al., *No evidence of association of two 5HT transporter gene polymorphisms and attention deficit hyperactivity disorder.* Psychiatr Genet, 2003. 13(2): p. 107-10.

[33] Fisher, S.E., et al., *A genomewide scan for loci involved in attention-deficit/hyperactivity disorder.* Am J Hum Genet, 2002. 70(5): p. 1183-96.

[34] Smalley, S.L., et al., *Genetic linkage of attention-deficit/hyperactivity disorder on chromosome 16p13, in a region implicated in autism.* Am J Hum Genet, 2002. 71(4): p. 959-63.

[35] Hebebrand, J., et al., *A genome-wide scan for attention-deficit/hyperactivity disorder in 155 German sib-pairs.* Mol Psychiatry, 2006. 11(2): p. 196-205.

[36] Winsberg, B.G. and D.E. Comings, *Association of the dopamine transporter gene (DAT1) with poor methylphenidate response.* J Am Acad Child Adolesc Psychiatry, 1999. 38(12): p. 1474-7.

[37] Roman, T., et al., *Dopamine transporter gene and response to methylphenidate in attention-deficit/hyperactivity disorder.* Pharmacogenetics, 2002. 12(6): p. 497-9.

[38] Kirley, A., et al., *Association of the 480 bp DAT1 allele with methylphenidate response in a sample of Irish children with ADHD.* Am J Med Genet B Neuropsychiatr Genet, 2003. 121B(1): p. 50-4.

[39] Langley, K., et al., *No support for association between the dopamine transporter (DAT1) gene and ADHD.* Am J Med Genet B Neuropsychiatr Genet, 2005. 139B(1): p. 7-10.

[40] Stein, M.A. and J.J. McGough, *The pharmacogenomic era: promise for personalizing attention deficit hyperactivity disorder therapy.* Child Adolesc Psychiatr Clin N Am, 2008. 17(2): p. 475-90, xi-xii.

In: Attention Deficit Hyperactivity Disorder (ADHD)
Editors: Stuart M. Gordon and Aileen E. Mitchell
ISBN 978-1-60741-581-7

Chapter 13

Motor Ability and Adaptive Behavior in Children with Attention Deficit Hyperactivity Disorder

***Hui-Yi Wang*[1] *and Tzu-Hsiu Huang*[2]**

[1]Department of Physical Therapy, College of Health Science, Kaohsiung Medical University, Kaohsiung, Taiwan

[2]Department of Rehabilitation, Chung-Ho Memorial Hospital, Kaohsiung Medical University, Kaohsiung, Taiwan

Abstract

Attention Deficit Hyperactivity Disorder (ADHD) is a common neuropsychiatric disorder with characteristics of inattention, hyperactivity and/or poor impulse control. Previous studies had also reported children with ADHD exhibit below average performance in adaptive functioning. In recent years, motor difficulties in children with ADHD have been addressed. Researchers found these children have poor postural adjustment, inadequate motor timing and force use. Given evidence of the deficits of adaptive functioning and motor ability, the aim of this study was to investigate the association between these two fields in children with ADHD.

The study group consisted of 25 children with ADHD, 19 males and 6 females, aged from 4.6 to 8.6 years (mean age 6.5 years, SD 1.2 years). The participants were recruited from a rehabilitation department of a teaching hospital. All the children were diagnosed by a pediatrician as meeting the Diagnostic and Statistical Manual of Mental Disorders-Fourth Edition Text Revision (DSM-IV) criteria for ADHD. The Movement Assessment Battery for Children (MABC), a standardized motor function assessment, was administrated by three physical therapists. MABC consists of three subtests: manual dexterity, ball skill, and static dynamic balance. The Chinese version of Adaptive Behavior Scales was used to assess the adaptive function of the children. This scale is a semi-structure parent-reported questionnaire, which consists of two parts for assessing adaptive behaviors in 10 life domains and mal-adaptive behaviors in other two life domains.

Nine (36%) children had significant motor impairments whereas seven (28%) children were in borderline. Ten (40%) children had definite adaptive problems in more than one adaptive domain. The children with impaired motor ability had significant poorer behaviors in the adaptive domains of communication and socialization. Regarding the subtest performances, children who had more impaired ability in manual dexterity performed worse behaviors in the adaptive domains of home living, socialization and self-direction. The results also showed children with poorer ball skill were associated with worse home-living behavior. Moreover, children who had more impaired balance exhibited poorer performance in the social behavior.

The results of this study offer evidences of motor problems and adaptive dysfunction in 25 children with ADHD. We found significant correlation between motor ability and adaptive functioning in these children, especially in the adaptive domains of self-direction, home-living and socialization. Identification of motor difficulties may have important implications for the type of support needed for effective management in the adaptive dysfunction in children with ADHD.

Introduction

Attention Deficit Hyperactivity Disorder (ADHD) is a common neuropsychiatric disorder. The diagnostic criteria of ADHD defined in the Diagnostic and Statistical Manual of Mental Disorders-Fourth Edition Text Revision (DSM-IV-TR) require the symptoms of inattention, hyperactivity and/ or impulsivity.[1] There must be clear evidence of clinically significant impairment in social, academic, or emotional functioning.[2, 3] ADHD can have significant impacts on multiple domains of health-related quality of life in children and adolescents.[4] Some difficulties in attention and self-regulation (e.g. inability to establish and maintain a routine, poor discipline) may also persist into adult years.[5]

Since ADHD will lead to functional difficulties, researchers have examined adaptive functions in children with ADHD. Adaptive function has been defined as the performance in daily activities, and is highly related to social and cultural demands. It is well recognized that proper adaptive function is age-related and suitable for social expectation. [6] Individuals should perform appropriate behaviors in adequate life aspects; otherwise they are considered deficient in adaptive functioning. Adaptive function is usually measured in terms of various life aspects, [7] such as self help skills (i.e., dressing and bathing, etc.), independence (i.e., functions well at home and in the community, etc.), self-knowledge (i.e., aware of body parts, personal identity, etc.), motor skills, social knowledge (i.e., recognizes and uses time, knows major community resources, etc.), and communication skills with others. Children who experience dysfunction in adaptive behavior would face the difficulties in successfully participating in home life and schooling.

Previous studies had reported below average performance in adaptive functioning among children with ADHD. [8, 9] Stein and colleagues examined adaptive functioning in children with ADHD by using the Vineland Adaptive Behavior Scales. [6] Participants in their study had significantly below average adaptive functioning in the areas of socialization, communication and daily living. In another study, [10] the adaptive function in children with ADHD were investigated by using the Adaptive Behavior Scale. Poorer performance in adaptive function was found significantly associated with higher levels of inattention or hyperactivity.

In recent years, researchers and clinical professionals are more interested in motor difficulties in children with ADHD. Since the 1970s, a syndrome of neurodevelopmental dysfunction, called "DAMP" (deficits in attention, motor control, perception) was noted in some children with poor attention.[11] These children experience obvious motor deficits. DAMP was also observed in about half of individuals with ADHD. [11] It was therefore deduced by some researchers that at least half of the children with ADHD have motor problems.[12, 13] Regarding the specificity of gross motor and fine motor deficits, excessive associated movements, inadequate force use and poor postural control were found in children with ADHD.[13-16] For example, a study investigated the timing and force control and found children with ADHD exhibited excessive grip force.[17] Such motor problems of poor postural adjustment, inadequate motor timing and force control may have negative impacts on daily life because managing daily life is not only associated with cognitive function and executive function, but also relies on motor ability. On the other hand, problems of lower social maturity were observed in children with ADHD, especially in their self-help and self-direction abilities.[18] However, social maturity was not significantly associated with fine motor skills but the ability of static-dynamic balance.

From a clinical practice perspective, it is necessary to identify factors associated with adaptive behaviors in children with ADHD, especially when it is necessary to deal with the child's mal-adaptations. The relationships between motor ability and adaptive function in these children are still not well examined. Through remedying and promoting children's motor ability, clinicians should be helpful to offer useful strategies to manage the difficulties in adaptive skills for children with ADHD. Thus, the aim of this study was to investigate the association between the performance of adaptive function and motor ability in children with ADHD.

Material and Method

Participants

The study group consisted of 25 children with ADHD aged between 4.6 and 8.6 years (mean age 6.5 years, SD 1.2 years). There were 19 boys and 6 girls. The participants were recruited from the rehabilitation department of a teaching hospital. All the children were diagnosed by a pediatrician as meeting the DSM-IV criteria for ADHD. Parents or guardians gave written informed consent. The study was approved by the Human Experiment and Ethics Committee of the hospital.

Measures

Motor Function Assessment

The Movement Assessment Battery for Children (MABC) [19] is a standardized motor function assessment tool currently used on children with ADHD,[14, 15, 20] and is available in four age bands (4-6, 7-8, 9-10, and 11-12 years). In this study, two of the age band forms (4-6, and 7-8 years) were administrated. The assessment for each age band consists of 8 items belonging to three performance subtests, which are manual dexterity (MD, 3 items), ball skill (BS, 2 items), and static dynamic balance (SDB, 3 items). Each item is rated on a 0-5 scale. The sum of scores for each subtest is calculated. Higher subtest score indicates poorer motor performance. A Total Impairment score (TIS) is then derived from the sum of the three subtest scores, translated into percentile scores in comparison with the normative data reported on the MABC manual. Higher percentile of TIS indicates better motor ability. Children with TIS lower than the fifth percentile are considered with definite motor problems; children with TIS between the 5th and 15th percentile demonstrate a degree of difficulty that is borderline.[19] The above four scores, TIS (in percentile rank) and the three subtest impairment scores (MD, BS, and SDB) were used for data analysis.

Adaptive Functioning Measurement

The Chinese Adaptive Behavior Scale (CABS) [21] is specially designed to assess the adaptive function of Taiwanese children aged from 5 to 15 years. It is a standardized test rated on a 0-4 scale and has good test-retest reliability. Higher item scores reflect better performance in adaptive function. The questionnaire can either be filled out by teachers familiar with the child's everyday life, or completed by an experienced instructor after interviewing the child's main caretaker. The CABS includes two parts. Part one consists of ten domains of adaptive function; they are domains of communication (20 items), self-care (20 items), home living (20 items), socialization (20 items), community use (20 items), self-direction (19 items), health and safety (20 items), functional academics (20 items), leisure (20 items), and work (20 items). Part two has two domains of mal-adaptive behaviors: internalizing (mal-adaptation to stay alone, 15 items) and externalizing (mal-adaptation to accompanists, 15 items). The sum of the item scores in each domain is translated to an age-related percentile score that is a domain score, and compared with the normative data on the CABS manual. Children with a domain score lower than the ninth percentile are considered with delayed adaptive function. Children with a domain score between 10 and 25 percentiles are considered as below average but within normal range of adaptive function. In Part Two of CABS, the items measure the frequency and intensity of mal-adaptive behaviors. Therefore, higher scores in mal-adaptive domains reflect poorer performance. Children with percentile score in these two domains above the 91st percentile are with impaired adaptive skills and abnormal behaviors. Children between the 75 and 90 percentiles are approximately abnormal.

Procedures of Assessments

Three physical therapists conducted the motor function assessment. Prior to the commencement of the study, inter-rater reliability was examined. The measurements demonstrated good to excellent interrater reliability with ICC (2, 1) values ranging from .89 to .95. CABS was administrated to parents also by the three therapists. All the children completed both the motor and adaptive function assessments.

Data Analysis

All statistics were calculated with SPSS V14. Pearson correlation was used to examine the correlation between motor ability and adaptive functioning. According to the TIS on the motor assessment, the children were classified into three groups: normal, borderline, and impaired motor ability. Group differences in adaptive function were analyzed using analyses of variance followed by Scheffe post hoc tests. Statistical significance was defined as $p \leq 0.05$.

Results

Scores of Motor Ability and Adaptive Functioning

The TIS on the motor assessment showed that 9 children (36%) were below the fifth percentile, having delayed motor ability. Seven children (28%) scored between 5th and 15th percentile, hence were within borderline range of motor ability. The remained 9 children had scores within the normal range. The mean TIS and subtest scores are shown in Table 1.

Regarding the adaptive function assessment, four children had impaired performance in more than two domains, and six had impairments in one domain.

Table 1. Scores (Mean±SD) on motor assessment in the three level groups [a] of children

TIS and subtest scores	Total n=25	Normal gr. n=9 (36%)	Borderline gr. n=7 (28%)	Impaired gr. n=9 (36%)
Total Impairment Score (TIS) [b]	14.1±19.3	30.9±24.2	8.9±3.5	1.4±0.7
Manual Dexterity (MD) [c]	6.6±4.3	3.6±2.5	6.4±2.9	9.8±4.6
Ball Skill (BS) [c]	5.0±2.7	3.2±2.5	4.9±2.4	7.0±1.9
Static-Dynamic Balance (SDB) [c]	3.2±3.4	0.3±0.6	2.3±2.9	6.7±2.3

SD: standard deviation, gr.: group

a: Normal gr.: TIS percentile rank >15%, Borderline gr.: TIS percentile rank 5%-15%, Impaired gr.: TIS percentile rank <5%;

b: in percentile rank c: item raw score

Table 2 displays the percentage of children in each of the three levels of adaptive function across the 12 adaptive domains. The results show that in the socialization domain, none of the children were in the impaired range. On the other hand, 16% had impairment in the self-care domain and 20% had impairment in the functional academics domain. In the maladaptive behavior section, almost all the children exhibited impaired performances in both of the internalizing and externalizing mal-adaptive domains.

Table 2. The children (number and percentage) distributing on the three levels of adaptive function [a] across the 12 domains of adaptive function

Domains of Adaptive function	Normal level no. (%)	Below average no. (%)	Impaired level no. (%)
Communication	22 (88)	2 (8)	1 (4)
Self-care	15 (60)	6 (24)	4 (16)
Home Living	17 (68)	7 (28)	1 (4)
Socialization	24 (96)	1 (4)	0 (0)
Community Use	21 (84)	3 (12)	1 (4)
Self-direction	18 (72)	5 (20)	2 (8)
Health and Safety	22 (88)	2 (8)	1 (4)
Functional academics	17 (68)	3 (12)	5 (20)
Leisure	23 (92)	1 (4)	1 (4)
Work	14 (56)	9 (36)	2 (8)
Maladaptive behavior			
Internalizing	0 (0)	0 (0)	25 (100)
Externalizing	0 (0)	1 (4)	24 (96)

a: Normal level: score percentile rank >25%
Below average level: score percentile rank 10%-25%
Impaired level: score percentile rank <9%

Adaptive Functioning Across Groups with Different Levels of Motor Ability

The 25 children were classified into three groups according to the levels of motor ability based on the TIS. The adaptive domain scores in these three groups are showed in Table 3. There were significant differences among the groups in the adaptive domains of communication, home living, and socialization ($p<0.05$). The Scheffe post hoc analysis further revealed that compared to children with normal motor ability, children with impaired motor ability had significantly lower percentiles in the adaptive domains of communication ($p<0.05$) and socialization ($p<0.01$). There was no significant difference across groups in home living adaptive domain.

Table 3. The 12 domain scores [a] (mean±SD) on the adaptive function assessment in the three motor ability level groups [b] of children

Domains of Adaptive function	Total children n=25	Levels of motor ability [b] Normal gr. n=9	Borderline gr. n=7	Impaired gr. n=9	F -value
Communication	58.7±26.6	75.2±23.4	56.7±25.3	43.8±23.0	3.96*
Self-care	38.0±27.8	41.6±33.0	32.7±20.4	38.7±29.6	0.19
Home Living	53.2±27.7	71.1±20.6	45.9±30.2	41.1±24.9	3.65
Socialization	61.4±22.5	76.0±14.2	64.7±19.6	44.2±21.3	6.81**
Community Use	53.0±24.6	51.9±28.1	57.2±25.2	50.8±23.1	0.13
Self-direction	43.0±26.3	55.3±24.8	45.2±30.4	28.9±19.1	2.62
Health and Safety	54.6±24.4	51.9±22.9	56.4±25.8	56.0±27.4	0.08
Functional Academics	47.5±28.7	51.2±28.4	48.7±32.1	42.8±29.3	0.19
Leisure	60.2±25.2	65.3±19.2	62.4±32.9	53.3±25.2	0.53
Work	40.4±27.8	47.6±31.2	35.3±24.3	37.1±28.5	0.46
Maladaptive Behavior					
Internalizing	86.6±10.9	92.2±8.8	87.6±7.7	80.2±12.2	3.34
Externalizing	88.4±18.3	86.9±27.1	94.1±4.3	85.4±14.8	0.47

SD: standard deviation, gr.: group
a: score in percentile
b: Normal gr.: TIS percentile rank >15%, Borderline gr.: TIS percentile rank 5%-15%,
Impaired gr.: TIS percentile rank <5%;
F-valve in ANOVA, significant difference between normal gr. and impaired gr.: *p< .05, ** p< .01

Associations of Scores in the Three Motor Subtests with Scores of Adaptive Functioning

To examine the relationship between the children's motor ability and their adaptive behaviors in more detail, the correlation of the motor subtest scores and the adaptive domain scores were analyzed. There were significant negative associations between the manual dexterity subtest score and the domain scores of home living (r=-0.468, p=0.018), socialization (r=-0.489, p=0.013) and self-direction (r=-0.413, p=0.040), respectively (Table

4). As higher subtest score indicates poorer motor performance, these data revealed that children who had more impaired ability in manual dexterity performed worse behaviors in the adaptive domains of home living, socialization and self-direction.

Regarding the result of ball skill subtest, children with higher score in this subtest were found to have lower adaptive domain of home living (r=-0.563, p=0.003), i.e. poorer ball skill was associated with worse home-living behavior.

Significant correlation was also found between the motor subtest of static/dynamic balance and the adaptive domain of socialization (r=-0.413, p=0.040); children who had more impaired balance exhibited poorer performance in the social behavior.

Table 4. Pearson correlation coefficient (r) for scores on the three motor subtests and domain scores of the adaptive behaviors and maladaptive behaviors

	Three motor subtests		
Domains of Adaptive function	Manual Dexterity (MD)	Ball Skill (BS)	Static Dynamic Balance (SDB)
Communication	-.266	-.363	-.291
Self-care	-.241	-.389	.026
Home Living	-.468*	-.563**	-.345
Socialization	-.489*	-.382	-.413*
Community Use	-.226	-.055	.026
Self-direction	-.413*	-.269	-.358
Health and Safety	-.279	.047	.066
Functional Academics	-.249	-.262	-.120
Leisure	-.247	-.184	-.044
Work	-.022	.081	.005
Maladaptive Behavior			
Internalizing	-.178	-.334	-.331
Externalizing	.007	.146	.008

* $p < .05$ ** $p < .01$

Discussion

In this study, the adaptive function and motor ability in 25 children with ADHD were investigated. The adaptive behavior assessment revealed a great variety of performances in different domains of adaptive functioning among the participants. It indicates that children with ADHD would exhibit adaptive function ranging from nearly normal to mal-adaptive behaviors. Ten of the 25 children in this study had impaired adaptive performance in more than one adaptive domain. Except the two maladaptive behavior domains, the proportion of children having normal level behaviors in the domains of work, self-care, home living and functional academics was relatively low, between 56 and 68%. These results suggest that children with ADHD exhibit common impairments in occupational and educational functioning.[22, 23] Surprisingly, for socialization, another common domain identified with deficit in ADHD children,[6, 9] all of the studied children except one in this study had normal level behavior. In another social-related domain, the communication domain, our result shows that there was also relatively high proportion of the children (22 out of the 25 children, 88 %) exhibited normal level behaviors. These results may reveal that in children with ADHD, their performances of certain adaptive functioning are variable among different situations as well as different conditions of the children. The better performances in the social-related domains may be due to in part the effects of treatment intervention; since these children were recruited from a rehabilitation department of a teaching hospital. The treatment intervention may make a positive impact on the children's adaptive functioning, especially for the socio-communication abilities. Regarding another part of the result of adaptive behavior assessment, all the children had impaired behaviors in both mal-adaptive domains of internalizing (i.e. inattention, self-stimulating behaviors) and externalizing (i.e. poor impulsive control, conflicts with others). It implies that even though children with ADHD have the abilities to perform daily function activities, mal-adaptive behaviors are still their key symptoms.

Our results also provide evidence of motor impairments in children with ADHD. In this study, 36% of the participants had significant motor impairments whereas 28 percent were borderline cases. The high percentage of children with motor difficulties was also found in previous studies. [11-13] The outcome of motor assessment demonstrates that insufficient performances in all the three subtest assessments contribute to the impairments of the overall gross motor ability (Table 1).

In adaptive functioning, there were relatively high proportions of the children displaying normal level behaviors in the domains of socialization and communication. On the other hand, it is interesting to note that in these two domains, there were significant differences in scores between children with normal motor ability and those with impaired motor ability (Table 3). Children with impaired motor ability had significantly lower scores (i.e. poorer performances). Although both children with normal motor ability and children with impaired motor ability were within normal range in the socialization and communication domain scores, the above result might still imply that there is a significant trend of association between the ability level of gross motor and social-related adaptive functioning in children with ADHD.

There were three main significant findings in relation to the correlations between the children's adaptive functioning and their performance on the individual motor subtests (Table 4). First, the children's manual dexterity ability was significantly associated with their adaptive performances in the domains of home living, socialization, and self-direction. Regarding these adaptive functioning on the CABS assessment, [21] home living describes household independence such as executing house chores, using tools and home appliance, and arranging daily schedule. Socialization behavior reflects the ability to start and end the interaction with others appropriately, to recognize emotion response, to regulate self behaviors, and to accept peers. In addition, self-direction is associated with making decisions appropriately, problem-solving and self-advocate. Motor ability of manual dexterity represents the abilities to use the hands, which include the functions of speed and sureness of each hand movement, coordination of two hands, and hand-eye coordination.[19]A child who cannot perform sufficient manual dexterity skills would fail in important learning experience, and is also hard to participate in peer playing and interaction. The finding in this study increases our understanding of a particular relationship between manual dexterity and adaptive behaviors of home living, socialization and self-direction respectively.

Another significant finding in this study was the correlation between the ability of the children's ball skills and their home living adaptive behaviors. The ability of ball skills refers to the movements of manipulating, throwing and catching an object, such as a ball. A child who executes a task of ball activity can reflect her/his abilities of timing, force control and body parts using.[24] These motions might be essential competences involved in homing living skills.

The third finding of correlation analysis was the significant association between the children's static/dynamic balance ability and their socialization behaviors. This result is similar to the finding in Kaneko's study.[18] Static/dynamic balance ability requires a child to maintain balance in a static posture and move actively in a variety of ways. This finding gives rise to an intensely interesting issue that how the ability of balance and socialization behaviors relate to each other. Several prior researches have studied balance-related performances, including postural stability and gait patterns in children with ADHD. [25-27] These researches discussed the fields of neural network configuration and sensory information processing in order to address the nature as well as possible mechanisms associated with balance control in ADHD children. Some studies on motor control in children with ADHD focused on a specific deficit, the executive dysfunction. [28, 29] Executive function is an umbrella term that incorporates the complex cognitive process required to perform goal-directed tasks.[30] It consists of three core domains: response selection/inhibition, flexibility, and planning/working memory. Children with ADHD were found to have impairments in response inhibition (inhibition of a pre-potent response and self-monitoring) and planning on working memory task.[30, 31] The association of socialization and executive function had been examined.[32] The results reported significant correlation between socialization and aspect of planning/working memory in children with typical development as well as in children with autism spectrum disorders. However, no such correlation held within the ADHD group of children. Further research will be needed to ascertain the complex connecting relationships among socialization, executive function, and special motor skills, such as balance control in children with ADHD.

From the clinical perspective, diagnosis of ADHD is only part of a comprehensive assessment of functioning for children with ADHD. Examination of motor ability is also crucial. ADHD cannot be cured but the core symptoms and associated impairments can be actively managed by a combination of approaches. Identification of their motor difficulties may have important implications for the type of support needed for effective management in the adaptive dysfunction in these children.

The limitation of this study was the symptoms of inattention and hyperactivity were not studied; hence the severity of the symptoms could not be correlated with the performance of motor ability and adaptive functioning. Moreover, a larger sample size of participants is needed in future study for further analyzing additional variables such as mental age and type of ADHD associating to motor ability and adaptive functioning in children with ADHD.

References

[1] American Psychiatric Association. Diagnostic and Statistical Manual of Mental Disorders: DSM-IV-TR 4th edn. Washington: American Psychiatric Association, 2000.

[2] Biederman J. Attention- deficit/hyperactivity disorder: A selective overview. *Biol Psychiatry* 2005; 57: 1215-20.

[3] Barkley RA. Issues in the diagnosis of attention-deficit/hyperactivity disorder in children. *Brain Dev* 2003; 25: 77-83.

[4] Klassen AF, Miller A, Fine S. Health-related quality of life in children and adolescents who have a diagnosis of attention-deficit/hyperactivity disorder. *Pediatrics* 2004; 114: e541-7.

[5] Wolf LE, Wasserstein J. Adult ADHD. Concluding thoughts. *Ann N Y Acad Sci* 2001; 931: 396-408.

[6] Stein MA, Szumowski E, Blondis TA, Roizen NJ. Adaptive skills dysfunction in ADD and ADHD children. *J Child Psychol Psychiatry* 1995; 36: 663-70.

[7] Barkley RA, Fischer M, Smallish L, Fletcher K. Young adult outcome of hyperactive children: adaptive functioning in major life activities. *J Am Acad Child Adolesc Psychiatry* 2006; 45: 192-202.

[8] Sukhodolsky DG, do Rosario-Campos MC, Katsovich L, Pauls DL, Peterson BS, King RA, et al. Adaptive, emotional, and family functioning of children with obsessive-compulsive disorder and comorbid attention deficit hyperactivity disorder. *Am J Psychiatry* 2005; 162: 1125-32.

[9] Nijmeijer JS, Minderaa RB, Buitelaar JK, Mulligan A, Hartman CA, Hoekstra PJ. Attention-deficit/hyperactivity disorder and social dysfunctioning. *Clin Psychol Rev* 2008; 28: 692-708.

[10] Muir-Broaddus JE, Rosenstein LD, Medina DE, Soderberg C. Neuropsychological test performance of children with ADHD relative to test norms and parent behavioral ratings. *Arch Clin Neuropsychol* 2002; 17: 671-89.

[11] Gillberg C. Deficits in attention, motor control, and perception: a brief review. *Arch Dis Child* 2003; 88: 904-10.

[12] Piek JP, Pitcher TM, Hay DA. Motor coordination and kinaesthesis in males with attention-deficit-hyperactivity disorder. *Dev Med Child Neurol* 1999; 41: 159-65.

[13] Pitcher TM, Piek JP, Hay DA. Fine and gross motor ability in males with ADHD. *Dev Med Child Neurol* 2003; 45: 525-35.

[14] Flapper BCT, Houwen S, Schoemaker MM. Fine motor skills and effects of methylphenidate in children with attention-deficit-hyperactivity disorder and developmental coordination disorder. *Dev Med Child Neurol* 2006; 48: 165-9.

[15] Miyahara M, Piek J, Barrett N. Accuracy of drawing in a dual-task and resistance-to-distraction study: Motor or attention deficit? *Hum Mov Sci* 2006; 25: 100-9.

[16] Jucaite A, Fernell E, Forssberg H, Hadders-Algra M. Deficient coordination of associated postural adjustments during a lifting task in children with neurodevelopmental disorders. *Dev Med Child Neurol* 2003; 45: 731-42.

[17] Pitcher TM, Piek JP, Barrett NC. Timing and force control in boys with attention deficit hyperactivity disorder: Subtype differences and the effect of comorbid developmental coordination disorder. *Hum Mov Sci* 2002; 21: 919-45.

[18] Kaneko F and Okamura H. Study on the social maturity, self-perception, and associated factors, including motor coordination, of children with attention deficit hyperactivity disorder. *Phys Occup Ther Pediatr* 2005; 25: 45-58.

[19] Henderson SE, Sugden DA. *Movement Assessment Battery for Children*. London: The Psychological Corporation; 1992.

[20] Watemberg N, Waiserberg N, Zuk L, Lerman-Sagie T. Developmental coordination disorder in children with attention-deficit-hyperactivity disorder and physical therapy intervention. Dev Med Child Neurol 2007; 49: 920-5.

[21] Hsu HL. *Chinese Adaptive Behavior Scale-Manual.* Taipei: Special Education Center at National Taiwan Normal University, 2004. [in Chinese]

[22] Stavro GM, Ettenhofer ML, Nigg JT. Executive functions and adaptive functioning in young adult attention-deficit/hyperactivity disorder. *J Int Neuropsychol Soc* 2007; 13: 324-34.

[23] Biederman J, Petty CR, Fried R, Kaiser R, Dolan CR, Schoenfeld S, et al. Educational and occupational underattainment in adults with attention-deficit/hyperactivity disorder: a controlled study. *J Clin Psychiatry* 2008; 69: 1217-22.

[24] Haywood KM, Getchell N. *Life span Motor Development.* 3rd ed. Champaign: Human Kinetics; 2001.

[25] Buderath P, Gartner K, Frings M, Christiansen H, Schoch B, Konczak J, et al. Postural and gait performance in children with attention deficit/hyperactivity disorder. Gait Posture 2008; [Epub ahead of print]

[26] Leitner Y, Barak R, Giladi N, Peretz C, Eshel R, Gruendlinger L, et al. Gait in attention deficit hyperactivity disorder: effects of methylphenidate and dual tasking. *J Neurol* 2007; 254: 1330-8.

[27] Cheng J, Wang YF. Comparison of postural control between normal and attention deficit hyperactivity disorder boys. *Beijing Da Xue Xue Bao* 2007; 39: 531-4.

[28] Livesey D, Keen J, Rouse J, White F. The relationship between measures of executive function, motor performance and externalising behaviour in 5- and 6-year-old children. *Hum Mov Sci* 2006; 25: 50-64.

[29] Roth RM, Saykin AJ. Executive dysfunction in attention-deficit/hyperactivity disorder: cognitive and neuroimaging findings. *Psychiatr Clin North Am* 2004; 27: 83-96, ix.

[30] Piek JP, Dyck MJ, Nieman A, Anderson M, Hay D, Smith LH, et al. The relationship between motor coordination, executive functioning and attention in school aged children. *Arch Clin Neuropsychol* 2004; 19: 1063-76.

[31] Piek JP, Dyck MJ, Francis M, Conwell A. Working memory, processing speed, and set-shifting in children with developmental disorder and attention-deficit-hyperactivity disorder. *Dev Med Child Neurol* 2007; 49: 678-83.

[32] Happé F, Booth R, Charlton R, Hughes C. Executive function deficits in autism spectrum disorders and attention-deficit/hyperactivity disorder: Examining profiles across domains and ages. *Brain Cogn* 2006; 61: 25-39.

In: Attention Deficit Hyperactivity Disorder (ADHD)
Editors: Stuart M. Gordon and Aileen E. Mitchell
ISBN 978-1-60741-581-7

Chapter 14

Attention Deficit Hyperactivity Disorder and Persons with Intellectual Disability

Eli Carmeli**[*1] **and Joav Merrick**[2,3,4,5]

[1]Department of Physical Therapy, Sackler Faculty of Medicine, Stanley Steyer School of Health Professions, Tel Aviv University, Ramat Aviv;
[2]National Institute of Child Health and Human Development, Office of the Medical Director, Division for Mental Retardation, Ministry of Social Affairs, Jerusalem,
[3]Zusman Child Development Center, Soroka University Medical Center, Beer-Sheva, Israel,
[4]Interuniversity College for Health and Development, Castle of Seggau, Graz, Austria,
[5]Kentucky Children's Hospital, University of Kentucky, Lexington, United States

Abstract

In this chapter we want to demonstrate a correlation between social skills and attention deficit hyperactivity disorder (ADHD) among adolescents with intellectual disability (ID). In a recent pilot study of adolescents dually diagnosed with mild intellectual disabilities and comorbid pathology of ADHD we defined three age-and IQ-match groups (males, n=12 in each group) with group I – composed of adolescent diagnosed with mild ID, group II - adolescents diagnosed with ADHD, and group III - adolescents diagnosed with ID and ADHD. The instruments used in the study were Wechsler Intelligence Scale for Children (WISC, according to the chronological age of the subjects) and the short version of the Developmental Behavior Checklist (DBC). We found that comorbidity was a factor differentiating. ADHD strongly increased the impairment of social skills, while behavioral disorders were less damaging in ID performance. The WISC and DBC instruments should be used with confidence in clinical

* Correspondence: Professor Eli Carmeli, PhD, Department of Physical Therapy, Sackler Faculty of Medicine, Stanley Steyer School of Health Professions, Tel Aviv University, IL- 69978 Ramat Aviv, Israel. Tel: 972 46405434; E mail: elie@post.tau.ac.il and Professor Joav Merrick, MD, MMedSci, DMSc, Medical Director, Division for Mental Retardation, Ministry of Social Affairs, POBox 1260, IL-91012 Jerusalem, ISRAEL. Tel: 972-2-6708122; Fax: 972-2-6703657; Mobile: 972-50-6223832; E-mail: jmerrick@zahav.net.il .

and service settings, to allow a better assessment of co-occurrence morbidity in adolescents with ID. The interactions between intellectual disability and psychopathology behavior highlight the need to plan a more accurate diagnosis and appropriate rehabilitative intervention program, essential for improving the quality of life of the ID population.

Introduction

Little is know about the prevelence of attention-deficit/hyperactivity disorder (ADHD) and persons with intellectual disability (ID), even though some attempts have been made to set objective outlines and criteria for psychiatric disorders in the population of persons with ID [1,2], but the question of the validity of ADHD in the ID population is still confusing and debatable. ADHD is a psychiatric condition in adolescence, which may exist in intellectual disability [3]. Research has shown that ADHD is usually diagnosed in childhood with symptoms such as hyperactivity, forgetfulness, mood shifts, poor impulse control and distractibility. There is much controversy surrounding the diagnosis of ADHD, such as whether the diagnosis denotes a cognitive development disorder or neurological dysfunction. Bower and Parsons [4] showed that the frontal lobe, basal ganglia interconnections, and the central aspects of the cerebellum may be involved in ADHD. The cerebellum which is believed to play a role in short-term memory, attention, impulse control, emotion, high ability to schedule and plan tasks have been shown to be smaller in those who have ADHD [5]. Pearson et al [6] indicated that adolescents with ID are at high risk for ADHD.

Previous studies indicated that the prevalence of psychopathology in adolescents with ID was approximately four times higher than in the general population. Yet, the available evidence was inconsistent regarding the prevalence of behavioral and emotional disturbances in persons with mild ID. The co-occurrence between ID and behavioral disturbances such as mood changes, anxiety, and communication disorders is a challenge to differentiate and to modify the mutual impact among them. Thus, if ADHD is a valid psychiatric disorder in adolescents with ID, clinicians may not employ an overlap diagnosis and may help to apply accurate treatment of individuals with both ID and ADHD.

In order to try to detect any difference among group means, and thus to demonstrate any existent relationship between social skills and ADHD represented by maladaptive behaviors we have recently conducted a small pilot study [7]. The current study sought to indicate the extent to which symptom differences could discriminate ID individuals from ADHD individuals and from ID and ADHD. Any advancement to our knowledge of how ADHD affects the presence of behavior among adolescent with ID could influence how we should address the series of signs and symptoms.

Experiences from Our Pilot Study

Our study (7) was conducted in residential care centers and hostels for persons with ID in Israel with participants attending a special education school divided into three groups. All participantss from groups 1 and 2 were selected from a residential care center, while group I were 12 individual males, diagnosed as having mild ID. Ages ranged from 8 to 16 years (mean age 12.4 ±2.2). The subjects of group II composed of 12 individuals diagnosed with ADHD. Age ranged from 8 to 16 years (mean age 13.1 ±1.9). The subjects of group III composed of 12 individuals diagnosed as mild ID and comorbid pathology as ADHD from two hostels. Ages ranged from 8 to 16 years (mean age 12.8 ±2.1). The diagnoses were formulated according to the criteria of the mild intellectual disability – code no 317.00 (DSM-IV-R). The range of the general IQ level was from 57.22 to 64.70. All subjects diagnosed with ADHD routinely used methylphenidate (i.e., Ritalin). Each child was assessed in detail by a multidisciplinary team comprising of pediatrician, sociologist, clinical psychologist, and special educator. The pediatrician took a detailed clinical history and performed a neurological examination.

The instruments used were the Wechsler Intelligence Scale for children (WISC) [8] and the Developmental Behavior Checklist (DBC) [9]. The tests were administrated by a qualified clinical psychologist. The WISC determines the level of 12 items and able to estimate intelligence (i.e. cognitive ability), verbal and nonverbal (performance) and global (full scale) IQ scores. The DBC is composed of 96-items or symptoms standardized teacher/sociologist report of behavioral problems in children with ID from 4 to 16 years of age. This test measures psychopathology in six domains: withdrawn, self absorbed, anxiety, social problems, attention, and aggressive behavior. Each item was scored on a 3-point Likert Scale. The global total behavior problem score (TBPS) was also included with a cut-off score of 48.

What Did We Find?

Analyses of variance showed differences in ADHD group and ID+ADHD. In the WISC 12 items, significant differences were found for the items understanding, information, calculation, digital span, block design and labyrinth (see table 1). Significant Bonferroni post-hoc test showed that in the above items, ID+ADHD have the highest mean scores, while the lowest scores were found in all the items in the ADHD group. The mean scores of the ID group were average and non significant from the other two groups.

In the Developmental Behavior Checklist (DBC) 96-items (see table 2), ID+ADHD has the highest means scores, and significant comparing the ADHD group in two items: Self absorbed (t=3.14) and anti-social behavior (t=2.97). On the basis of a TBPS score, the ID+ADHD group was over the cut-off point, which indicated a clinical significance. In both test instruments, the score of ID group was comparable to ADHD score, and there was no difference between groups.

Discussion

Our study [7] confirmed the fact that ADHD often coexist with ID and differential diagnosis is therefore crucial.

Table 1. Differences in WISC items between means of the three groups

Item	ID	ADHD	ID+ADHD	ANOVA (df 2,9)
	n=12	n=12	n=12	*F*
Understanding	7.29	6.71	9.11	2.64*
Information	6.54	4.35	8.82	3.78*
Similarity	6.89	5.22	9.07	1.57
Calculation	5.31	3.99	8.14	3.26*
Digital span	4.98	4.02	8.30	5.21*
Vocabulary	19.57	15.32	20.19	1.88
Picture arrangement	7.77	4.99	12.31	2.02
Picture completion	12.76	9.84	15.08	1.11
Object congregation	11.02	9.79	13.53	0.99
Block design	8.97	5.95	14.79	3.10*
Labyrinth	9.68	8.86	10.13	1.33
Coding	16.27	14.67	22.48	1.85

(.05) F= (2,9) = 4.26
Significant Bonferroni post-hoc test, (* $p < .05$)
Understanding - ID+ADHD > ADHD (t=3.24)
Information - ID+ADHD > ADHD (t=3.14)
Calculation - ID+ADHD > ADHD (t=3.04)
Digital span - ID+ADHD > ADHD (t=2.97)
Block design - ID+ADHD > ADHD (t=2.97)

Table 2. Differences in Developmental Behavior Checklist (DBC) items between means of the three groups

Item	ID	ADHD	ID+ADHD	ANOVA (df 2,94)
	n=12	n=12	n=12	*F*
Withdrawn	4.02	4.98	5.14	1.21
self absorbed	10.23	9.21	12.76	2.56*
anxiety	8.34	7.25	9.85	1.83
anti-social	2.31	1.12	2.79	2.63*
behavior	7.72	6.77	7.29	1.02
attention	13.16	12.89	14.21	1.81
aggressive		45.78	42.22	52.04
behavior				
TBPS				

(.05) F= (2,94) = 3.11
Significant Bonferroni post-hoc test (* $p < .05$)
TBPS - Total Behavior Problem Score (cut off score 48)
Self absorbed - ID+ADHD > ADHD (t=3.14)
Anti-social behavior - ID+ADHD > ADHD (t=2.97)

In that study we looked for some specific patterns of behavioral differences in ID+ADHD comparing ID and ADHD subjects. In both test instruments (i.e., WISC and DBC), where social skills were measured, the ID+ADHD group had the highest score level.

In agreement with previous research [10], we can claim that the ID+ADHD individuals showed a greater impairment in cognitive and social skills compared to the ID or ADHD individuals.

The two instruments measured a total of 18 domains indicating cognitive, emotional, and social skills. In seven domains the ID+ADHD individuals demonstrated a significant difference from the ADHD individuals. Understanding, information, calculating, digital span and block design were cognitive skills requiring memory ability. Moreover, the behavioral profile, demonstrated by DBC, indicated that in self absorbtion and social skills the ID+ADHD individuals were shortcoming. In ID and ADHD populations, in all ages, the learning and retention, as measured by WISC is challenging not only secondary to cognitive impairment, but perhaps due to lack of motivation and interest, a sedentary life style, limited narrative language skills, slow reaction time, and reduction in attention performances requested from the questionnaire [11]. We assume that those limitations contributed substantially to their failure of learning and retention task.

As stated by previous investigators [12] the co-occurrence of ADHD and ID impaired less the area of motor skills, verbal communication, visual spatial skills and behavior under stressful condition. The impact of ADHD on ID individuals was mainly on skills requiring judgment, conclusion, memory and reminiscence. However, there was little evidence of gender and age difference, and no strong associations with domains of adaptive behavior (socialization, communication, and daily living skills).

The ultimate goals of treatment for persons with ID are to improve both cognitive and communication skills, and to integrate these into social and community activity. The interactions between intellectual disability and psychopathology behavior highlight the needs to plan a more accurate diagnosis and appropriate rehabilitative intervention program, essential for the improving of the quality of life of ID. Jou et al [13] stated that psycho-stimulants might be effective and well-tolerated in the diagnosis and treatment of ADHD in adults with ID.

There were some limitations to our study (7) due to the fact that participants came from two different supporting facilities; one was a residential care center specialized in the ID population, whereas the other facility was a hostel specialized in the ADHD population. This could introduce a bias toward one group. In addition, only in two items out of six items from the DBC used to evaluate behavioral profiles we found significant differences. Moreover, the numbers of individuals that participated were small preventing us from drawing firm conclusions from our finding of a consistent behavioral pattern differentiating between ID, ADHD and ID+ ADHD.

Conclusions

The experience from our pilot study (7) support previous research and suggest that ADHD may be a valid psychiatric diagnosis for children with intellectual disabilities. However, larger prospective open-label studies and eventually double-blind placebo-controlled studies are needed to confirm these findings. Thus, a great deal more research is needed to explore the phenomenology of ADHD in intellectual disability and to develop an evidence base for psychosocial intervention.

References

[1] Walters AS, Barrett RP, Knapp LG, Borden MC. Suicidal behavior in children and adolescents with mental retardation. Res Dev Disabil 1995;16(2):85-96.

[2] Masi G, Mucci M, Favilla L, Poli P. Dysthymic disorder in adolescents with intellectual disability. J Intellect Disabil Res 1999;43(Pt 2):80-7.

[3] Handen BL, Janosky J, McAuliffe S. Long-term follow-up of children with mental retardation/borderline intellectual functioning and ADHD. J Abnorm Child Psychol 1997;25(4):287-95.

[4] Bower JM, Parsons LM. Rethinking the "lesser brain". Sci Am 2003; 289(2):50-7.

[5] Geurts HM, Verte S, Oosterlaan J, Roeyers H, Sergeant JA. How specific are executive functioning deficits in attention deficit hyperactivity disorder and autism? J Child Psychol Psychiatry 2004; 45(4):836-54.

[6] Pearson DA, Santos CW, Roache JD, Casat CD, Loveland KA, Lachar D, Lane DM, Faria LP, Cleveland LA. Treatment effects of methylphenidate on behavioral adjustment in children with mental retardation and ADHD. J Am Acad Child Adolesc Psychiatry 2003; 42(2):209-16.

[7] Carmeli E, Klein N, Sohn M. The implications of having attention-deficit/hyperactivity disorder in male adolescents with intellectual disability. Int JAdolesc Med Health 2007;19(2)209-14.

[8] Wechsler D. Wechsler Intelligence Scale for Children, 4th Ed (WISC-IV®). San Antonio, TX: Harcourt Assessment, 2003.

[9] Mohr C, Tonge BJ, Einfeld SL. The development of a new measure for the assessment of psychopathology in adults with intellectual disability. J Intellect Disabil Res 2005;49(Pt 7):469-80.

[10] Hastings RP, Beck A, Daley D, Hill C. Symptoms of ADHD and their correlates in children with intellectual disabilities. Res Dev Disabil 2005;26(5):456-68.

[11] Abbeduto L, Short-Meyerson K, Benson G, Dolish J. Relationship between theory of mind and language ability in children and adolescents with intellectual disability. J Intellect Disabil Res 2004;48(Pt 2):150-9.

[12] Di Nuovo SF, Buono S. Psychiatric syndromes comorbid with mental retardation: Differences in cognitive and adaptive skills. J Psychiatr Res 2006 May 11 [Epub ahead of print]

[13] Jou R, Handen B, Hardan A. Psychostimulant treatment of adults with mental retardation and attention-deficit hyperactivity disorder. Australas Psychiatry 2004;12(4):376-9.

Index

A

B

C

D

E

F

G

H

I

N

O

P

Q

R

S

T